PEDIATRIC AND OBSTETRICAL ANESTHESIA

DEVELOPMENTS IN
CRITICAL CARE MEDICINE AND ANESTHESIOLOGY

Volume 30

The titles published in this series are listed at the end of this volume.

PEDIATRIC AND OBSTETRICAL ANESTHESIA

Papers presented at the 40th Annual Postgraduate Course in Anesthesiology, February 1995

edited by

T. H. STANLEY AND P. G. SCHAFER

University of Utah School of Medicine,
Department of Anesthesiology,
Salt Lake City, Utah, U.S.A.

SPRINGER SCIENCE+BUSINESS, MEDIA, B.V.

A C.I.P. Catalogue record for this book is available from the Library of Congress.

ISBN 978-0-7923-3346-3   ISBN 978-94-011-0319-0 (eBook)
DOI 10.1007/978-94-011-0319-0

Printed on acid-free paper

TABLE OF CONTENTS

Preface

Patrick G. Schafer, M.D.

Pediatric and Obstetrical Anesthesia contains the Refresher Course manuscripts of the presentations of the 40th Annual Postgraduate Course in Anesthesiology which took place at The Cliff Conference Center in Snowbird, Utah, February 24-28, 1995. The chapters reflect recent advances in the physiology, pharmacology, and anesthetic management of patients with central nervous system disease. There are also chapters which deal with central nervous system trauma and with brain protection. Each of the chapters is written by an authority in the field and has been edited only to the extent that was necessary to produce a coherent book. No effort has been made to provide a uniform presentation or style.

The purposes of the textbook are to 1) act as a reference for the anesthesiologists attending the meeting, and 2) serve as a vehicle to bring many of the latest concepts in anesthesiology to others within a short time of the formal presentation. Each chapter is a brief but sharply focused glimpse of the interests in anesthesia expressed at the conference. This book and its chapters should not be considered complete treatises on the subjects addressed but rather attempts to summarize the most salient points.

This textbook is the thirteenth in a continuing series documenting the proceedings of the Postgraduate Course in Salt Lake City. We hope that this and the past and future volumes reflect the rapid and continuing evolution of anesthesiology in the late twentieth century.

J. Michael Badgwell, M.D.
Department of Anesthesiology, Texas Tech University Health Sciences
Center, Lubbock, Texas, U.S.A.

Frederic A. Berry, M.D.
Department of Anesthesiology, University of Virginia Health Sciences
Center, Charlottesville, Virginia, U.S.A.

David J. Birnbach, M.D.
Department of Anesthesiology, Columbia University, St. Luke's —
Roosevelt Hospital Center, New York, New York, U.S.A.

Steven L. Clark, M.D.
Department of Perinatology, LDS Hospital, Salt Lake City, Utah, U.S.A.

D. Ryan Cook, M.D.
Department of Anesthesiology, University of Pittsburgh School of
Medicine, Children's Hospital of Pittsburgh, Pittsburgh, Pennsylvania,
U.S.A.

Mieczyslaw Finster, M.D.
Department of Anesthesiology, Columbia University College of
Physicians and Surgeons, New York, New York, U.S.A.

Charles P. Gibbs, M.D.
Department of Anesthesiology, University of Colorado Health Sciences
Center, Denver, Colorado, U.S.A.

Raafat S. Hannallah, M.D.
Department of Anesthesiology, George Washington School of Medicine,
Children's Hospital, Washington, D.C., U.S.A.

Paul R. Hickey, M.D.
Department of Anesthesia, Harvard Medical School, Children's Hospital,
Boston, Massachusetts, U.S.A.

Jerrold Lerman, M.D., FRCPC
Department of Anaesthesiology , Hospital for Sick Children, Toronto,
Ontario, Canada

Andrew M. Malinow, M.D.
Department of Anesthesiology, University of Maryland Medical System,
Baltimore, Maryland, U.S.A.

Gerard W. Ostheimer, M.D.
Department of Anesthesia, Harvard Medical School, Brigham and
Women's Hospital, Boston, Massachusetts, U.S.A.

Jeffrey P. Phelan, M.D.
Department of Anesthesiology, Queen of the Valley Hospital, West
Covina, California, U.S.A.

Linda J. Rice, M.D.
Department of Anesthesia, Hartford Hospital, Hartford, Connecticut,
U.S.A.

PHYSIOLOGIC ADAPTATION DURING PREGNANCY

G. W. Ostheimer

Pregnancy involves major physiologic and anatomic adaptation by all of the maternal organ systems. The anesthesiologist caring for the pregnant patient must understand these physiologic changes in order to provide safe analgesia and anesthesia to the mother and enable safe delivery of the fetus.

CARDIOVASCULAR SYSTEM

CARDIAC OUTPUT

Oxygen consumption increases during pregnancy, and maternal cardiac output rises to meet the demand (Table 1) (1). The rise in cardiac output is a result of increased heart rate and decreased afterload, as stroke volume does not change appreciably during normal pregnancy (2). Cardiac output rises most rapidly during the second trimester (Figure 1) and then remains steady until term, when labor and uteroplacental transfusion of blood into the intravascular system cause further increase in cardiac output.

BLOOD VOLUME

Blood volume increases by 35% during pregnancy compared with the nonpregnant state (3). The stimulus for this change is controversial. Increased mineralocorticoid levels during pregnancy may predispose to progressive sodium and water retention with consequent enlargement of the intravascular space (the "overfill" hypothesis). Alternatively, primary enlargement of this space owing to hormonal (prostaglandin, progesterone) vasodilation and placental arteriovenous shunting may be the stimulus for secondary renal sodium and water retention (the "underfill" hypothesis) (4). Recent evidence seems to favor primary peripheral vasodilation early in the first trimester (underfill) as the cause of subsequent blood volume expansion (5).

1

T.H. Stanley and P.G. Schafer (eds.), Pediatric and Obstetrical Anesthesia, 1-26.
© *1995 Kluwer Academic Publishers.*

Table 1. Maternal cardiovascular alterations at term. Adapted from Mashini et al (2), and Skaredoff and Ostheimer (56), with permission.

Variable	Change	Rate (%)
Cardiac output	↑↑↑↑	40
Stroke volume	±↑	0-30
Heart rate	↑↑	15
Systolic blood pressure	↓	0-5 mmHg
Diastolic blood pressure	↓↓	10-20 mmHg
Total peripheral resistance	↓↓	15
Central venous pressure	+	0
Pulmonary wedge pressure	-	0
Ejection fraction	-	0

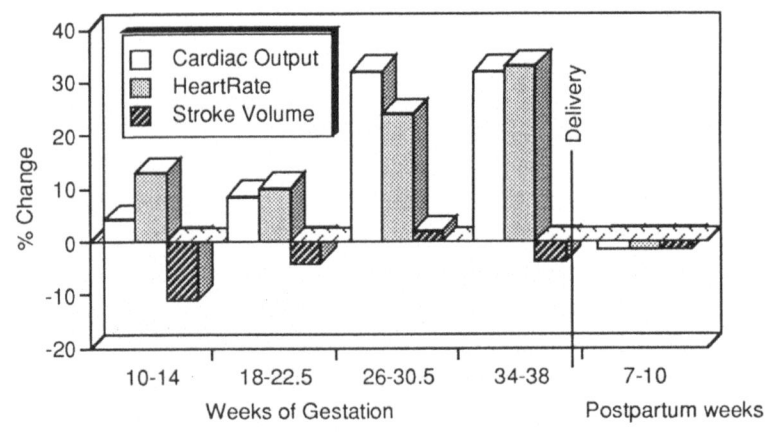

Figure 1.   Hemodynamic changes during pregnancy. Adapted from Mashini et al (2), with permission.

UTERINE SIZE AND VASCULARITY

The gravid uterine blood flow is 20-40 times above the nonpregnant level, accounting for 20% of the maternal cardiac output at term. Uterine vascular resistance is markedly reduced during gestation, producing a low-pressure circuit in "parallel" with a maternal circulation characterized by reduced systemic vascular resistance.

The enlarged uterus produces mechanical compression surrounding vascular structures, known as aortocaval compression, or the "maternal supine hypotensive syndrome" (6). In the supine position, compression of the inferior vena cava decreases venous return, resulting in decreased stroke volume and hypotension; compression of the aorta further decreases uterine perfusion and may result in fetal distress. Normal maternal compensatory responses to aortocaval compression consist of tachycardia and lower-extremity vasoconstriction.

THE PERICARDIUM

Recent noninvasive studies have demonstrated a high incidence of asymptomatic pericardial effusion during normal pregnancy (7). The stimulus is unknown, as plasma volume and protein fraction changes do not seem to correlate with the development of such effusion (5).

VASCULAR TONE

Normal parturients are less responsive to vasopressor and chronotropic agonists (8,9). Epinephrine, isoproterenol, and angiotensin II all show dose-related blunting of effect during pregnancy. Down-regulation of α- and β-adrenergic receptors has been postulated as the cause of these phenomena. However, the presence of vasodilator prostaglandins may play a role as well, since 1) inhibitors of prostaglandin synthesis have been shown to reverse vascular unresponsiveness to catecholamines, and 2) toxemic patients who have an abundance of vasoconstricting prostaglandin (e.g., thromboxane) are more sensitive to exogenous catecholamines.

CLINICAL IMPLICATIONS

Aortocaval compression should always be avoided. Parturients should not be allowed to rest in the supine position, but rather be encouraged to maintain uterine displacement by a right or (preferably) left lateral tilt of the pelvis (Figure 2). Sympathetic blockade due to spinal or epidural anesthesia interferes with the mechanisms that compensate for aortocaval compression, sometimes causing profound hypotension in the absence of adequate uterine displacement and intravascular volume expansion. Conditions involving a particularly large uterus (e.g., multiple gestation, polyhydramnios, or diabetes mellitus) predispose to the risk and consequences of aortocaval compression.

Engorgement of the epidural vasculature (Batson's plexus) makes puncture or cannulation of an epidural vein more likely than in the non-

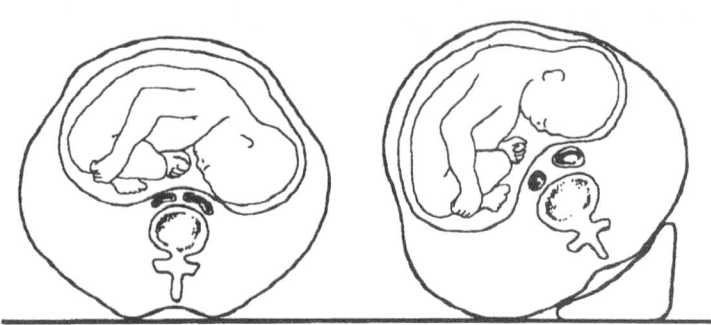

Figure 2. Aortocaval decompression with left lateral tilt.

pregnant patient during initiation of epidural anesthesia. Likewise, negative pressure in the epidural space may not be consistently found in the parturients (10), theoretically rendering the "hanging drop" technique for identification of the epidural space less successful in the pregnant patient than in nonpregnant patients.

Patients with cardiac disease may tolerate pregnancy poorly. The increased blood volume and decreased systemic resistance may cause decompensation in patients with stenotic valvular lesions and may worsen right-to-left shunting in the presence of uncorrected congenital heart defects. In contrast, parturients with regurgitant valvular lesions usually do quite well during pregnancy. Although coronary artery disease is rare among women of childbearing age, a gradual trend to older parturients may increase the incidence of myocardial ischemia, infarction, or both, during gestation (11). The hypermetabolic demands of pregnancy suggest that invasive monitoring be considered in parturients with known or suspected atherosclerotic, spastic, or thrombotic coronary artery disease. In addition, the differential diagnosis of hemodynamic instability from any cardiac etiologic factor should include echocardiography evaluation to rule out pericardial effusion.

RESPIRATORY SYSTEM

THE UPPER AIRWAY

Whereas generalized peripheral edema is a common nusiance in pregnancy, edematous changes of the upper airway may be life threatening. Mucous membranes become extremely friable during the third trimester, and manipulation of the upper airway, such as may occur during insertion of nasal airways or nasogastric tubes, or during nasotracheal intubation, should be done with great care to avoid severe bleeding. Toxemic patients are particularly susceptible to airway and vocal cord edema (12). The possibility of technically difficult intubation requiring small-diameter endotracheal tubes (i.e., 6.0 mm or less) should always be kept in mind when caring for such patients.

RESPIRATORY MECHANICS

The expanding uterus produces cephalad displacement of the diaphragm; thus, functional residual capacity (FRC) is decreased (13). Total lung capacity, vital capacity, and inspiratory capacity all remain unchanged, however, because of compensatory subcostal widening and enlarging of the thoracic anteroposterior diameter (14). The increased oxygen consumption of pregnancy is compensated by a 70% increase in alveolar ventilation at term (15). This is accomplished by increases in both tidal volume (40%) and respiratory rate (15%). Enhancement of tidal volume is largely due to rib cage volume displacement and less so to abdominal (diaphragmatic) movement (14). The rise in alveolar ventilation exceeds the oxygen demands of the parturient and is probably a result of elevated progesterone levels, which increases the ventilatory response to carbon dioxide (Table 2) (16).

Table 2. Maternal respiratory alterations at term. Adapted from Skaredoff and Ostheimer (56), with permission.

Variable	Change	Rate (%)
Minute ventilation	↑↑↑↑	50
Alveolar ventilation	↑↑↑↑↑	70
Tidal volume	↑↑↑	40
Respiratory rate	↑	15
Closing volume	±↓	0
Airway resistance	↓↓	36
Vital capacity	±	0
Inspiratory lung capacity	±	0
Functional residual capacity	↓↓	20
Total lung capacity	±	0
Expiratory reserve volume	↓↓	20
Residual volume	↓↓	20
Oxygen consumption	↑↑	20

GAS EXCHANGE

Ventilatory augmentation produces a respiratory alkalosis with compensatory renal excretion of bicarbonate and, hence, partial pH correction (15). Oxygenation is improved during normal pregnancy; arterial PO_2 values are typically slightly higher than in the nongravid state (Table 3). Physiologic dead space at term is decreased (17). It is likely that increased cardiac output with favorable ventilation-perfusion matching in upper lung zones accounts for both the increased PO_2 values and the decreased dead space.

Table 3. Acid base values in pregnancy vs. the nonpregnant state.

Variable	Nonpregnant state	Pregnancy
pH	7.38-7.42	7.38-7.42
PaO2 (mmHg)	90-100	100-110
PaCO2 (mmHg)	35-45	28-32

CLINICAL IMPLICATIONS

The decreased FRC is usually of little concern to the normal parturient. However, conditions that decrease closing volume (otherwise unchanged in normal pregnancy), such as smoking, obesity, or kyphoscoliosis, may result in airway closure and increasing hypoxemia as pregnancy progresses (18). The relationship between FRC and closing volume may be further aggravated by the positions assumed during birth (Trendelenburg, lithotomy, and supine) and by induction of general anesthesia (19). One should, therefore, have a low threshold for administration of supplemental oxygen to the parturient in labor, particularly during episodes of fetal distress or FRC, implying that acute oxygenation (denitrogenation) can occur more rapidly in the parturient than in the nonpregnant woman, and indeed this is the case (20). However, the marked increase in oxygen consumption contributes to the frighteningly rapid development of maternal hypoxemia during periods of apnea (21). The decrease in dead space serves to enhance further the reliability of noninvasive respiratory monitoring (capnography and/or mass spectrometry), as the gap between end-tidal and arterial gas measurements narrows (22).

GASTROINTESTINAL SYSTEM

Elevated levels of circulating progesterone decrease gastrointestinal motility, decrease food absorption, and lower esophageal sphincter pressure (23). In addition, elevated gastrin levels (of placental origin) result in more acidic gastric contents (24). The enlarged uterus increases intragastric pressure and decreases the normal oblique angle of the gastroesophageal junction.

CLINICAL IMPLICATIONS

These gastrointestinal tract alterations mean that the parturient should always be considered to have a full stomach, regardless of the actual number of hours elapsed since the last meal. Consequently, pregnant patients should always be considered at risk for aspiration of gastric contents (Mendelson syndrome), and measures should be taken to minimize this risk. Moreover, pain, anxiety, and treatment with narcotic analgesics serve to retard further gastric emptying during labor (25). Maternal "bearing down" efforts and the lithotomy position during the second stage of labor and delivery, coupled with incompetence of the lower esophageal sphincter mechanisms, make silent regurgitation and pulmonary aspiration more common than we often realize.

Our practice is to require oral administration of 30 ml of a nonarticular antacid (0.3 mol/L sodium citrate or its equivalent) before the initiation of any anesthetic. This agent rapidly decreases the acidity of gastric contents and helps ameliorate the consequences of aspiration. Histamine receptor (H_2) antagonists such as cimetidine (Tagamet) or ranitidine (Zantac) may be administered orally the evening before, and orally or intravenously the morning of, an elective procedure. Metoclopramide (Reglan) stimulates gastric emptying, increases lower esophageal sphincter tone, and serves as a centrally acting antiemetic. Metoclopramide has been very useful in parturients who have eaten a large meal shortly before arriving at the labor suite, as well as in diabetic patients, whose disease results in inherently slow gastric emptying.

HEMATOLOGIC SYSTEM

Both plasma volume and erythrocyte mass increase above prepregnant values, but the increase in the former far exceeds the increase in the latter. A "dilutional" anemia therefore ensues (3) (Table 4). Blood viscosity and oxygen content both decrease. Platelet count is usually

Table 4. Maternal hematologic alterations at term. From Skaredoff and Ostheimer (56), with permission.

Variable	Change	Rate (%)
Blood volume	↑↑↑	35
Plasma volume	↑↑↑↑	45
Erythrocyte volume	↑↑	20
Blood urea nitrogen	↓↓↓	33
Plasma cholinesterase	↓↓	20
Total protein	↑	18
Albumin	↓	14
Globulin	±	0
AST, ALT, LDH	↑	
Cholesterol	↓	
Alkaline phosphatase (produced by placenta)	↑↑	

AST, aspirate aminotransferase; ALT, alanine aminotransferase; LDH, lactate dehydrogenase.

elevated, as are coagulation factors I, VII, X, and XII. Thrombocytopenia may, however, be seen in some normal pregnant patients in the absence of any other hematopathology (26,27). Systemic fibrinolysis is slightly decreased from normal levels.

CLINICAL IMPLICATIONS

The physiologic "anemia of pregnancy" (normal hematocrit of 35%) is usually of little concern to the normal parturient, as increases in cardiac output serve actually to increase oxygen delivery to tissues. The increase in coagulation factors (Table 5) renders pregnancy a "hypercoaguable" state, with a consequent increase in the incidence of thrombotic events (e.g., deep venous and cortical vein thrombosis). Enhanced clotting, coupled with the expanded blood volume, affords teleological protection to the parturient against the effects of bleeding at the time of delivery.

RENAL SYSTEM

Renal hemodynamics undergo profound changes during gestation (28). Marked increases in renal plasma flow (80% above normal) occur by the middle of the second trimester and then decline slightly by term. Glomerular filtration rate (GFR) increases to 50% above prepregnant values by the 16th gestational week and remains so until delivery (Figure

Table 5. Coagulation factors and inhibitors during normal pregnancy. From
Shnider and Levinson (57), with permission.

Factor	Nonpregnant	Late pregnancy
Factor I (fibrinogen)	200-450 mg/dl	400-650 mg/dl
Factor II (prothrombin)	75-125%	100-125%
Factor V	75-125%	100-150%
Factor VII	75-125%	150-200%
Factor VIII	75-125%	200-500%
Factor IX	75-125%	100-150%
Factor X	75-125%	150-250%
Factor XI	75-125%	50-100%
Factor XII	75-125%	100-200%
Factor XIII	75-125%	35-75%
Antithrombin III	85-110%	75-100%
Antifactor Xa	85-110%	75-100%
Platelets		Slight ↑
Fibrinolysis		Slight ↓

3). Consequently, 24-hour creatine clearance values are elevated, a change
discernible as early as the eighth week of gestation. Glycosuria is common
in normal pregnancy, owing to both alteration in tubular reabsorptive
capacity and the increased load of glucose presented by the increased GFR.
While these changes are noted in early pregnancy, implying a hormonal
stimulus, the exact mechanism is as yet unknown. Increased levels of
aldosterone, cortisol, and human placental lactogen all contribute to the
multifactorial renal adaptations to pregnancy. Progesterone causes dilation of the renal pelvis and ureters. Hence, the incidence of urinary tract
infections is increased, particularly after instrumentation of the urinary
bladder (29).

CLINICAL IMPLICATIONS

Laboratory determinations of renal function are so altered that great
care must be exercised when "normal" nonpregnant values are applied to
the pregnant woman. For example, "normal" values of blood urea nitrogen and creatinine in a preeclamptic or diabetic patient may actually indicate serious renal compromise; in contrast, such values may indicate
hypovolemia in a parturient with otherwise normal renal function.

Serum electrolyte values are unchanged during pregnancy.
Expansion of plasma volume must therefore be accompanied by

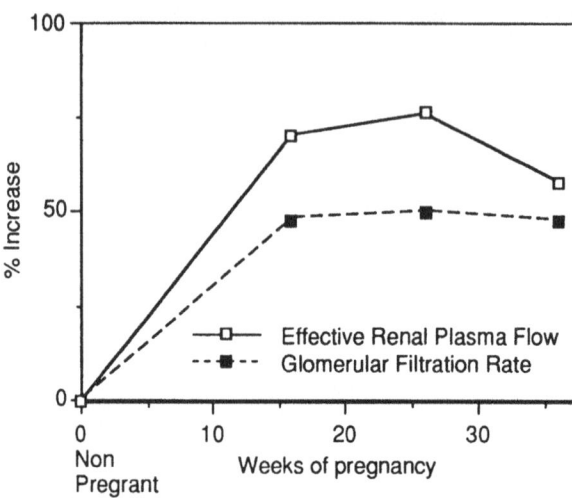

Figure 3. Renal function during pregnancy. Redrawn from Davison (28), with permission.

electrolyte retention. A primary resetting of thirst and vasopressin osmo-receptors allows the pregnant woman to maintain internal homeostasis during this volume-expanded state (i.e., the threshold for antidiuretic hormone secretion is reset at a lower level of plasma sodium, thus allowing volume expansion without accompanying diuresis). The antecedent stimulus for this adaptation has yet to be elucidated (28).

CENTRAL NERVOUS SYSTEM

Emotional, social, and cultural factors all contribute to the parturient's psychological milieu during labor and delivery (31-34). Pregnancy is a stressful experience, and wide mood swings during gestation, delivery, and the postpartum period can be expected. A hormonal basis for this emotional lability has been proposed, inasmuch as progesterone and endogenous endorphins act as both neurotransmitters and analgesics. Progesterone and endorphins also serve to decrease minimal alveolar concentration (MAC) of all inhaled anesthetic agents (35,36). In addition, reduced enzymatic degradation of opioids at term contributes to elevated pain thresholds (37).

Reduced doses of local anesthetic agents are required for spinal and epidural anesthesia compared with doses for nonpregnant patients (38). Vascular congestion in the epidural space contributes to the decreased local anesthetic requirement through three mechanisms:

1. Reduced volume in the epidural space facilitates spread of a given dose of local anesthetic over a wider number of dermatomes.
2. Increased pressure within the epidural space facilitates dural diffusion and higher cerebrospinal fluid levels of local anesthetic.
3. Venous congestion of the lateral foramina decreases egress of local anesthetic via the dural root sleeves.

The respiratory alkalosis of pregnancy may enhance local anesthetic action by increasing the relative concentration of uncharged local anesthetic molecules, which facilitates penetration through neural membranes. This decreased requirement for local anesthetic is seen as early as the first trimester. Hormonal changes may be operative as well, since progesterone has been shown to correlate with enhanced conduction blockade in isolated nerve preparations (39,40).

MISCELLANEOUS

MUSCULOSKELETAL

Placental production of the hormone relaxin stimulates generalized ligamentous relaxation (41). Particularly notable is the widening of the pelvis in preparation for fetal passage. A resultant "head-down" tilt is seen when the parturient assumes the lateral position, and compensation should be made when the anesthesiologist performs regional anesthesia (Figure 4).

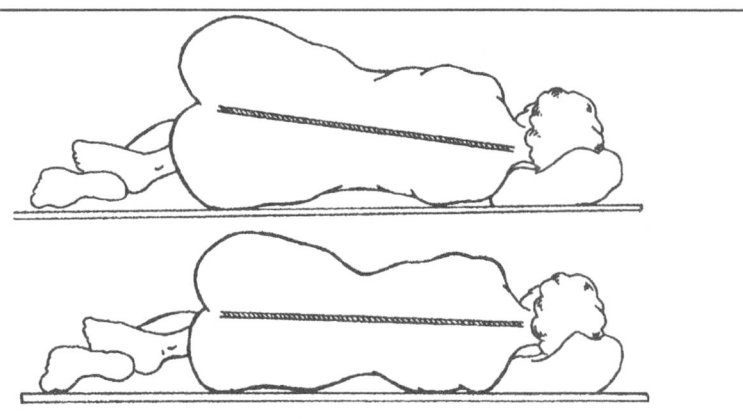

Figure 4. Pelvic widening and resultant "head-down" tilt in the lateral position during pregnancy. (Upper panel, pregnant).

Generalized vertebral collagenous softening, coupled with the burden of a gravid uterus, increases the lumbar lordosis. Technical difficulty with regional anesthesia may result. In addition, these changes account for the high incidence of back pain and sciatica during pregnancy, complaints which, per se, do not represent contraindications to regional anesthesia (42). Stress fractures of the weight-bearing bony pelvis have also been noted, especially during difficult deliveries (43).

DERMATOLOGIC

Hyperpigmentation of the face, neck (chloasma or "mask of pregnancy"), and abdominal midline (linea nigra) are due to the effects of melanocyte-stimulating hormone (MSH), a congener of adrenocorticotropic hormone (ACTH). Levels of MSH increase markedly during the first trimester and remain elevated until after delivery (44).

MAMMARY

Breast enlargement is typical in normal pregnancy and is a result of human placental lactogen secretion. Enlarged breasts in an obese parturient with a short neck may lead to difficult laryngoscopy and intubation. Use of a short-handled laryngoscope can be extremely helpful in these patients (Figure 5) (45).

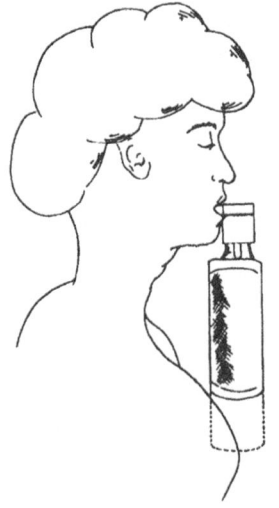

Figure 5. Use of the short-handled laryngoscope for the large-breasted parturient. Dotted line indicates a traditional laryngoscope handle impinging on breast tissue.

OCULAR

Conjunctival vasospasm and subconjunctional hemorrhage are occasionally seen, especially during maternal expulsive efforts and in preeclamptic patients (46). The retina may manifest focal vascular spasm, detachment, and retinopathy associated with hypertensive disorders. Central serous choriodopathy, or a breakdown of the blood-retina barrier, may occur even in the absence of hypertension.

Intraocular pressure is lower during pregnancy—perhaps a result of progesterone and relaxin effects (which facilitate aqueous outflow) and human chorionic gonadotropin (which depresses aqueous humor production). Corneal thickening, a manifestation of the generalized edema of pregnancy, may produce mild visual disturbances and contact lens intolerance during gestation (47).

INTRAPARTUM CHANGES

Active labor magnifies many of the physiologic variables already altered during gestation. Although the rigors of labor are usually well tolerated, the limited reserves of the term parturient may sometimes be stressed in ways not beneficial to mother or fetus.

CARDIOVASCULAR SYSTEM

Cardiac output during active labor rises to approximately twice prelabor values, with the maximal increase seen in the immediate postdelivery period (Figure 6). The rise in cardiac output is multifactorial. First, pain and anxiety during labor increase maternal circulating catecholamines, with a resultant tachycardia and increased stroke volume (48). Second, uterine contractions result in cyclic autotransfusion and increased central blood volume. This augmentation of preload in the setting of normal (or hyperdynamic) ventricular function contributes to increased cardiac output via Frank-Starling mechanisms.

Adequate regional anesthesia can ameliorate many of the pain-mediated hemodynamic consequences of labor. Uterine contractions, however, will still cause transient autotransfusions of blood with elevation of central vascular pressures.

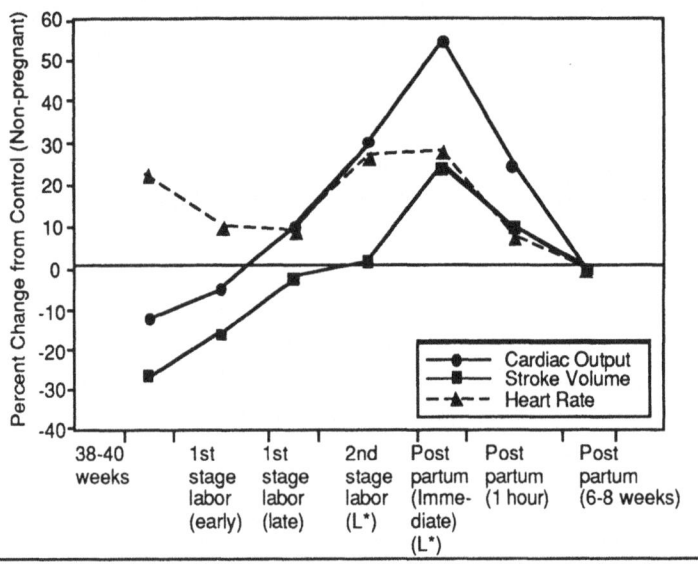

Figure 6. Cardiovascular alterations during labor. Redrawn from Shnider and Levinson (57), with permission.

RESPIRATORY SYSTEM

Hyperventilation is common during labor. This may be a natural response to pain or the result of various prepared childbirth methods in which repetitive, panting breathing techniques are used. Hyperventilation during labor in the setting of an already lowered maternal $PaCO_2$ at term may result in dangerous degrees of alkalemia. Women who have received narcotic analgesics during labor may alternate periods of hyperventilation with marked hypoventilation between concentrations, resulting in wide swings in $PaCO_2$ (49). The uterine vascular response to hypocarbia is vasoconstriction and subsequent decreased placental perfusion (50). Thus the potential for fetal hypoxemia exists during episodes of maternal alkalemia, particularly if a fetus is already compromised for other reasons.

Regional anesthesia during labor obviates the need for "breathing techniques" and eliminates pain-induced hyperventilation, so patients with marginal placental reserve (from preeclampsia, diabetes, postmature pregnancy, or small abruptio placentae, for example) are strong candidates for epidural anesthesia during labor.

METABOLIC EFFECTS

The homeostatic milieu that develops during gestation undergoes marked changes during labor. Metabolic acidosis may occur for several reasons. First, prolonged labor, especially in the setting of inadequate intravenous hydration, sometimes contributes to elevated lactate and pyruvate levels (51). Second, muscular activity, due to pain, shivering, or respiratory muscle demands, adds to acidic metabolites in the maternal circulation. Third, maternal alkalemia may predispose to compensatory acid retention. Overall maintenance of normal acid-base status during labor is accomplished by the balance of what may be markedly altered (vs. nonpregnant) levels of acidemic and alkalemic mediators. Thus, situations that further aggravate pH balance (e.g., dehydration, vomiting, ketoacidosis, hypothermia, hemorrhage) may be poorly tolerated by the gravida in labor.

The common markers of physiologic stress (epinephrine, norepinephrine, and cortisol) all increase during labor (52,53). The magnitude of this increase is blunted by regional anesthesia.

PUERPERAL RESOLUTION

Cardiac output rises sharply immediately after birth, as sustained contraction of the emptied uterus results in autotransfusion of 500-750 ml blood, coincident with elimination of the placental arteriovenous shunt. The immediate postpartum period is a high-risk time for decompensation in patients with certain cardiac disease states (particularly stenotic valvular lesions or pulmonary hypertension). Cardiac output gradually returns to nonpregnant levels by 2-4 weeks after delivery (3).

Uterine evacuation and involution promote rapid resolution of many of the pulmonary changes induced by mechanical compression of the diaphragm and lungs by the gravid uterus. The FRC and residual volume quickly return to normal. The gradual decline in blood progesterone levels is mirrored by a slow rise in arterial PCO_2, and alveolar ventilation returns to normal by 2-3 weeks postpartum (54).

Postpartum diuresis is common; this diuretic phase contributes to gradual decline in plasma volume, although red cell mass remains constant. Thus, the "dilutional" anemia of pregnancy resolves, and the hematocrit rises to nonpregnant levels in 2-4 weeks. Excessive blood loss at delivery markedly alters the course of hematologic resolution. The

GFR, blood urea nitrogen, and creatinine levels return to normal in 1-3 weeks (28).

Mechanical effects of the gastrointestinal tract rapidly resolve by 2-3 days postpartum. However, elevated levels of progesterone persist and may delay gastric emptying for several weeks. Precautions to minimize the risk and consequences of acid aspiration should therefore be taken if surgery with anesthesia is planned during this period (55).

THE DIFFICULT AIRWAY AND THE MANAGEMENT OF FAILED INTUBATION

Difficult airway management is one of the principal risks of general anesthesia for cesarean delivery. Gibbs (58) has estimated that difficult intubations are encountered in 5% of obstetric general anesthetics. Difficulty intubating the trachea may lead to hypoxemia, hypoventilation, and aspiration of gastric contents. The "Report on Confidential Inquiry into Maternal Deaths" in England and Wales for the years 1979-1981 revealed that 14% of deaths related to anesthesia were from anoxia and 10% were from aspiration associated with difficult intubation (59).

Three factors contribute to the complexity of airway management in obstetric anesthesia. First, altered gastrointestinal physiology during pregnancy places every parturient at risk for possible regurgitation and acid aspiration. Second, the time required for airway management and induction of general anesthesia may be critical in obstetric emergencies such as fetal distress or maternal hemorrhage. Third, airway anatomy may be altered in pregnancy. For example, patients with pregnancy-induced hypertension (PIH) may have edema of the upper airway (60,61).

PREOPERATIVE EVALUATION

Although the time required for preoperative evaluation in the parturient requiring an emergent operation may be limited, complete evaluation of the airway is essential. Mallampati et al (62) has shown in a prospective study that a classification system based on the ability to preoperatively visualize the soft palate, uvula, and faucial pillars accurately predicts difficult intubation.

Patients are divided into three classes:

Class 1: Faucial pillars, soft palate, and uvula can be visualized.

Class 2: Faucial pillars and soft palate can be visualized, but uvula is masked by the base of the tongue.

Class 3: Only soft palate can be visualized.

In addition to anatomic factors, the influence of physiologic changes associated with normal or complicated pregnancy must be considered. For example, upper airway edema can be seen with PIH, and with prolonged labor. In addition, breast enlargement associated with pregnancy can interfere with insertion of the laryngoscope (63).

If difficult intubation is suspected, the patient should be intubated while conscious. An alternative is to perform direct laryngoscopy under topical anesthesia. If the larynx can be visualized, intubation can be performed after induction of general anesthesia. If it is not visualized, awake intubation or regional anesthesia should be used.

TECHNIQUES FOR DIFFICULT INTUBATION

When possible, intubation by direct laryngoscopy is preferred because it is rapid, effective, and provides visual confirmation of placement of the endotracheal tube in the trachea (64). In our practice, we equip each operating room with MacIntosh #3 and #4 blades, a Miller #3 blade and a short laryngoscope handle for use in obese or large-breasted patients.

A second technique for difficult intubation is blind nasal intubation. This technique is relatively contraindicated in obstetric patients because it can cause nasal bleeding, which may hamper subsequent attempts at intubation. The risk of bleeding is particularly high in the parturient because the mucous membranes become very friable in late pregnancy. A second limitation of this technique is that it may be time consuming. Compared to orotracheal intubation using direct laryngoscopy or the lighted stylet, blind nasal intubation requires more time to perform, requires more attempts, and has a lower overall success rate (65,66).

A third approach to intubation of the parturient with a difficult airway involves the lighted stylet. This technique, which utilizes the position of transilluminated light to localize the tip of the styleted endotracheal tube in the airway, is easily learned. When compared to intubation by direct laryngoscopy the lighted stylet is equally as fast and requires only slightly more attempts (67). However, these comparisons were made in patients not preselected as having difficult airways, so further evaluation is necessary before this technique can be recommended for routine use in the parturient with a difficult airway.

A very powerful method for endotracheal intubation is fiberoptic endoscopy. Although this technique can be extremely valuable, its use may be limited by three factors. First, many anesthesiologists are not sufficiently experienced with fiberoptic endoscopy to utilize it for a difficult intubation. Second, the necessary equipment is expensive and complex, and may not be available in all obstetric operating rooms. Third, the time required for intubation in the most difficult cases may be longer than is desirable in an emergent situation (68).

A fifth approach to intubation of the difficult airway is the retrograde method (69). Reported success rates are high, but failures do occur. In addition, the time required for intubation has not been critically evaluated. However, most anesthesiologists are familiar with cricothyroid puncture and, with proper preparation, should be capable of using the technique.

The use of regional anesthesia for the patient with a difficult airway is controversial. Ideally, it avoids airway manipulation. However, complications of the regional anesthetic technique or intraoperative development of inadequate anesthesia may require emergent intubation. The utility of regional anesthesia for the patient with a difficult airway requiring cesarean delivery has been reviewed (69). It was suggested that continuous spinal anesthesia may be the safest and most reliable regional technique. However, for cesarean delivery, use of a single-dose spinal anesthetic or utilization of a previously placed epidural catheter may also be lifesaving.

THE DIFFICULT AIRWAY AND OBSTETRIC EMERGENCIES

A difficult and controversial issue is the management of anesthesia for cesarean delivery when the mother has a difficult airway and the fetus is in distress. True fetal distress is usually managed by cesarean delivery after rapid-sequence induction of general anesthesia. However, rapid-sequence induction is contraindicated in a patient with a suspected difficult airway because it can result in an anesthetized, paralyzed patient who cannot be intubated. Therefore, even in the setting of fetal distress, time must be taken to safely perform awake laryngoscopy, awake intubation, infiltration anesthesia, or major regional anesthesia. Regional anesthetic options include single-dose spinal anesthesia, continuous spinal anesthesia, or utilization of a pre-existing epidural catheter. Although the time required for these procedures may put the fetus at risk, the bulk of medical and legal doctrine favors overlooking the fetus before putting the mother at risk. In addition, the condition of an asphyxiated fetus may worsen if the mother becomes hypoxemic or hyperbaric. If a patient is suspected of having a difficult airway, the situation should be discussed with the obstetrician and patient early in labor. In this way, the obstetrician may elect less-emergent cesarean delivery at the earliest suspicion of fetal distress. In this manner, potential conflicts can be anticipated and avoided, and the patient and surgeon will not have unrealistic expectations.

MANAGEMENT OF FAILED INTUBATION

If intubation fails, the lungs should be ventilated while cricoid pressure remains applied. The prompt decision to abandon the first intubation attempt and ventilate the lungs by mask is critical. Scott has argued that patients do not die from failure to intubate, they die from failure to stop trying to intubate (70). The hemoglobin saturation of the parturient at term will decline very rapidly when the patient is apneic because oxygen consumption is increased and the functional residual capacity is decreased during pregnancy. In addition, prolonged attempts at intubation may provoke retching, vomiting, and subsequent aspiration of gastric contents.

Further attempts at intubation should be limited and well conceived, in order to minimize airway trauma. Alternative methods, such as the lighted stylet or fiberoptic endoscope, should be considered. Additional anesthetic or neuromuscular-blocking agents should not be administered unless: 1) successful intubation is considered to be certain with an additional attempt, or 2) it is elected to proceed with general anesthesia and mask ventilation.

If intubation fails, one must decide whether to awaken the patient and employ an alternative anesthetic approach, such as awake intubation or regional anesthesia, or to proceed with general anesthesia and mask ventilation. If the fetus does not require emergent cesarean delivery for distress, the patient should be allowed to awaken. If the fetus is at risk, the decision must be based upon the clinical situation and the philosophy of the individual practitioner.

Some authors propose the use of lateral or head-down positions, laryngeal masks, esophageal obturator airways, or gastric suctioning in managing failed intubation. We do not routinely utilize these maneuvers because changes in patient position or manipulation of the pharynx and esophagus might interfere with ventilation, alter the competency of the lower esophageal sphincter, or stimulate retching and/or vomiting.

FAILURE OF INTUBATION AND VENTILATION

If the trachea cannot be intubated and the lungs cannot be ventilated via mask, two options exist: the lungs can be ventilated using transtracheal jet ventilation, or an airway can be established by cricothyroidotomy.

The utility of transtracheal jet ventilation in the management of the difficult airway has recently been reviewed (71). This technique has been shown to provide excellent oxygenation and ventilation in experimental animals, in elective surgical patients, and in patients with complete upper airway obstruction. Using a driving pressure of 50 psi, a gas flow of 500 ml/sec can be delivered through a 16-gauge catheter. This gas flow is sufficient for adequate ventilation.

If transtracheal jet ventilation is utilized, it may be continued until either the patient regains consciousness, the airway is secured by orotracheal and nasotracheal intubation, or cricothyroidotomy or tracheotomy is performed. Although transtracheal jet ventilation is a very useful technique, it does not provide protection of the airway from aspiration of gastric contents, a significant concern in the parturient.

Cricothyroidotomy is more complex and invasive than transtracheal jet ventilation but has three potential advantages. First, insertion of a cuffed tube protects the airway from aspiration. Second, insertion of an appropriately sized tube allows tracheal suctioning. Third, there may be less likelihood of barotrauma and emphysema than with transtracheal jet ventilation. Therefore, this technique should be considered, particularly if prolonged ventilatory support is anticipated.

Although cricothyroidotomy is an invasive procedure, it is one which every anesthesiologist should be prepared to perform. Many approaches and techniques have been described. Although several adjunctive or percutaneous devices have been developed, none have found widespread use. (See Figure 1).

What is the place for the laryngeal mask airway in parturients that cannot be intubated? Unfortunately, the place for the laryngeal mask is still being defined. Brain (72) states he is aware of it being "lifesaving" on a number of occasions with failed intubation (73,74). Since the laryngeal mask cannot guarantee against aspiration, it must be viewed as a device to help provide oxygenation and avoid hypoxia. Heath has shown (75) that the laryngeal mask can be used as a guide for intubation, but this usage requires some experience with the laryngeal mask. More information will be developed on this device in the future.

CARDIAC ARREST IN THE PARTURIENT

Cardiac arrest in late pregnancy or during delivery is a rare event. Unfortunately, when it occurs, maternal survival is very low because the etiology of the arrest is not often reversed and the physiologic changes present in late pregnancy often hamper effective cardiopulmonary resuscitative efforts.

Some causes of cardiac arrest in the parturient at term include:
1. airway problems
2. "total" spinal anesthetic
3. local anesthetic toxicity from unintentional intravascular injection
4. trauma
5. embolism-amniotic, thrombus.

PHYSIOLOGIC CHANGES OF PREGNANCY AS THEY RELATE TO CARDIOPULMONARY RESUSCITATION

Term pregnant patients are at a distinct disadvantage during cardiac arrest. They become hypoxic more readily because of a 20% decrease in their functional residual capacity and a 20% increase in their resting oxygen consumption (76). The enlarged uterus, along with the resultant upward displacement of the abdominal viscera, will decrease compliance during controlled ventilation. The most serious problem is the effect of aortocaval compression in the supine position. During closed chest cardiac compression (CCCC) in adults, the best cardiac output that can be achieved is between one-fourth to one-third of normal. Although many factors contribute to this, poor venous return to the heart is of paramount importance. At term, the vena cava is completely occluded in 90% of supine pregnant patients, resulting in as much as a 70% decrease in cardiac stroke volume. Therefore, it is essential that lateral displacement of the gravid uterus be initiated at once during cardiopulmonary resuscitation of the pregnant patient.

TREATMENT OF MATERNAL CARDIAC ARREST

The resuscitation of a pregnant patient at term is unlikely to be successful unless vena caval compression is eliminated. To accomplish this, a "wedge" must be placed under the right hip to displace the gravid uterus to the left. Rees and Willis (77) have shown that effective CCCC can be accomplished with a patient tilted at a 30-degree angle to the left. CPR should begin immediately by securing the airway and following current ACLS guidelines. If aggressive CPR with a properly positioned patient is not successful after a short interval, immediate cesarean delivery must be performed as soon as possible (78-80). This procedure will immediately relieve the vena caval obstruction from the gravid uterus and increase the chance of survival for both the infant and the mother. CPR must be continued throughout the procedure until spontaneous and effective cardiac activity occurs. Controlled ventilation may have to be continued for a longer period of time. This aggressive approach to management will increase survival rates for mothers and newborns.

REFERENCES

1. Pernoll ML, Metcalf J, Schlensler TL: Oxygen consumption at rest and during exercise in pregnancy. Respir Physiol 22:285, 1975
2. Mashini IS, Albazzaz SJ, Fadel HE: Serial noninvasive evaluation of cardiovascular hemodynamics during pregnancy. Am J Obstet Gynecol 156:208, 1987
3. Ueland K: Maternal cardiovascular hemodynamics. VII: Intrapartum blood volume changes. Am J Obstet Gynecol 126:671, 1976
4. Shrier RW, Durr JA: Pregnancy: An overfill or underfill state. Am J Kidney Dis 9:284, 1987
5. Schrier RW: Pathogenesis of sodium and water retention in high-output and low-output cardiac failure, nephrotic syndrome, cirrhosis, and pregnancy. N Eng J Med 319:1127, 1988
6. Eckstein KL, Marx GF: Aortocaval compression: Incidence and prevention. Anesthesiology 40:381, 1965
7. Enein M, Zina AA, Kassem M et al: Echocardiography of the pericardium in pregnancy. Obstet Gynecol 69:851, 1987
8. Paller MS: Decreased pressor responsiveness in pregnancy: Studies in experimental animals. Am J Kidney Dis 9:308, 1987
9. De Simone CA, Leighton BL, Norris MC et al: The chronotropic effect of isoproterenol is reduced in term pregnant women. Anesthesiology 69:626, 1988
10. Messih MNA: Epidural space pressures during pregnancy. Anaesthesia 36:775, 1981
11. Kirz DS, Dorchester W, Freeman RK: Advanced maternal age; the mature gravida. Am J Obstet Gynecol 152:7, 1985
12. Bletka M, Hlavat JV, Trakova M: Volume of whole blood and absolute amount of serum proteins in the early stages of late toxemia of pregnancy. Am J Obstet Gynecol 106:10, 1970
13. Knuttgen HG, Emerson K: Physiologic response to pregnancy at rest and during exercise. J Appl Physiol 36:549, 1975

14. Gilroy RJ, Mangura BT, Lavietes MH: Rib cage and abdominal volume displacements during breathing in pregnancy. Am Rev Respir Dis 137:668, 1988
15. Prowse CM, Gaenster EA: Respiratory and acid-base changes during pregnancy. Anesthesiology 26:381, 1965
16. Tyler JM: The effects of progesterone on the respiration of patients with emphysema and hypercapnea. J Clin Invest 39:34, 1960
17. Shankar KB, Moseley H, Vemula V et al: Physiological dead space during general anesthesia for caesarean section. Can J Anaesth 34:373, 1987
18. Leontie EA: Respiratory disease in pregnancy. Med Clin North Am 62:111, 1974
19. Bevan DR, Holdcroft A, Loh L et al: Closing volume and pregnancy. Br Med J [Clin Res] 1:13, 1974
20. Russell GN, Smith CL, Snowdon SL et al: Preoxygenation and the parturient patient. Anaesthesia 42:346, 1987
21. Archer GW, Marx GF: Arterial oxygen tension during apnea in parturient women. Br J Anaesth 46:358, 1974
22. Bhavanishankaat K, Moseley H, Kumar Y et al: Arterial to end-tidal carbon dioxide tension difference during anaesthesia for tubal ligation. Anaesthesia 42:482, 1987
23. Lind LJ, Smith AM, McIver DK et al: Lower esophageal sphincter pressures in pregnancy. Can Med Assoc J 98:571, 1968
24. Attia RR, Ebeid AM, Fisher JE et al: Maternal, fetal and placental gastrin concentrations. Anaesthesia 37:18, 1982
25. O'Sullivan GM, Sutton AJ, Thompson SA et al: Noninvasive measurement of gastric emptying in obstetric patients. Anesth Analg 66:505, 1987
26. O'Brien WF, Saba HI, Knuppel RA et al: Alterations in platelet concentration and aggregation in normal pregnancy and preeclampsia. Am J Obstet Gynecol 155:486, 1986
27. Burrows RF, Kelton JG: Incidentally detected thrombocytopenia in healthy mothers and their infants. N Engl J Med 319:142, 1988
28. Davison JM: Overview of kidney function in pregnant women. Am J Kidney Dis 9:248, 1987
29. Bellina JH, Dougherty CM, Mickal A: Ureteral dilation in pregnancy. Am J Obstet Gynecol 108:356, 1970
30. Datta S, Kitzmiller JL, Naulty JS et al: Acid-base status of diabetic mothers and their infants following spinal anesthesia for cesarean section. Anesth Analg 61:662, 1982
31. Stewart DE: Psychiatric symptoms following attempted natural childbirth. Can Med Assoc J 127:713, 1982
32. Lee RV, D'Alauro F, White LM et al: Southeast Asian folklore about pregnancy and parturition. Obstet Gynecol 71:643, 1922
33. Senden IP, Wetering VD, Eskes TK et al: Labor pain: A comparison of parturients in a Dutch and American teaching hospital. Obstet Gynecol 71:541, 1988

34. Colman AD: Psychological state during first pregnancy. Am J Orthospychiatry 39:788, 1969
35. Palahniuk RJ, Shnider SM, Eger EI: Pregnancy decreases the requirement for inhaled anesthetic agents. Anesthesiology 41:82, 1974
36. Goland RS, Wordlaw SL, Stark RI et al: Human plasma endorphin during pregnancy, labor and delivery. J Clin Endocrinol Metab 52:74, 1981
37. Lyrenas S, Nyberg F, Lindberg BO et al: Cereborspinal fluid activity of dynorphin-converting enzyme at term pregnancy. Obstet Gynecol 72:54, 1988
38. Datta S, Hurley RJ, Naulty JS et al: Plasma and cerebrospinal fluid progesterone concentrations in pregnant and nonpregnant women. Anesth Analg 69:950, 1986
39. Datta S, Lambert DH, Gregus J et al: Differential sensitivities of mammalian nerve fibers during pregnancy. Anesth Analg 62:1070, 1983
40. Flanagan HL, Datta S, Lambert DH et al: Effect of pregnancy on bupivacaine-induced conduction blockade in the isolated rabbit vagus nerve. Anesth Analg 66:123, 1987
41. Kemp BE, Niall HD: Relaxin. Vitam Horm 41:79, 1985
42. Berg G, Hammar M, Moller J et al: Low back pain during pregnancy. Obstet Gynecol 71:71, 1988
43. Moran JJ: Stress fractures in pregnancy. Am J Obstet Gynecol 158:1274, 1988
44. Diczfalusy E, Troen P: Endocrine functions of the human placenta. Vitam Horm 19:229, 1961
45. Datta S, Briwa J: Modified laryngoscope for endotracheal intubation of obese partients. Anesth Analg 60:120, 1981
46. Weinreb RN, Lu A, Key T: Maternal ocular adaptations during pregnancy. Obstet Gynecol Surv 42:471, 1987
47. Weinreb RN, Lu A, Besson C: Corneal thickness in pregnancy. Am J Opthalmol 105:258, 1988
48. Jones CM, Greiss FC: The effect of labor on maternal and fetal circulating catecholamines. Am J Obstet Gynecol 194:149, 1982
49. Huch A, Huch R, Lindmark G et al: Transcutaneous oxygen measurements in labor. J Obstet Gynaecol Br Commonw 81:608, 1974
50. Moya F, Morishima HO, Shnider SM et al: Influence of maternal hyperventilation on the newborn infant. Am J Obstet Gynecol 90:76, 1965
51. Zador G, Willeck-Lund G, Nillson BA: Acid-base changes associated with labor. Acta Obstet Gynecol Scand (suppl) 34:41, 1974
52. Lederman RP, McCann DS, Work B: Endogenous plasma epinephrine and norepinephrine in last trimester pregnancy and labor. Am J Obstet Gynecol 129:5, 1977
53. Maltau JM, Eielsen OV, Stotcke KT: Effect of stress during labor on the concentration of cortisol and esteriol in maternal plasma. Am J Obstet Gynecol 134:681, 1979

54. Cugell DW: Pulmonary function in pregnancy. I. Serial observations in normal women. Am Rev Tuberc 67:568-1953
55. James CF, Gibbs CP, Banner TE: Postparum perioperative risk of pulmonary aspiration. Abstracts of scientific papers. Society for Obstetric Anesthesia and Perinatology. Vancouver, Canada, May, 1983
56. Skaredoff MN, Ostheimer GW: Physiological changes during pregnancy; effects of major regional anesthesia. Reg Anesth 6:28, 1981
57. Shnider S, Levinson G: Anesthesia for obstetrics. 2nd edition. Baltimore, Williams & Wilkins, 1987
58. Gibbs CP: Gastric aspiration: prevention and treatment. Clin Anesthesiol 4:47-52, 1986
59. Turnbull AC, Tindall VR, Robson G et al: Report on confidential enquiries into maternal deaths in England and Wales 1979-1981. London, Her Majesty's Stationary Office, 1986, pp 85-87
60. Brock-Utne JG, Downing JW, Seedat F: Laryngeal oedema associated with preeclampsic toxemia. Anaesth 32:556-558, 1977
61. Jouppila R, Joupilla P, Hollmen A: Laryngeal oedema as an obstetric anesthesia complication. Acta Anaesthesiol Scand 24:97-98, 1980
62. Mallampati SR, Gatt SP, Gugino LD et al: A clinical sign to predict difficult intubation: A prospective study. Can Anaes Soc J 32:429-434, 1985
63. Latto IP: Management of difficult intubation. In Latto IP, Rosen M, eds. Difficulties in tracheal intubation. London: Balliere Tindall, 99-141, 1985
64. Gold MI, Buechel DR: A method of blind nasal intubation for the conscious patient. Anesth Analg 39:257-263, 1960
65. Fox DJ, Castro T, Rastrelli AJ: Comparison of intubation techniques in the awake patient: The Flexi-lum surgical light (lightwand) versus blind nasal approach. Anesthesiology 66:69-71, 1987
66. Ellis DG, Jakymec A, Kaplan RM et al: Guided orotracheal intubation in the operating room using a lighted stylet: A comparison with direct laryngoscopic technique. Anesthesiology 64:823-826, 1986
67. Ovasappian A, Yelich S, Dykes MHM et al: Fiberoptic nasotracheal intubation—incidence and causes of failure. Anesth Analg 62:692-695, 1983
68. Dhara SS: Guided blind endotracheal intubation. Anaesth 35:81, 1980
69. Malan TP, Johnson MD: The difficult airway in obstetric anesthesia: Techniques for airway management and the role of regional anesthesia. J Clin Anesth 1:104-110, 1988
70. Scott DB: Endotracheal intubation: Friend or foe? Br Med J 292:157, 1986
71. Benumof JL, Scheller MS: The importance of transtracheal jet ventilation in the management of the difficult airway. Anesthesiology 71:769-778, 1989
72. Brain AIJ: Use of the laryngeal mask in obstetric anesthesia. In Van Zundert A, Ostheimer GW, eds. Pain relief and anesthesia in obstetrics. London, Churchill-Livingstone, 1994

73. Chadwick IS, Vohra A: Anaesthesia for cesarean section using the laryngeal airway. Anaesthesia 44:261-262, 989

74. McClune S, Moore J: Laryngeal mask airway for caesarean section. Anaesth 46:227-228, 1990

75. Heath ML: Endotracheal intubation through the laryngeal mask— helpful when laryngoscopy is difficult or dangerous. Eur J Anaesth 4:41-45, 1991

76. Zakowski MI, Ramanathan S: CPR in pregnancy. Cur Rev Clin Anesth (review) 10:106-111, 1990

77. Rees GAD, Willis BA.: Resuscitation in late pregnancy. Anaesth 43:347-349, 1988

78. Oates S, Williams GL, Rees GAD: Cardiopulmonary resuscitation in late pregnancy. Br Med J 297:404-405, 1988

79. Marx G.: Cardiopulmonary resuscitation of late pregnant women. Anesthesiology 56:156, 1982

80. O'Connor RL, Sevarino FB: Cardiopulmonary arrest in the pregnant patient: A report of a successful resuscitation. J Clin Anesth 6:66-68, 1994

CARDIAC DISEASE IN PREGNANCY*

S. L. Clark

Pregnancy brings about profound alterations in the maternal cardio-vascular system. The pregnant patient with normal cardiac function accommodates such physiologic changes without difficulty. However, in the presence of significant cardiac disease, pregnancy can be extremely haz-ardous and may result in decompensation and death. Indeed, in the pres-ence of cardiac disease involving pulmonary hypertension, pregnancy car-ries a risk of maternal mortality (30-50%) exceeding that which is associ-ated with any other systemic disease. This chapter focuses on the interac-tion between structural cardiac disease and pregnancy.

COUNSELING THE PREGNANT CARDIAC PATIENT

Prior to 1973, the Criteria Committee of the New York Heart Association (NYHA) recommended cardiac disease classification based on clinical function (Classes I-IV). Although such a classification is useful in discussing the pregnant cardiac patient, up to 40% of patients developing congestive heart failure and pulmonary edema during pregnancy are func-tional Class I prior to pregnancy; indeed, in one review, the majority of maternal deaths during pregnancy occurred in patients who were initially Class I or II (1). For such reasons, the older functional classification largely has been abandoned and replaced by a more complex descriptive system encompassing etiologic, anatomic, and physiologic diagnosis (2). Despite this reclassification, the older and simpler functional classification remains prognostically useful when comparing the performance of indi-viduals with uniform etiologic and anatomic diagnoses (for example, all patients with rheumatic mitral stenosis). Further, the severity of maternal symptoms has been shown to be directly proportional to adverse perinatal outcome, irrespective of the type or duration of cardiac disease (3).

*Clark SL: Structural cardiac disease in pregrancy. *Critical Care Obstetrics*, II ed. Chpt. 7. SL Clark, DB Cotton, GD Hankins and JP Phelan, eds. Blackwell Scientific Publications, Boston, MA, U.S.A., 1991. Reproduced with permission.

T.H. Stanley and P.G. Schafer (eds.), Pediatric and Obstetrical Anesthesia, 27-49.
© 1995 *Kluwer Academic Publishers.*

Counseling the pregnant cardiac patient about her prognosis for successful pregnancy is complicated by recent advances in medical and surgical therapy, fetal surveillance, and neonatal care. Such advances render invalid many older estimates of maternal mortality and fetal wastage. Table 1 represents a synthesis of current maternal mortality estimates for various types of cardiac disease. Both counseling and general management approaches are based on this classification. Group I includes conditions that, with proper management, should have negligible maternal mortality (<1%). Cardiac lesions in Group II carry a 5-15% risk of maternal mortality, either secondary to the cardiac disease itself, or because of associated thromboembolic phenomena and the need for anticoagulation during pregnancy. In individual cases, and after appropriate counseling, this risk may prove acceptable to some women. Patients with cardiac lesions in Group III are subject to a mortality risk exceeding 25%. In all but exceptional cases, this risk proves unacceptable to the patient, and prevention or interruption of pregnancy should be recommended strongly.

Table 1. Mortality Risk Associated with Pregnancy

Group I—Mortality <1%	Group II—Mortality 5-15%	Group III—Mortality 25-50%
Atrial septal defect	Mitral Stenosis with Atrial Fibrillation	Pulmonary hypertension
Ventricular septal defect	Artificial valve	Coarctation of aorta, complicated
Patent ductus arteriosus*	Mitral stenosis, NyHA Class III and IV	Marfan syndrome with aortic involvement
Pulmonic tricuspid disease	Aortic stenosis	
Corrected tetralogy of Fallot	Coarctation of aorta, uncomplicated	
Porcine valve	Uncorrected tetralogy of Fallot	
Mitral stenosis, NYHA Class I and II	Previous myocardial infarction	
	Marfan's Syndrome with normal aorta	

*Uncomplicated

CONGENITAL CARDIAC DISEASE

The relative frequency of congenital, as opposed to acquired, heart disease is changing (1). Rheumatic fever is uncommon in the United States, and more patients with congenital cardiac disease now survive to reproductive age. In a review in 1954, the ratio of rheumatic-to-congenital heart disease seen during pregnancy was 16:1; by 1967, this ratio had changed to 3:1 (4,5). In the subsequent discussion of specific cardiac lesions, no attempt is made to duplicate existing comprehensive texts regarding physical diagnostic, electrocardiographic, and radiographic findings of specific cardiac lesions. (For a comprehensive discussion of diagnostic findings, see Braunwald E., ed.: Heart Disease, 5th edition. Philadelphia, W.B. Saunders Co., 1988.) Rather, the discussion presented here focuses on aspects of cardiac disease that are unique to pregnancy.

ATRIAL SEPTAL DEFECT (ASD)

Atrial septal defect (ASD) is the most common congenital lesion to be seen during pregnancy and, in general, it is asymptomatic (6,7). The two significant potential complications that are seen with ASD are arrhythmias and heart failure. Although atrial arrhythmias are not uncommon in patients with ASD, their onset generally occurs after the fourth decade of life; thus such arrhythmias are unlikely to be encountered in the pregnant woman. In ASD patients with arrhythmias, atrial fibrillation is most common; however, supraventricular tachycardia and atrial flutter also may occur (8). Initial therapy is with digoxin; less commonly, propranolol, quinidine, or even cardioversion may be necessary. The hypervolemia associated with pregnancy results in an increased left-to-right shunt through the ASD; thus a significant burden is imposed on the right ventricle. Although this additional burden is tolerated well by most patients, congestive failure and death with ASD have been reported (9-12). In contrast to the high-pressure/high-flow state seen with ventricular septal defect (VSD) and patent ductus arteriosus (PDA), ASD is characterized by high pulmonary blood flow associated with normal pulmonary artery pressures. Because pulmonary artery pressures are low, the development of pulmonary hypertension is unusual. The vast majority of patients with ASD tolerate pregnancy, labor, and delivery without complication. Neilson et al (9) reported 70 pregnancies in 24 patients with ASD; all patients had an uncomplicated ante- and intrapartum course. Intrapartum management of patients with ASD is outlined at this chapter's conclusion. Prophylaxis against subacute bacterial endocarditis is perhaps the most important consideration (Table 2).

VENTRICULAR SEPTAL DEFECT (VSD)

Ventricular septal defect may occur as an isolated lesion or in conjunction with other congenital cardiac anomalies, including tetralogy of

Table 2. Subacute Bacterial Endocarditis Prophylaxis*
Ampicillin 2 gm IV plus Gentamicin sulfate 1.5 mg/kg IM or IV
Vancomycin 1 gm IV plus Gentamicin sulfate 1.5 mg/kg IM or IV[†]

*Administer every 8 hr for up to 3 doses, beginning 1/2 to 1 hour prior to delivery. IV = intravenous, IM = intramuscular
[†]For patients allergic to penicillin.

Fallot, transposition of the great vessels, and coarctation of the aorta. The size of the septal defect is the most important determinant of clinical prognosis during pregnancy. Small defects are tolerated well; larger defects are associated more frequently with congestive failure, arrhythmias, or the development of pulmonary hypertension. In addition, a large VSD often is associated with some degree of aortic regurgitation, which can add to the risk of congestive failure. Pregnancy, labor, and delivery generally are tolerated well by patients with uncomplicated VSD (12). Schaefer et al (10) compiled a series of 141 pregnancies in 56 women with VSD. The only two maternal deaths were in women whose VSD was complicated by pulmonary hypertension (Eisenmenger syndrome). Although very rarely indicated, successful primary closure of a large VSD during pregnancy has been reported (13). Intrapartum management of patients with uncomplicated VSD, ASD, or PDA involves principally fluid restriction and prophylaxis against endocarditis.

PATENT DUCTUS ARTERIOSIS (PDA)

Although patent ductus arteriosis is one of the most common congenital cardiac anomalies, its almost universal detection and closure in the newborn period makes it uncommon during pregnancy (14,15). As with uncomplicated ASD and VSD, most patients are asymptomatic, and PDA generally is tolerated well during pregnancy, labor, and delivery. As with a large VSD, however, the high-pressure/high-flow left-to-right shunt associated with a large, uncorrected PDA can lead to pulmonary hypertension. In such cases, the prognosis becomes much worse. In one study of 18 pregnant women who died of congenital heart disease, 3 had PDA; however, all of these patients had secondary severe pulmonary hypertension (11). The continuous "machinery" murmur of PDA is known well; however, the murmur may disappear following the development of pulmonary hypertension.

EISENMENGER SYNDROME

Eisenmenger syndrome develops when, in the presence of a congenital left-to-right shunt, progressive pulmonary hypertension leads to shunt reversal or bidirectional shunting. Although the syndrome can occur with ASD, VSD, or PDA, the low-pressure/high-flow shunt seen with ASD is far less likely to result in pulmonary hypertension and shunt reversal than is the condition of high pressure and high flow seen with VSD and PDA. Whatever the etiology, pulmonary hypertension carries a grave prognosis during pregnancy. During the antepartum period, the decreased systemic vascular resistance associated with pregnancy increases the likelihood or degree of right-to-left shunting. Pulmonary perfusion then decreases; this decrease results in hypoxemia and deterioration of maternal and fetal condition. In such a patient, systemic hypotension leads to decreased right ventricular filling pressures; in the presence of fixed pulmonary hypertension, such decreased right-heart pressures may be insufficient to perfuse the pulmonary arterial bed. This insufficiency may result in sudden, profound hypoxemia and death. Such hypotension can result from hemorrhage or complications of conduction anesthesia and can lead to sudden death (16-19). Such an occurrence is the principal clinical concern in the intrapartum management of patients with pulmonary hypertension.

Maternal mortality in the presence of Eisenmenger syndrome is reported as 30-50% (17,18). In a review of the subject, Gleicher et al (17) reported a 34% mortality associated with vaginal delivery and a 75% mortality associated with cesarean section. Eisenmenger syndrome associated with VSD appears to carry a higher mortality risk (65%) than that associated with PDA or ASD (33%). In addition to the previously discussed problems associated with hemorrhage and hypovolemia, thromboembolic phenomena occur, and they have been associated with up to 43% of all maternal deaths in Eisenmenger syndrome (17). However, Pitts et al (20) reported an increased mortality associated with prophylactic peripartum heparinization. Sudden delayed postpartum death, occurring 4-6 weeks after delivery, also has been reported on several occasions (17,21). Although the pathophysiology of this condition is unknown, such deaths may involve a rebound worsening of pulmonary hypertension associated with the loss of pregnancy-associated hormones.

Because of the high mortality associated with continuing pregnancy, abortion is the preferred management for the woman with pulmonary hypertension of any etiology. Dilatation and curettage in the first trimester or dilatation and evacuation in the second trimester are the methods of choice. Hypertonic saline and F-prostaglandins are contraindicated, the latter due to documented maternal oxygen desaturation that accompanies the use of these agents (22). The hemodynamic effects of E-prostaglandins in patients with pulmonary hypertension are not documented, but a 65% increase in cardiac output has been demonstrated in association with those agents in normal pregnancy patients (23). This hemodynamic effect, and the lack of immediate reversibility of this agent, should be considered when contemplating the use of E-prostaglandins in a pregnant patient with cardiac disease.

For a patient with a continuing gestation, hospitalization for the duration of pregnancy is often appropriate. Continuous administration of O_2, the pulmonary vasodilator of choice, is mandatory. In cyanotic heart disease of any etiology, fetal outcome correlates well with maternal hematocrit, and successful pregnancy is unlikely with a hematocrit >65%. Maternal arterial partial pressure of oxygen (paO_2) should be maintained at a level of 70 mm Hg or above (24). Third trimester fetal surveillance with ultrasound and antepartum testing is important because at least 30% of the fetuses will be growth retarded (17). Overall fetal wastage with Eisenmenger syndrome is reported to be up to 75%.

Pulmonary artery catheterization is recommended during the intrapartum period. Placement and maintenance of the pulmonary artery catheter often is difficult in the presence of pulmonary hypertension. In such cases, we have used successfully a catheter with an accessory lumen. Following placement, a guide wire is introduced to provide the necessary rigidity to maintain the catheter in place. In a number of cases, simultaneous cardiac imaging with ultrasound also has been helpful in catheter placement. During labor, uterine contractions are associated with a decrease in the ratio of pulmonary-to-systemic blood flow (Qp/Qs) (25). Pulmonary artery catheterization and serial arterial blood gas determinations allow the clinician to detect and treat early changes in cardiac output, pulmonary artery pressure, and shunt fraction. We have used a fiberoptic pulmonary artery catheter in conjunction with an oximeter to detect early changes in mixed venous O_2 saturation during the successful intrapartum management of patients with pulmonary hypertension. Because the primary concern in such patients is the avoidance of hypotension, any attempt at preload reduction (i.e., diuresis) must be undertaken with great caution even in the face of initial fluid overload. We prefer to manage such patients on the "wet" side; therefore, we maintain a preload margin against unexpected blood loss, even at the risk of some degree of pulmonary edema (21). Intrapartum management is described in more detail at the conclusion of this chapter.

Anesthesia for patients with pulmonary hypertension is controversial. Theoretically, conduction anesthesia, with its accompanying risk of hypotension, should be avoided. However, there are several reports of its successful use in patients with pulmonary hypertension of different etiologies (18,25,26). The use of epidural or intrathecal morphine sulfate, a technique devoid of effect on systemic blood pressure, has been described by Abboud et al (27) and represents perhaps the best approach to anesthetic management of these difficult patients.

COARCTATION OF THE AORTA

Coarctation of the aorta accounts for 9% of all congenital cardiac disease. The most common site of coarctation is the origin of the left subclavian artery. Associated anomalies of the aorta and left heart, including VSD and PDA, are common, as are intracranial aneurysms of the circle of Willis (28). Coarctation is usually asymptomatic. Its presence is suggested by hypertension confined to the upper extremities, although Goodwin (27) cites data suggesting a generalized increase in peripheral resistance throughout the body. Resting cardiac output may be increased; however, increased left atrial pressure with exercise suggests occult left ventricular dysfunction. Aneurysms also may develop below the coarctation or involve the intercostal arteries, and they may lead to rupture. In addition, ruptures without prior aneurysm formation have been reported (29).

Over 400 patients have been reported with coarctation during pregnancy, with maternal mortality ranging from 0% to 17% (19,29-31). Fifty percent of fatalities occurred during the first pregnancy. In a review of 200 pregnant women with coarctation of the aorta before 1940, Mendelson (32) reported 14 maternal deaths and recommended routine abortion and sterilization of these patients. Deaths in this series were from aortic dissection and rupture, congestive heart failure, cerebral vascular accidents, and bacterial endocarditis. Six of the 14 deaths occurred in women with associated lesions. In contrast to this dismal prognosis, a more recent series by Deal and Wooley (30) reported 83 pregnancies in 23 women with uncomplicated coarctation of the aorta. All were NYHA Class I or II prior to pregnancy. In these women, there were no maternal deaths or permanent cardiovascular complications. In one review, aortic rupture was more likely to occur in the third trimester, prior to labor and delivery (33). Thus patients who have coarctation of the aorta that is uncomplicated by aneurysmal dilation or associated cardiac lesions, and who enter pregnancy as Class I or II, have a good prognosis and a minimal risk of complications or death. On the other hand, in the presence of aortic or intervertebral aneurysm, known aneurysm of the circle of Willis, or associated cardiac lesions, the risk of death may approach 15%; therefore, therapeutic abortion must be considered strongly.

TETRALOGY OF FALLOT

Tetralogy of Fallot refers to the cyanotic complex of VSD, overriding aorta, right ventricular hypertrophy, and pulmonary outflow tract stenosis. Most cases of tetralogy of Fallot are corrected during infancy or childhood. Several published reports attest to the relatively good outcome of pregnancy in patients with corrected tetralogy of Fallot or transposition of the great vessels (34-37). In a review of 55 pregnancies in 46 patients, there were no maternal deaths among 9 patients with correction prior to pregnancy; however, there was a 15% mortality with an uncorrected lesion (35). In patients in whom the VSD is uncorrected, the decline in SVR that accompanies pregnancy can lead to worsening of the right-to-left shunt. This condition can be aggravated further by systemic hypotension as a result of peripartum blood loss. A poor prognosis has been related to prepregnancy hematocrit exceeding 65%, history of syncope or congestive failure, electrocardiographic evidence of right ventricular strain, cardiomegaly, right ventricular pressure in excess of 120 mm Hg, and peripheral O_2 saturation below 80% (34).

PULMONIC STENOSIS

Pulmonic stenosis is a common congenital defect. Although obstruction can be valvular, supravalvular, or subvalvular, the degree of obstruction, rather than its site, is the principal determinant of clinical performance. A transvalvular pressure gradient exceeding 80 mm Hg is considered severe and mandates surgical correction. A compilation (totaling 106 pregnancies) of three series of patients with pulmonic stenosis revealed no maternal deaths (9-11). With severe stenosis, right heart failure can occur; fortunately, this is usually less severe clinically than is the left heart failure associated with mitral or aortic valve lesions.

FETAL CONSIDERATIONS

Perinatal outcome in patients with cyanotic congenital cardiac disease correlates best with hematocrit; successful outcome in patients with a hematocrit exceeding 65% is unlikely. Such patients have an increased risk of spontaneous abortion, intrauterine growth retardation, and stillbirth. Maternal partial pressure of oxygen (pO_2) below 70 mmHg results in decreased fetal O_2 saturation (24); thus paO_2 should be kept above this level during pregnancy, labor, and delivery. Serial antepartum sonography for the detection of growth retardation and antepartum fetal heart rate testing are mandatory in any patient with significant cardiac disease. Of equal concern in patients with congenital heart disease is the risk of fetal congenital cardiac anomalies (Table 3). Although this risk was previously felt to be on the order of 5%, recent data suggest that the actual risk may be as high as 10%, or even higher in women whose congenital lesion involves ventricular outflow obstruction (38). In such women, fetal echocardiography is indicated for prenatal diagnosis of congenital cardiac defects. Of special interest is the fact that affected fetuses appear to

Table 3. Congenital Heart Defects in 372 Offspring of 233 Mothers with Congenital Cardiac Anomalies

Defect in infant	Obstruction		Left-to-right shunts				Cyanotic		
	LHO	RHO	PDA	VSD	ASD	Misc.	Cyan.	Rep.	Total
AS	9*	1	1	1					12
PS		3*	1			2	1*	1*	8
PS+ASD		1*							1
PPS	1							1*	2
PDA	1	1	3*	1			1		7
VSD	1	3		9*	3	1	1*		18†
VSD + PS				5*					5
ASD			1	1	1*			1	4
MVP		1							1
Complex					2				2
Total									60

*Concordant anomalies.
†Seven ventricular septal defects closed: AS = aortic; ASD = atrial septal defect; LHO = left heart outflow obstruction; MVP = mitral valve prolapse; PDA = patient ductus arteriosus; PPS = peripheral pulmonary valve stenosis; PS = pulmonary stenosis; Rep. = repaired; RHO = right heart outflow obstruction; VSD = ventricular septal defect (From Whitteranore R, Hobbins JC, Engle MA: Pregnancy and its outcome in women with and without surgical treatment of congenital heart disease. Am J Cardiol 50:645, 1982. Reproduced with permission.

be concordant for the maternal lesion in only 50% of cases. In mothers with uncorrected congenital cardiac malformations, premature delivery also appears to be a significant risk (39).

ACQUIRED CARDIAC LESIONS

Acquired valvular lesions generally are rheumatic in origin, although endocarditis secondary to intravenous drug abuse occasionally may be involved, especially with right-heart lesions. During pregnancy, maternal morbidity and mortality with such lesions result from congestive failure or arrhythmias. Pulmonary edema is the leading cause of death in rheumatic heart disease patients during pregnancy (1). Szekely et al (1) found that the risk of pulmonary edema in pregnant patients with rheumatic heart disease increases with increasing age and length of gestation. The onset of atrial fibrillation during pregnancy carried with it a higher risk of both right and left ventricular failure (63%) than did fibrillation with onset prior to gestation (22%). In addition, the risk of systemic embolization after the onset of atrial fibrillation during pregnancy appears to exceed that associated with onset in the nonpregnant state (1). Counseling the patient with severe rheumatic cardiac disease about the advisability of initiating or continuing pregnancy, the physician also must consider the long-term prognosis of the underlying disease. For up to 44 years, Chesley (40) followed 134 women who had functionally severe rheumatic heart disease and had completed pregnancy. He reported a mortality of 6.3% per year but concluded that in patients who survived the gestation, maternal life expectancy was not shortened by pregnancy.

Intrapartum management of select patients who have valvular disease and/or pulmonary hypertension has been facilitated by the use of the pulmonary artery catheter. In determining which patients may benefit from such invasive monitoring, we have found the older NYHA functional classification to be useful. Patients who reach term as Class I or II generally tolerate properly managed labor without invasive monitoring. Patients who are or have been Class III or IV, or those in whom pulmonary hypertension is present or suspected, may benefit from pulmonary artery catheterization during the intrapartum period.

PULMONIC AND TRICUSPID LESIONS

Isolated right-sided valvular lesions of rheumatic origin are uncommon; however, such lesions are seen with increased frequency in intravenous drug abusers, where they are secondary to valvular endocarditis. Pregnancy-associated hypervolemia is far less likely to be symptomatic with right-sided lesions than with those involving the mitral or aortic valves. In a review of 77 maternal cardiac deaths, Hibbard (11) reported none associated with isolated right-sided lesions. Even following complete tricuspid valvectomy for endocarditis, pregnancy, labor, and delivery generally are tolerated well. Cautious fluid administration is the mainstay of labor and delivery management in such patients. In general, invasive hemodynamic monitoring during labor and delivery is not indicated.

MITRAL STENOSIS

Mitral stenosis is the most common rheumatic valvular lesion encountered during pregnancy (21). It can occur as an isolated lesion or in conjunction with aortic or right-sided lesions. The principal hemodynamic aberration involves ventricular diastolic filling obstruction, resulting in a relatively fixed cardiac output. If the pregnant patient is unable to accommodate the volume fluctuations associated with normal pregnancy, labor, and delivery, pulmonary edema will result.

Cardiac output in patients with mitral stenosis is largely dependent on two factors. First, these patients depend on adequate diastolic filling time; thus, although in most patients tachycardia is a clinical sign of underlying hemodynamic instability, in patients with mitral stenosis, the tachycardia itself, regardless of etiology, can become a significant contributing factor to hemodynamic decompensation. During labor, such tachycardia can accompany the exertion of pushing or be secondary to pain or anxiety. Such a patient may exhibit a rapid and dramatic fall in cardiac output and blood pressure. This fall compromises maternal as well as fetal wellbeing. In order to avoid hazardous tachycardia, the physician should consider oral beta-blocker therapy for any patient with severe mitral stenosis who enters labor with a pulse exceeding 90 beats per minute (bpm). In patients who are not initially tachycardiac, acute control of tachycardia is only rarely necessary.

A second important consideration in patients with mitral stenosis is left ventricular preload. In the presence of mitral stenosis, pulmonary capillary wedge pressure is not an accurate reflection of left ventricular filling pressures. Such patients often require high-normal or elevated pulmonary capillary wedge pressure in order to maintain adequate filling pressure and cardiac output. Any preload manipulation (i.e., diuresis)

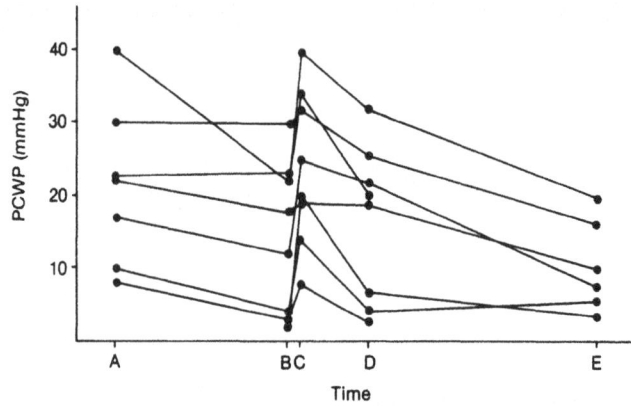

Figure 1.   Intrapartum alterations in pulmonary capillary wedge pressure (PCWP) in
8 patients with mitral stenosis. **A:** first stage labor. **B:** second-stage labor.
15-30 min before delivery. **C:** 5-15 min postpartum. **D:** 4-6 hr postpartum.
E: 18-24 hr postpartum (from Clark SL, Phelan JP, Greenspoon J, et al (10)
Produced with permission

therefore must be undertaken with extreme caution and careful attention
to maintenance of cardiac output (21).

Potentially dangerous intrapartum fluctuations in cardiac output
can be minimized by using epidural anesthesia (41); however, the most
hazardous time for these women appears to be the immediate postpartum
period (21). Such patients often enter the postpartum period already operating at maximum cardiac output and cannot accommodate the volume
shifts that accompany delivery. A 1985 study of patients with severe
mitral stenosis found that a postpartum rise in wedge pressure of up to 16
mm Hg could be expected in the immediate postpartum period (Figure 1).
Because frank pulmonary edema generally does not occur with wedge
pressures below 28-30 mm Hg, it follows that the optimal predelivery
wedge pressure for such patients is 14 mm Hg or lower, as indicated by
pulmonary artery catheterization (21,42). Such a preload may be appropri-
ated cautiously by intrapartum diuresis and with carefully attentive maintenance of adequate cardiac output. Active diuresis is not always necessary
in patients who enter labor with evidence of only mild fluid overload. In
such patients, simple fluid restriction and the associated sensible and
insensible fluid losses that accompany labor can result in a significant fall
in wedge pressure prior to delivery (21).

Previous recommendations for delivery in patients with cardiac
disease have included the liberal use of midforceps to shorten the second

stage of labor. In cases of severe disease, cesarean section with general anesthesia also has been advocated as the mode of delivery least likely to result in hemodynamic compromise (43). If intensive monitoring of intrapartum cardiac patients cannot be carried out in the manner described here, the recommendation for elective cesarean section may be valid. However, with the aggressive management scheme presented, experience suggests that vaginal delivery is safe even in patients with severe disease and pulmonary hypertension (21). Additionally, my colleagues and I have usually found it unnecessary to resort to midforceps deliveries for other than standard obstetric indications.

MITRAL INSUFFICIENCY

Hemodynamically significant mitral insufficiency is usually rheumatic in origin and most commonly occurs in conjunction with other valvular lesions. This lesion generally is tolerated well during pregnancy, and congestive failure is an unusual occurrence. A more significant risk is the development of atrial enlargement and fibrillation. There is evidence to suggest that the risk of developing atrial fibrillation is increased during pregnancy (1). Because of this increased risk, some authors have recommended prophylactic digitalization during pregnancy for patients with significant mitral insufficiency (44). In Hibbard's (11) review of 28 maternal deaths associated with rheumatic valvular lesions, no patient died with complications of mitral insufficiency unless there was coexisting mitral stenosis.

Congenital mitral valve prolapse is much more common during pregnancy than is rheumatic mitral insufficiency and has been reported in up to 17% of healthy women ages 17-35. However, when strict diagnosis criteria are applied, the prevalence of this condition is probably closer to 2% (45,46). Generally, it is asymptomatic. The midsystolic click and murmur associated with congenital mitral valve prolapse syndrome are characteristic; however, the intensity of this murmur, as well as that associated with rheumatic mitral insufficiency, may decrease during pregnancy because of decreased systemic vascular resistance (47). Endocarditis prophylaxis during labor and delivery is recommended for rheumatic mitral insufficiency, as well as for the more common mitral valve prolapse syndrome when associated with a murmur or regurgitation.

AORTIC STENOSIS

Aortic stenosis is most commonly of rheumatic origin and usually occurs in conjunction with other lesions. Less often, it can occur congenitally and represents 5% of all congenital cardiac lesions. In contrast to mitral valve stenosis, aortic stenosis generally does not become hemodynamically significant until the orifice has diminished to one-third or less of normal. The major problem experienced by patients with valvular aortic stenosis is maintenance of cardiac output. Because of the relative hypervolemia associated with gestation, such patients generally tolerate pregnancy well. However, with severe disease, cardiac output will be relatively fixed and, during exertion, may be inadequate to maintain coronary artery or cerebral perfusion. This inadequacy can result in angina, myocardial infarction, syncope, or sudden death. Thus marked limitation of physical activity is vital to patients with severe disease. If activity is limited and the mitral valve is normal, pulmonary edema will be rare during pregnancy.

Delivery and pregnancy termination appear to be the times of greatest risk for patients with aortic stenosis (48). The maintenance of cardiac output is crucial; any factor leading to diminished venous return will cause an increase in the valvular gradient and diminished cardiac output. The literature suggests that pregnancy termination may be especially hazardous in this regard and carries a mortality of up to 40% (48). Hypotension resulting from blood loss, ganglionic blockade from epidural anesthesia, or supine vena cava occlusion by the pregnant uterus can result in severe hypotension.

The cardiovascular status of patients with aortic stenosis is complicated further by the frequent coexistence of ischemic heart disease; thus death associated with aortic stenosis can occur secondary to myocardial infarction rather than as a direct complication of the valvular lesion itself (48). The overall reported mortality associated with aortic stenosis in pregnancy is 17%, although more recent data suggest an improved maternal outcome (49). Patients with valvular gradients exceeding 100 mm Hg are at greatest risk. Pulmonary artery catheterization allows precise hemodynamic assessment and control during labor and delivery. Because hypovolemia is a far greater threat to the patient than pulmonary edema, the wedge pressure should be maintained at or near 16 mm Hg to maintain a margin of safety against unexpected peripartum blood loss. The management of aortic stenosis in pregnancy has recently been reviewed by Easterling et al (49).

AORTIC INSUFFICIENCY

Aortic insufficiency is most commonly rheumatic in origin and, as such, is associated almost invariably with mitral valve disease. Aortic insufficiency generally is tolerated well during pregnancy because the increased heart rate seen with advancing gestation decreases time for regurgitant flow during diastole. In Hibbard's evaluation of 28 maternal rheumatic cardiac deaths (11), only 1 was associated with aortic insufficiency in the absence of concurrent mitral stenosis. Endocarditis prophylaxis during labor and delivery is indicated.

PERIPARTUM CARDIOMYOPATHY

Peripartum cardiomyopathy is defined as cardiomyopathy developing in the last month of pregnancy or the first 6 months postpartum in a woman without previous cardiac disease and after exclusion of other causes of cardiac failure (50). It is therefore a diagnosis of exclusion that should not be made without a concerted effort to identify valvular, metabolic, infectious, or toxic causes of cardiomyopathy. Much of the current controversy surrounding this condition is the result of unusual culturally mandated peripartum customs involving excessive sodium intake and may represent, as such, simple fluid overload (51,52). In the United States, the peak incidence of peripartum cardiomyopathy occurs in the second postpartum month, and there appears to be a higher incidence among older, multiparous black females (51). Other suggested risk factors include twinning and pregnancy-induced hypertension. In some cases, a familial recurrence pattern has been reported (52). The condition is manifest clinically by increasing fatigue, dyspnea, and peripheral or pulmonary edema. Physical examination reveals classic evidence of congestive heart failure, including jugular venous distention, rales, and an S_3 gallop. Cardiomegaly and pulmonary edema are found on chest x-ray, and the electrocardiogram often demonstrates left ventricular and atrial dilatation, and diminished ventricular performance. In addition, up to 50% of patients with peripartum cardiomyopathy may manifest evidence of pulmonary or systemic embolic phenomena. Overall mortality ranges from 25% to 50% (51,52).

The histologic picture of peripartum cardiomyopathy involves nonspecific cellular hypertrophy, degeneration, fibrosis, and increased lipid deposition. Although some reports have documented the presence of a diffuse myocarditis, it must be questioned whether such cases represent the same syndrome.

Because of the nonspecific clinical and pathologic nature of peripartum cardiomyopathy, its existence as a distinct entity has been questioned by some (53). Proof of its existence is supported primarily by epidemiologic evidence suggesting that 80% of cases of idiopathic cardiomyopathy in women of child-bearing age occur in the peripartum period (51,52). Such an epidemiologic distribution could be attributed also to an exacerbation of underlying subclinical cardiac disease related to the hemodynamic changes accompanying normal pregnancy (53). However, as such changes are maximal in the third trimester of pregnancy and return to normal within a few weeks postpartum, such a pattern does not explain the peak incidence of peripartum cardiomyopathy occurring, in most reports, during the second month postpartum (51,52). Nevertheless, the diagnosis of peripartum cardiomyopathy remains primarily a diagnosis of exclusion and cannot be made until underlying conditions, including chronic hypertension, valvular disease, and viral myocarditis, have been excluded.

Although nutritional, hormonal, and autoimmune etiologies all have been suggested, substantial backing for any of these theories is lacking. In one case, an autoimmune phenomenon clearly seemed involved because there was transplacental passage of antibody and subsequent stillbirth (54).

Therapy includes digitalization, diuretics, sodium restriction, and prolonged bed rest. In refractory cases, concomitant afterload reduction with hydralazine or nitrates may be useful. Early endomyocardial biopsy has been suggested to identify a subgroup of patients who have a histologic picture of inflammatory myocarditis and who may be responsive to immunosuppressive therapy. Such patients may represent up to 29% of women with peripartum cardiomyopathy (55). Echocardiographic features of patients with peripartum cardiomyopathy have been described by Aroney et al (56).

A notable feature of peripartum cardiomyopathy is its tendency to recur with subsequent pregnancies. Several reports have suggested that prognosis for future pregnancies is related to heart size. Patients whose cardiac size returned to normal within 6-12 months had an 11-14% mortality in subsequent pregnancies; those patients with persistent cardiomegaly had a 40-80% mortality (49). Thus pregnancy is definitely contraindicated in all patients with persistent cardiomegaly; the 11-14% risk of maternal mortality with subsequent pregnancy seen in patients with normal heart size would seem, in most cases, to be unacceptable, as well.

HYPERTROPHIC CARDIOMYOPATHY

Hypertrophic cardiomyopathy is an autosomal, dominantly inherited condition with variable penetrance. This condition most commonly becomes clinically manifest in the second or third decade of life; thus it often may be first manifest during pregnancy. Detailed physical and echocardiographic diagnostic criteria have been described elsewhere. Hypertrophic cardiomyopathy involves primarily left ventricular hypertrophy, typically involving the septum to a greater extent than the free wall. The hypertrophy results in obstruction to left ventricular outflow and secondary mitral regurgitation, the two principle hemodynamic concerns of the clinician (57). Although the increased blood volume associated with normal pregnancy should enhance left ventricular filling and improve hemodynamic performance, this positive effect of pregnancy is counterbalanced by the fall in arterial pressure and the vena cava obstruction that are found in late pregnancy. In addition, tachycardia resulting from pain or fear in labor diminishes left ventricular filling and aggravates the relative outflow obstruction, an effect also resulting from second-stage Valsalva maneuver.

From this discussion, it can be seen that the keys to successful management of the peripartum period in patients with hypertrophic cardiomyopathy involve avoidance of hypotension (resulting from conduction anesthesia or blood loss) and tachycardia, as well as labor in the left lateral recumbent position. The use of forceps to shorten the second stage also has been recommended. As with most other cardiac disease, cesarean section of these patients should be reserved for obstetric indications only.

Despite the potential hazards, maternal and fetal outcome in patients with hypertrophic cardiomyopathy is generally excellent (58). In a 1979 report of 54 pregnancies in 23 patients, no maternal or neonatal deaths occurred (59). Although beta-blocking agents once were used routinely in these patients, currently they are reserved for patients with angina, recurrent supraventricular tachycardia, or occasional beta-blocker-responsive arrhythmias. Antibiotic prophylaxis against subacute bacterial endocarditis is recommended.

MARFAN SYNDROME

Marfan syndrome is an autosomal dominant disorder characterized by generalized weakness of connective tissue; the weakness results in skeletal, ocular, and cardiovascular abnormalities. The increased risk of maternal mortality during pregnancy stems from aortic root and wall involvement, which may result in aneurysm formation, rupture, or aortic dissection. Fifty percent of aortic aneurysm ruptures in women under age 40 occur during pregnancy (29). Rupture of splenic artery aneurysms also occurs more frequently during pregnancy (29). Sixty percent of patients with Marfan syndrome have associated mitral or aortic regurgitation (60). Although some authors feel pregnancy is contraindicated in any woman with documented Marfan syndrome, prognosis is best individualized and should be based on echocardiographic assessment of aortic root diameter and postvalvular dilation. It is important to note that enlargement of the aortic root is not demonstrable by chest x-ray until dilation has become pronounced (60). Women with an abnormal aortic valve or aortic dilation may have up to a 50% pregnancy-associated mortality; women who lack these changes and have an aortic root diameter of less than 40 mm have a mortality of less than 5% (61). Even in patients meeting these echocardiographic criteria, however, special attention must be given to signs and symptoms of aortic dissection because even serial echocardiographic assessment is not invariably predictive of complications (62). The routine use of oral beta-blockers to decrease pulsatile pressure on the aortic wall has been recommended (63). If cesarean section is performed, retention sutures should be used because of generalized connective tissue weakness.

MYOCARDIAL INFARCTION

Coronary artery disease is uncommon in women of reproductive age; therefore, myocardial infarction in conjunction with pregnancy is rare. In a review of 68 reported cases, myocardial infarction during pregnancy was associated with a 35% mortality rate (64). Only 13% of patients were known to have had coronary artery disease prior to pregnancy. Two-thirds of the women suffered infarction in the third trimester; mortality for these women was 45%, as compared to 23% in those suffering infarction in the first or second trimesters. Thus it appears that the increased hemodynamic burden imposed on the maternal cardiovascular system in late pregnancy may unmask latent coronary artery disease in some women and worsen the prognosis for patients suffering infarction. Fetuses from surviving women appear to have an increased risk of spontaneous abortion and unexplained stillbirth.

Antepartum care of women with prior myocardial infarction revolves around bed rest to minimize myocardial oxygen demands. In women with angina, nitrates have been used without adverse fetal effects. Delivery within 2 weeks of infarction is associated with increased mortality; therefore, if possible, attempts should be made to allow adequate convalescence prior to delivery. If the cervix is favorable, cautious induction under controlled circumstances and after a period of hemodynamic stabilization is optimal. Labor in the lateral recumbent position, the administration of O_2, pain relief with epidural anesthesia, and hemodynamic monitoring with a pulmonary artery catheter are essential. Additional considerations in managing the pregnant patient with coronary artery disease have recently been reviewed by Graber (65).

CARDIOVASCULAR SURGERY

There are numerous reports of cardiovascular surgery during pregnancy; this surgery includes successful correction of most types of congenital and acquired cardiac disease and coronary artery bypass surgery (66). Early reports of closed mitral valve commissurotomy during pregnancy were favorable and indicated a maternal death rate of 1-2% and perinatal loss at or near 10% (67). Subsequently, this procedure has been replaced by open valvuloplasty, with equally favorable results.

Initial reports of cardiopulmonary bypass during pregnancy were not nearly as favorable, indicating a fetal wastage of up to 33%. Initiation of cardiopulmonary bypass is followed generally by fetal bradycardia, correctable by high flow rates (68,69). With the use of continuous electronic fetal heart rate monitoring, flow rate can be adjusted to avoid or correct fetal hypoperfusion and bradycardia, and thus fetal mortality can be reduced to less than 10%. Maternal mortality is, of course, highly dependent on the specific nature of the procedure being performed and does not appear to be increased significantly by pregnancy. High-flow/high-pressure normothermic perfusion and continuous electronic fetal heart rate monitoring appear to be optimal for the fetus (66).

REFERENCES

1. Szekely P, Turner R, Snaith L: Pregnancy and the changing pattern of rheumatic heart disease. Br Heart J 35:1293, 1973
2. The Criteria Committee of the New York Heart Association: Nomenclature and criteria for diagnosis of diseases of the heart and great vessels. 8th edition. New York, New York Heart Association, Inc, 1979

3. Jindal VN, Dhall GI, Vasishta K et al: The effect of maternal cardiac disease on perinatal outcome. AVST NZ J Obstet Gynecol 28:113, 1988

4. Ullery JC: Management of pregnancy complicated by heart disease. Am J Obstet Gynecol 67:834, 1954

5. Niswander KR, Berendes H, Dentschberger J et al: Fetal morbidity following potential anoxigenic obstetric conditions. V. Organic heart disease. Am J Obstet Gynecol 98:871, 1967

6. Etheridge MJ, Pepperell RJ: Heart disease and pregnancy at the Royal Women's Hospital. Med J Aust 2:277, 1971

7. Veran FX, Cibes-Hernandez JJ, Pelegrina I: Heart disease in pregnancy. Obstet Gynecol 34:424, 1968

8. Ellison CR, Sloss CJ: Electrocardiographic features of congenital heart disease in the adult. In Roberts WC, ed. Congenital heart disease in adults. Philadelphia, FA Davis Co, 1979, p 119

9. Neilson G, Galea EG, Blunt A: Congenital heart disease and pregnancy. Med J Aust 30:1086, 1970

10. Schaefer G, Arditi LI, Solomon HA et al: Congenital heart disease and pregnancy. Clin Obstet Gynecol 11:1048, 1968

11. Hibbard LT: Maternal mortality due to cardiac disease. Clin Obstet Gynecol 18:27, 1975

12. Mendelson CL: Cardiac disease in pregnancy. Philadelphia, FA Davis Co, 1960, p 151

13. Zitnick RS, Brandenburg RO, Sheldon R et al: Pregnancy and open heart surgery. Circulation 39:157, 1969

14. Szekely P, Julian DG: Heart disease and pregnancy. Curr Probl Cardiol 4:1, 1979

15. Kelly DT: Patent ductus arteriosis in adults. In Roberts WC, ed. Congenital heart disease in adults. Philadelphia, FA Davis Co, 1979, p 321

16. Knapp RC, Arditi LI: Pregnancy complicated by patent ductus arteriosus with reversal of flow. NY J Med 67:573, 1967

17. Gleicher N, Midwall J, Hochberger D et al: Eisenmenger's syndrome and pregnancy. Obstet Gynecol Surv 34:721, 1979

18. Pirlo A, Herren AL: Eisenmenger's syndrome and pregnancy. Anesth Rev 6:9, 1979

19. Sinnenberg RJ: Pulmonary hypertension in pregnancy. S Med J 73:1529, 1980

20. Pitts JA, Crosby WM, Basta LL: Eisenmenger's syndrome in pregnancy. Does heparin prophylaxis improve the maternal mortality rate? Am Heart J 93:321, 1977

21. Clark SL, Phelan JP, Greenspoon J et al: Labor and delivery in the presence of mitral stenosis: Central hemodynamic observations. Am J Obstet Gynecol 152:986, 1985

22. Hankins GDV, Berryman GK, Scott RT et al: Maternal arterial desaturation with 15-Methyl prostglandier F_2 alpha for uterine atony. Obstet Gynecol 72:367, 1988

23. Willis DC, Caton D, Levell P et al: Cardiac output response to prostaglandin E_2-induced abortion in the second trimester. Am J Obstet Gynecol 156:170, 1987

24. Sobrevilla LA, Cassinelli MT, Carcelen A et al: Human fetal and maternal oxygen tension and acid-base status during delivery at high altitude. Am J Obstet Gynecol 111:1111, 1971

25. Midwall J, Jaffin H, Herman MV et al: Shunt flow and pulmonary hemodynamics during labor and delivery in the Eisenmenger syndrome. Am J Cardiol 42:299, 1978

26. Spinnato JA, Kraynack BJ, Cooper MW: Eisenmenger's syndrome in pregnancy: Epidural anesthesia for elective cesarean section. N Engl J Med 304:1215, 1981

27. Abboud JK, Raya J, Noueihed R et al: Intrathecal morphine for relief of labor pain in a parturient with severe pulmonary hypertension. Anesthesiology 59:477, 1983

28. Taylor SH, Donald KW: Circulatory studies at rest and during exercise in coarctation, before and after correction. Br Heart J 22:117, 1960

29. Barrett JM, VanHooydonk JE, Boehm FH: Pregnancy-related rupture of arterial aneurysms. Obstet Gynecol Surv 37:557, 1982

30. Deal K, Wooley CF: Coarctation of the aorta and pregnancy. Ann Intern Med 78:706, 1973

31. Szekely P, Snaith L: Heart disease and pregnancy. Edinburgh and London, Churchill Livingstone, 1974, p 167

32. Mendelson CL: Pregnancy and coarctation of the aorta. Am J Obstet Gynecol 39:1014, 1940

33. Barash PG, Hobbins JC, Hook R et al: Management of coarctation of the aorta during pregnancy. J Thorac Cardiovasc Surg 69:781, 1975

34. Jacoby WJ: Pregnancy with tetralogy and pentology of Fallot. Am J Cardiol 14:866, 1964

35. Meyer EC, Tulsky AS, Sigman P et al: Pregnancy in the presence of tetralogy of Fallot. Am J Cardiol 14:874, 1964

36. Loh TF, Tan NC: Fallot's tetralogy and pregnancy: A report of a successful pregnancy after complete correction. Med J Aust 2:141, 1975

37. Sellers JD, Block FE, McDonald JS: Anesthetic management of labor in a patient with dextrocardia, congenitally corrected transposition. Wolff-Parkinson-White syndrome and congestive heart failure. Am J Obstet Gynecol 161:1001, 1989

38. Whittmore R, Hobbins JC, Engle MA: Pregnancy and its outcome in women with and without surgical treatment of congenital heart disease. Am J Cardiol 50:641, 1982

39. Sulovic V, Radunovic N, Pilic Z: Nonsurgically corrected congenital cardiac malformations in pregnant women. J Gynecol Obstet Biol Reprod 14:493, 1985

40. Chesley LC: Severe rheumatic cardiac disease and pregnancy: The ultimate prognosis. Am J Obstet Gynecol 136:552, 1980

41. Ueland K, Akamatsu TJ, Eng M et al: Maternal cardiovascular dynamics. IV. Cesarean section under epidural anesthesia without epinephrine. Am J Obstet Gynecol 114:775, 1972

42. Forrester JS, Swan HJC: Acute myocardial infarction: A physiological basis for therapy. Crit Care Med 2:283, 1974

43. Ueland K, Hansen J, Eng M et al: Maternal cardiovascular dynamics v. section under thiopental, nitrous oxide and succinylcholine anesthesia. Am J Obstet Gynecol 108:615, 1970

44. Ueland K: Rheumatic heart disease and pregnancy. In Elkayam Y, Gleicher N, eds. Cardiac problems in pregnancy. New York, Alan R. Liss, Inc, 1982, p 82

45. Wann LS, Grove JR, Hess TR et al: Prevalence of mitral valve prolapse by two-dimenstional echocardiography in healthy young women. Br Heart J 49:334, 1983

46. Perloff JK, Child JS, Edwards JE: New guidelines for the clinical diagnosis of mitral valve prolapse. Am J Cardiol 57:1124, 1986

47. Haas JM: The effect of pregnancy on the midsystolic click and murmur of the prolapsing posterior leaflet of the mitral valve. Am Heart J 92:407, 1976

48. Arias F, Pineda J: Aortic stenosis and pregnancy. J Reprod Med 20:229, 1978

49. Easterling TR, Chadwick HS, Otto CM et al: Aortic stenosis in pregnancy. Obstet Gynecol 72:113, 1988

50. Demakis JG, Rahimtoola SH, Sutton GC et al: Natural course of peripartum cardiomyopathy. Circulation 44:1053, 1971

51. Homans DC: Peripartum cardiomyopathy. N Engl J Med 312:1432, 1985

52. Veille JC: Peripartum cardiomyopathies: A review. Am J Obstet Gynecol 148:805, 1984

53. Cunningham FG, Pritchard JA, Hankins GDV et al: Peripartum heart failure: Idiopathic cardiomyopathy or compounding cardiovascular events? Obstet Gynecol 67:157, 1986

54. Rand RJ, Jenkins DM, Scott DG: Maternal cardiomyopathy of pregnancy causing stillbirth. Br J Obstet Gynecol 82:172, 1975

55. O'Connell JB, Costanzo-Nordin MR, Subraminian R et al: Peripartum cardiomyopathy: Clinical, hemodynamic, histologic and prognostic characteristics. J Am Coll Cardiol 8:52, 1986

56. Aroney C, Khafagi F: Peripartum cardiomyopathy: Echocardiographic features in five cases. Am J Obstet Gynecol 155:103, 1986

57. Kolibash AJ, Ruiz DE, Lewis RP: Idiopathic hypertrophic subaortic stenosis in pregnancy. Ann Intern Med 82:791, 1975

58. Shah DM and Sunderji SG: Hypertrophic cardiomyopathy and pregnancy: Report of a maternal mortality and review of the literature. Obstet Gynecol Surv 40:444, 1985

59. Oakley GDG, McGarry K, Limb DG et al: Management of pregnancy in patients with hypertrophic cardiomyopathy. Br Med J 1:1749, 1979

60. Pyeritz RE, McKusick VA: The Marfan syndrome: Diagnosis and management. N Engl J Med 300:772, 1979
61. Pyeritz RE: Maternal and fetal complications of pregnancy in the Marfan syndrome. Am J Med 71:784, 1984
62. Rosenblum NG, Grossman AR, Gabbe SG et al: Failure of serial echocardiographic studies to predict aortic dissection in a pregnant patient with Marfan's syndrome. Am J Obstet Gynecol 146:470, 1983
63. Slater EE, DeSanctis RW: Dissection of the aorta. Med Clin North Am 63:141, 1979
64. Hankins GDV, Wendel GD, Leveno KJ et al: Myocardial infarction during pregnancy: A review. Obstet Gynecol 65:139, 1985
65. Graber EA: When an OB patient has coronary artery disease. Contemp OB-GYN June:56, 1989
66. Bernal JM, Miralles PJ: Cardiac surgery with cardiopulmonary bypass during pregnancy. Obstet Gynecol Surv 41:1, 1986
67. Ueland K: Cardiovascular surgery and the OB patient. Contemp OB-GYN Oct:117, 1984
68. Koh KS, Friesen RM, Livingstone RA et al: Fetal monitoring during maternal cardiac surgery with cardiopulmonary bypass. CMAJ 112:1102, 1975
69. Werch A, Lambert HM, Cooley D et al: Fetal monitoring and maternal open heart surgery. South Med J 70:1024, 1977

ANESTHESIA FOR SEVERE PREECLAMPSIA

C. P. Gibbs

Preeclampsia is a syndrome of hypertension, proteinuria, and generalized edema occurring after the 20th week of gestation and usually abating within 48 hours of delivery. Pregnancy-induced hypertension (PIH) is the term used when proteinuria and/or edema are not present. However, the two terms are often used interchangeably.

Mild preeclampsia can be defined as follows: 1) Systolic blood pressure greater than 140, and diastolic blood pressure greater than 90. There is a rise in systolic blood pressure of 30 mm Hg or a rise in diastolic blood pressure of greater than 15 mm Hg. These readings must be present on at least two separate occasions or at least 6 hours apart. 2) Proteinuria greater than 0.3 g/liter on two random samples at least 6 hours apart. 3) Edema.

Severe preeclampsia is a significantly more serious disease and is identified by the following: 1) blood pressure 160/110 mm Hg or greater; 2) proteinuria greater than 5 grams per 24 hours; 3) urine output less than 500 ccs per 24 hours and a rising creatinine level; 4) pulmonary edema; 5) persistent cerebral or visual disturbances; 6) epigastric or right upper quadrant pain (indicating hepatic rupture); 7) hepatocellular damage; 8) severe thrombocytopenia or overt intravascular coagulation.

Eclampsia is preeclampsia with superimposed convulsions.

The Hellp Syndrome refers to a relatively new syndrome composed of hemolysis, elevated liver enzymes, and low platelets (1).

ETIOLOGY

The etiology of preeclampsia remains unknown. However, at least four theories have received considerable attention recently. They are:

1. An immune mechanism (2,3), which would help explain why preeclampsia is more common in prima gravidas than in multi gravidas.
2. Some sort of prostaglandin imbalance (4,5), in which there are too many vasoconstrictors and too few vasodilators.

51

T.H. Stanley and P.G. Schafer (eds.), Pediatric and Obstetrical Anesthesia, 51-63.
© *1995 Kluwer Academic Publishers.*

3. A calcium deficiency (6), which is principally supported by the fact that patients given supplemental calcium tend to develop preeclampsia less often than those not given calcium.

4. Placental hypoxia. Normally, the trophoblastic tissue of the placenta invades the uterine wall and spiral arteries. Thus the muscular coat of the spiral arteries are removed, which allows for maximal dilation of these arteries. This in turn allows for flow to increase to meet the demands of the growing fetoplacental unit, and a normal pregnancy results. It is proposed that in preeclamptic patients, the trophoblasts do not adequately invade the spiral arteries, and therefore they retain their muscular coats. Thus, there is no maximal dilation, and the fetoplacental unit gradually outgrows its blood supply. This then results in tissue hypoxia, which causes the release of endoperoxides. The endoperoxides cause endothelial damage, which results in the clinical picture of preeclampsia (7). Lipid peroxides are destructive to vascular endothelium, cause platelet aggregation, inhibit prostacyclin production, enhance thromboxane production, inhibit endothelium-derived relaxing factor, stimulate vascular contractility, and are found in increased concentrations during preeclampsia (8).

Injured endothelial cells (the injury caused by endoperoxides) decrease anticoagulant substances and vasodepressors, as well as cause a loss of fluid and proteins. They also stimulate procoagulant synthesis and stimulate activation of the clotting cascade at the site. Platelet-derived growth factor, a vasoconstrictor, is also increased (7).

MANIFESTATIONS

Whatever the etiology of preeclampsia, for the anesthesiologist's purposes, it is a disease of generalized vasoconstriction, and the vasoconstriction causes most of the manifestations that are of concern to the anesthesiologist. For the most part, they are as follows:

1. The severe preeclamptic patient is a critically ill patient and must be considered as such. If this concept is accepted, then the care and ultimate prognosis will be significantly improved.

2. Hypertension: generalized vasospasm produces an increased peripheral vascular resistance resulting in hypertension.
3. Leaky vessels—secondary to endothelial damage.
4. Decreased uterine blood flow usually in proportion to severity of disease (9,10).
5. Decreased glomerular filtration rate, which can lead to decreased urine output-Oliguria (11).
6. Hypovolemia: secondary to the generalized vasoconstriction and comparable to that seen in other hypertensive states. Pritchard measured blood volume in normal pregnant and toxemic pregnant women and found the blood volume in the toxemia patients to be 27% lower (12).
7. Generalized and cerebral edema occasionally resulting in pharyngolaryngeal edema and a difficult intubation (13,14).
8. Decreased colloid osmotic pressure (15-17). May also be due at least in part to impaired endothelium.
9. Coagulopathies (18-21):
    a. Decreased number of platelets—platelet count.
    b. Decreased function of platelets—bleeding time.
    c. Bleeding time and platelets do not always correlate.
    d. Decreased fibrinogen—fibrinogen level.
    e. May have PT, PTT, and clot time abnormal or normal.
10. Hypersensitivity to endogenous and exogenous vasopressor agents (22,23).
11. Hyperdynamic CV state—usually (i.e., increased CO, etc.) (24,25). *However, this is quite variable* (26).
12. Many problems become manifest in the postpartum period, particularly pulmonary edema and renal failure. Also, eclampsia frequently occurs in the postpartum period (27,28).
13. Causes of death: two common causes of death are cerebral hemorrhage and pulmonary edema (29).

OBSTETRIC MANAGEMENT

It is important for the anesthesiologist to understand obstetric treatment because some of it may influence the condition of the patient, as well as anesthetic management. Aspects of obstetric management that may be relevant to the anesthesiologist include the following:

1. Bed rest. Occasionally, bed rest alone will result in marked improvement in these pregnant patients. Blood pressure will come down, edema will diminish, and urine output will increase. Obstetricians may use agents such as morphine and/or phenobarbital to facilitate the patient remaining at bed rest.

2. Sedation, as above.

3. Antihypertensives: the most common agents used by obstetricians are hydralazine and methyldopa. Some are now using labetalol and calcium channel blockers.

4. Magnesium sulphate. This agent is particularly appropriate to the preeclamptic patient. It seems that every new aspect of its action helps explain why it is so successfully used in the preeclamptic patient. It can be characterized by the following:

    a. Anticonvulsant. This is the principal reason why magnesium sulphate is used in the treatment of preeclampsia. Although it does have some vasodilating effect, it is used primarily to prevent convulsions. If adequate blood levels are achieved, convulsions will not occur.

    b. Sedative--good for preeclamptic patients.

    c. Skeletal muscle relaxant: it blocks release of AcCh, decreases sensitivity of endplate, and stabilizes membranes.

    d. Tocolytic.

    e. Negative ionotrope.

    f. Increases prostocyclin production (30).

        1) Vasodilation.

        2) Inhibits platelet aggregation.

    g. Anti-angiotensin II activity (31).

    h. Excreted by kidney.

    i. Normal level: 1.5-2 mEq/l.

        1) Therapeutic Level: 4-6 mEq/l.

        2) Respiratory Depression: 12-15 mEq/l.

5. Aspirin (low-dose); it inhibits thromboxane (32-34). Several large studies now confirm that patients given low-dose aspirin prophylactically are considerably less likely to develop preeclampsia than those not given aspirin.

6. Plasmapheresis (35). This is a relatively new treatment plan which calls for plasma exchange in patients with the Hellp syndrome who do not get better by the third postpartum day. Studies indicate that when plasmapheresis is instituted, liver enzymes decrease and platelet counts increase. Occasionally, three episodes of plasmapheresis will be necessary.
7. Occasionally, diuretics for ↑ PCWP (36).
8. Recent studies indicate that immediate postpartum curettage, usually done under conscious sedation circumstances, may also improve blood pressure and urinary output in severely preeclamptic patients postpartum (37).

ANESTHETIC MANAGEMENT

MILD PREECLAMPSIA

The mildly preeclamptic patient is a totally different person from the severely preeclamptic one. The cardiovascular changes are not nearly as marked. Thus, although caution must be taken, these patients will usually tolerate either regional or general anesthesia for cesarean section and would probably benefit from regional anesthesia during labor to make the laboring process as comfortable as possible.

SEVERE PREECLAMPSIA

The most important aspect of dealing with these patients is to realize that many of them are critically ill. The contribution of the anesthesiologist to these patients is twofold: 1) to help evaluate and optimize the overall condition of the patient, and 2) to provide pain relief.

What kind of monitoring is necessary? An arterial line will be necessary for the patient whose infant is delivered by cesarean section under general anesthesia. Blood pressure swings are great during intubation and extubation. Thus potent vasodilating agents are necessary, and their use will require an arterial line. For the patient undergoing cesarean section with regional anesthesia, an arterial line is probably not mandatory but could be helpful. For the patient in labor, again, an arterial line is not mandatory but could be helpful. For the most part, the automated blood pressure devices are reasonably accurate and sufficient.

Regarding central line placement, most studies indicate that the central venous pressure does not reliably correlate with the pulmonary artery wedge pressure in individual patients. However, there is a fairly good correlation when the initial CVP measurement is less than 6-8 mm Hg (25,38). Therefore, in our institution, a pulmonary artery catheter is indicated in the following circumstances: persistent oliguria, an elevated CVP (>6-8 mm Hg), and pulmonary edema.

Regarding oliguria, a reasonable plan for management would include the administration of 500 cc saline over a 20-minute period, which can be repeated once if urine output does not increase. If the oliguria is not resolved after the second 500 cc bolus of saline, a pulmonary artery catheter is placed to guide additional fluid management or the patient is delivered expeditiously.

The question of whether or not one should administer fluid to these patients is somewhat controversial, although less so than previously. Some believe that these patients, who are usually volume depleted, should not have their volumes corrected (24,39). Their belief is that when these patients are given fluid replacement during labor, the fluid replacement will contribute to development of pulmonary edema postpartum. Others believe that the low volume should be corrected. Indeed, studies indicate that when volume is corrected, blood pressure and peripheral vascular resistance decrease while cardiac output increases (40). Also, blood flow velocity in the uterine circulation and the umbilical circulation increases when fluids are given (41). Nevertheless, in spite of these seemingly beneficent effects, there is some justification for the fear that fluids administered intrapartum can contribute to the pulmonary edema that is so frequently seen postpartum. Thus, a reasonable approach would be to try to get the central venous pressure or pulmonary capillary wedge pressure to a level that would be considered *low* normal. To do so, crystalloid can be administered at a rate of 125-175 cc/hour. If this does not result in sufficient volume replacement, then either 25% or 5% albumin can be given. In fact, if the patient has a very low albumin, and many of them will, one may wish to start with albumin as the replacement fluid. Albumin correlates very well with colloid osmotic pressure (42).

ANESTHESIA

LABOR AND VAGINAL DELIVERY

Lumbar epidural analgesia has been, and can be, used effectively (43). If regional analgesia is contraindicated or unacceptable, small incremental doses of narcotics can be used for labor; inhalational analgesia, small doses of narcotics, plus a pudendal block must suffice for vaginal delivery.

When regional anesthesia is utilized, the following technique is appropriate:

1. Check coagulation profile. If the patient has overt DIC or other grossly abnormal clotting factors, regional anesthesia is probably contraindicated, except perhaps in the instance when a difficult airway is expected. It is the patient with marginal coagulation defects that is the problem. In the past, because these patients could have both a decreased number of platelets and decreased functioning platelets (19,21), anesthesiologists would obtain a platelet count and a bleeding time to assess this particular coagulation defect. In the more recent past, it has been determined that the bleeding time is a particularly subjective test and almost never predictive of the coagulation status of the patient (20). Thus, most obstetric anesthesiologists no longer obtain bleeding times before instituting epidural anesthesia. On the other hand, most continue to get platelet counts. At our institution, we do not do epidural or regional anesthesia in the presence of a platelet count less than 100,000. Others will go as low as 50,000.

2. Optimize volume status and blood pressure as described above. (CVP should be at 6-8 mm Hg or pulmonary wedge pressure should be at 8-12 mm Hg.)

3. Electronic fetal monitoring: regional anesthesia should not be carried out in these patients without being aware of fetal status at all times.

4. The aim is to establish a segmental epidural block (i.e., a block that produces a band of analgesia at the T10-L1-2 level). The level should be achieved *slowly* to avoid hypotension.

5. Direct particular attention toward maintaining left uterine displacement. The *supine position* should be avoided.

6. Treat falling blood pressure *immediately* with fluids, exaggerated LUD, and *small* doses of ephedrine (5 mg IV). These patients are hypersensitive to vasopressor.

7. Dosage and choice of local anesthetics are the same as for other obstetric patients.

The advantages of regional anesthesia are that it provides good pain relief, decreases the stress response (44), increases uterine artery and umbilical artery flow velocity (41), lowers pressure and systemic vascular resistance (43), and increases intervillous blood flow (45). Thus regional anesthesia for Labor and Delivery is optimum.

Recently, intrathecal narcotics have been used, and they may prove helpful. They do, however, have a small incidence of hypotension, which was previously thought not to be the case (46). Also, they provide no analgesia for the second stage.

ANESTHESIA FOR CESAREAN SECTION

Regional anesthesia would seem to be the better choice over general anesthesia because it avoids the problems associated with intubation (i.e., the hypertensive response and the possibility of a difficult intubation secondary to laryngotracheal edema). Further, as with anesthesia for Labor and Delivery, regional anesthesia decreases the stress response and seems to be helpful for the fetus. When regional anesthesia is appropriate (i.e., not contraindicated) the lumbar epidural technique is chosen over the spinal technique because it is more controllable and the incidence of hypotension is less. The technique for lumbar epidural anesthesia is as follows:

1. Optimization and stabilization.

2. Test dose: 3 ccs 1.5% lidocaine. The use of 1:200,000 epinephrine is *controversial* (47). We do not use it in preeclampsia because, if the test dose is injected intravascularly, an increase in heart rate and blood pressure will ensue.

3. Loading dose: 15-20 ccs of 1.5% or 2% lidocaine, or 3% chloroprocaine, or 0.5% bupivacaine. These loading doses should be given as *incremental doses* of 5-6 ccs at a time.

4. Maintain left uterine displacement. Treat falling blood pressure immediately as described above for epidural anesthesia during labor.

In some patients, regional anesthesia will be inappropriate (i.e., in those patients with significant coagulapathies as described above). In these instances, general anesthesia is appropriate and can be done safely, as follows:

1. Again, optimize and stabilize as for regional anesthesia.

2. Prevent cardiovascular effects of laryngoscopy and intubation by administering an intravenous antihypertensive agent. Because these patients may become quite agitated on arrival in the operating room, these antihypertensive agents need to be started as preparation before the operation begins. Usually, however, it will suffice to begin a slow infusion at the time of preoxygenation. The slow infusion is maintained until a short time after intubation is accomplished. Prior to intubation, blood pressure is lowered by approximately 20%, and the goal is to maintain blood pressure at a level not exceeding those which existed before being brought to the operating room (48). Antihypertensive agents include:

   a. *Nitroprusside*. This agent is effective. Because the amount used is so small, and the duration of its use is so short, it is unlikely that toxicity will occur (49,50). The recent study by Ramanathan is testimony to the effectiveness of this agent when applied appropriately in these patients. Blood pressures were able to be maintained at levels not significantly different from pre-intubation levels (48).

   b. *Trimethaphan*. This is another short-acting antihypertensive agent that enjoys some popularity. Because it is at least partially destroyed by cholinesterases, it may potentiate the action of succinylcholine (51).

   c. *Nitroglycerin*. This agent is relatively free of complications, but its effectiveness in the preeclamptic patient has recently been questioned (52).

   d. *Labetalol*. This is effective and appears to be safe (53,54).

   e. *IV Lidocaine*. This can be made more helpful with proper timing. Three minutes prior to intubation may be optimal (55).

3. Be aware of the potential for pharyngeal-laryngeal edema (14). These patients have edema throughout their bodies, and this means that they may have edema of their airways. Thus a thorough and careful awake examination of the airway is indicated before a rapid-sequence induction is attempted.

4. Avoid ergot drugs because of hypersensitivity to vasopressors.

5. Perform awake extubation. The process requires use of the same drugs as for intubation.

6. Hodgkinson provides a good study for comparison with regional anesthesia (56). A recent retrospective study by Ramanathan is also informative (48).

POSTPARTUM MANAGEMENT

Remember that many of these patients get into trouble postpartum. Many patients will have a decreased urine output, and it is here where proper monitoring of volume status is most helpful. Without adequate knowledge of the central blood volume, the patient may be presumed to be in renal shutdown, when in reality she is severely volume depleted. Such a differentiation is most important to ensure proper treatment. Also remember that 70-80% of the preeclamptic patients who develop pulmonary edema will do so in the postpartum period (27,28). Thus it is imperative that the anesthesiologist not abandon these patients once the delivery process is over. The skills brought to the scene by the anesthesiologist are the very skills necessary for proper treatment of these patients at this time.

SUMMARY

The severely preeclamptic patient is a critically ill patient and must be treated as such. An understanding of the pathophysiology and manifestations of the disease will help the anesthesiologist contribute maximally to these patients' care. In most instances, regional anesthesia will be the anesthetic of choice for both labor and vaginal delivery, as well as cesarean section. However, a properly managed general anesthesia can be administered safely. Finally, these patients frequently get into trouble in the postpartum period and will continue to require critical care management.

REFERENCES

1. Sibai BM et al: Maternal-perinatal outcome associated with the syndrome of hemolysis, elevated liver enzymes, and low platelets in severe preeclampsia-eclampsia. Am J Obstet Gynecol 155:501-509, 1986

2. Symonds EM: Aetiology of preeclampsia: A review. J R Soc Med 73:871-875, 1980

3. Redman CWG: Immunologic factors in the pathogenesis of preeclampsia. Contrib Nephrol 25:120-127, 1981

4. Walsh SW: Preeclampsia: An imbalance in placental prostacyclin and thromboxane production. Am J Obstet Gynecol 152:335-340, 1985

5. Friedman SA: Preeclampsia: A review of the role of prostaglandins. OB/GYN 71:122-137, 1988

6. Kawasaki et al: Effect of calcium supplementation on the vascular sensitivity to Angiotensin II in pregnant woman. Am J Obstet Gynecol 153:576, 1985

7. Roberts JM et al: Preeclampsia: An endothelial cell disorder. Am J Obstet Gynecol 161:1200-1204, 1989

8. Hubel CA et al: Lipid peroxidation in pregnancy: New perspectives on preeclampsia. Am J Obstet Gynecol 161:1025-1034, 1989

9. Dixon HG et al: Choriodecidual and myometrial blood-flow. Lancet 2:369, 1963

10. Johnson T et al: Diffusion of radioactive sodium in normotensive and pre-eclamptic pregnancies. Br Med J 1:312, 1957

11. Clark SL et al: Severe preeclampsia with persistent oliguria: Management of hemodynamic subjects. Am J Obstet Gynecol 154:490, 1986

12. Pritchard JA et al: Clinical and laboratory observations on eclampsia. Am J Obstet Gynecol 99:754, 1967

13. Benedetti TJ et al: Cerebral edema in severe pregnancy-induced hypertension. Am J Obstet Gynecol 99:754, 1967

14. Heller PJ et al: Pharyngolaryngeal edema as a presenting symptom in preeclampsia. OB/GYN 62:523, 1983

15. Benedetti TJ et al: Studies of colloid osmotic pressure in pregnancy-induced hypertension. Am J Obstet Gynecol 135:308, 1979

16. Moise KJ, Cotton DB: Colloid osmotic pressure and pregnancy. In Clark SL, Cotton DB, Hankins GDV, Phelan JP, eds. Critical care obstetrics, 2nd edition. Boston, Blackwell Scientific Publications, 1991, pp 35-61

17. Bhatia RK et al: Mechanisms for reduced colloid osmotic pressure in preeclampsia. Am J Obstet Gynecol 157:106, 1987

18. Pritchard JA et al: Coagulation changes in eclampsia: Their frequency and pathogenesis. Am J Obstet Gynecol 124:855, 1976

19. Kelton JG et al: A platelet function defect in preeclampsia. OB/GYN 65:107, 1985

20. Gibson B et al: Thrombocytopenia in preeclampsia and eclampsia. Semin Thrombo Hemost 8:234-47, 1982

21. Ramanathan J et al: Correlation between bleeding times and platelet counts in women with preeclampsia undergoing cesarean section. Anes 71:188, 1989
22. Zuspan FP et al: Epinephrine infusions in normal and toxemic pregnancy. Am J Obstet Gynecol 90:88, 1964
23. Gant NF et al: A study of angiotension II pressor response throughout primigravid pregnancy. J Clin Invest 52:2682, 1973
24. Hankins GDV et al: Longitudinal evaluation of hemodynamic changes in eclampsia. Am J Obstet Gynecol 150:506-512, 1984
25. Clark SL et al: Clinical indications for pulmonary artery catheterization in the patient with severe preeclampsia. Am J Obstet Gynecol 158:453-458, 1988
26. Phelan JP et al: Severe Preeclampsia I Peripartum Hemodynamic Observations. Am J Obstet Gynecol 144:17, 1982
27. Benedetti TJ et al: Hemodynamic observations in severe preeclampsia complicated by pulmonary edema. Am J Obstet Gynecol 152:330-334, 1985
28. Sibai BM et al: Pulmonary edema in severe preeclampsia-eclampsia: Analysis of thirty-seven consecutive cases. Am J Obstet Gynecol 156:1174-1179, 1987
29. Govan ADT: The pathogenesis of eclamptic lesions. Patholigia et Microbiologia 24:S562, 1961
30. Watson K et al: Magnesium sulfate: Rationale for its use in preeclampsia. Proc Natl Acad Sci 83:1075, 1986
31. Fuentes A et al: Angiotension-converting enzyme activity in hypertensive subjects offer magnesium sulfate therapy. Am J Obstet Gynecol 156:1375, 1987
32. Spitz B et al: Low-dose aspirin. I. Effect on angiotensin II pressor responses and blood prostaglandin concentrations in pregnant women sensitive to angiotensin II. Am J Obstet Gynecol 159:1035-1043, 1988
33. Benigni A et al: Effect of low-dose aspirin on fetal and maternal generation of thromboxane by platelets in women at risk for pregnancy-induced hypertension. N Engl J Med 321:357-362, 1989
34. Schiff E et al: The use of aspirin to prevent pregnancy-induced hypertension and lower the ratio of thromboxane A_2 to prostacyclin in relatively high risk pregnancies. N Engl J Med 321:351-356, 1989
35. Martin NJ Jr.et al: Plasma exchange for preeclampsia. Am J Obstet Gynecol 162:126, 1990
36. Kirshon B et al: Role of volume expansion in severe preeclampsia. Surg Gynecol Obstet 167:367, 1988
37. Magann EF et al: Immediate postpartum curretage: Accelerated recovery from severe preeclampsia. Obstet Gynecol 81:502-506, 1993
38. Cotton DB et al: Cardiovascular alterations in severe pregnancy-induced hypertension: Relationship of central venous pressure to pulmonary capillary wedge pressure. Am J Obstet Gynecol 151:762-764, 1985

39. Pritchard JA et al: The Parkland Memorial Hospital protocol for treatment of eclampsia: Evaluation of 245 cases. Am J Obstet Gynecol 148:951, 1984

40. Groenendijk R et al: Hemodynamic measurements in preeclampsia: Preliminary observations. Am J Obstet Gynecol 150:232, 1984

41. Giles WB et al: The effect of epidural anaesthesia for caesarean section on maternal uterine and fetal umbilical artery blood flow velocity waveforms. Br J Obstet Gynecol 94:55-59, 1987

42. Nguyen HN et al: Peripartum colloid osmotic pressures: Correlation with serum proteins. OB/GYN 68:807, 1986

43. Newsome LR et al: Severe preeclampsia: Hemodynamic effects of lumbar epidural anesthesia. Anesth Analg 65:31, 1986

44. Abboud T et al: Sympathoadrenal activity, maternal, fetal, and neonatal responses after epidural anesthesia in the preeclamptic patient. Am J Obstet Gynecol 144:915, 1982

45. Joupilla P et al: Lumbar epidural analgesia to improve intervillous blood flow during labor in severe preeclampsia. OB/GYN 59:158, 1982

46. Cohen SE et al: Intrathecal sufentanil for labor analgesia—sensory changes, side effects, and fetal heart rate changes. Anesth Analg 77:1155-1160, 1993

47. Heller PJ et al: Use of local anesthetic with epinephrine for epidural anesthesia in preeclampsia. Anesthesiology 65:224, 1986

48. Ramanathan J et al: Anesthetic modification of hemodynamic and neuroendocrine stress responses to cesarean delivery in women with severe preeclampsia. Anesth Analg 73:772, 1991

49. Stempel JE et al: Use of sodium nitroprusside in complications of gestational hypertension. OB/GYN 60:533, 1982

50. Naulty J et al: Fetal toxicity of nitroprusside in the pregnant ewe. Am J Obstet Gynecol 139:78, 1981

51. Sosis M et al: In defiance of trimethaphan for use in preeclampsia. Anesthesiology 64:657, 1986

52. Longmire S et al: The hemodynamic effects of intubation during nitroglycerin infusion in severe preeclampsia. Am J Obstet Gynecol 164:551-556, 1991

53. Jouppila P et al: Labetalol does not alter the placental and fetal blood flow in maternal prostanoids in pre-eclampsia. Br J Obstet Gynecol 93:543, 1986

54. Ramanathan J et al: The use of labetalol for attenuation of hypertensive response to endotracheal intubation. Am J Obstet Gynecol 159:650, 1988

55. Tam S et al: Intravenous lidocaine: Optimal time of injection before tracheal intubation. Anesth Analg 66:1036, 1987

56. Hodgkinson R, Husain FJ, Hayashi RH: Systemic and pulmonary blood pressure during cesarean section in patients with gestational hypertension. Can Anaes Soc J 27:389, 1980

EFFECTS OF PREGNANCY ON LOCAL ANESTHETIC ACTION AND TOXICITY

M. Finster

It has been known since the early 1960s that the dose requirement for lumbar epidural or spinal anesthesia is reduced during pregnancy and parturition (1-3). This altered response to local anesthetics persists into the early puerperium (4,5). Engorgement of epidural veins resulting in decreased capacity of the spinal and epidural spaces was the commonly accepted explanation for this phenomenon until 1979, when it was noted that a facilitated spread of epidural analgesia occurs even during the first trimester of pregnancy, at a time when mechanical factors are unlikely to play a significant role (6). The authors proposed that hormonal changes of pregnancy, particularly the increase in progesterone levels, may alter the susceptibility of nerve membrane to local anesthetics. Datta et al found that indeed there was a significant correlation between lidocaine dose requirement for spinal anesthesia and CSF progesterone concentration (5). Less lidocaine was required in parturients and postpartum patients than in nonpregnant patients.

Increased susceptibility to local anesthetics during pregnancy was also noted in peripheral nerves. Lidocaine inhibited impulse conduction in median nerve fibers to a greater extent in pregnant than nonpregnant women (7). Similarly, conduction blockade, induced by exposure to bupivacaine, was greater and occurred more rapidly in A and C fibers of isolated vagus nerves obtained from pregnant rabbits than in nerves from nonpregnant animals (8,9). Administration of progesterone to rabbits, over a 4-day period, increased the susceptibility of excised vagus nerve to bupivacaine (10), but an acute nerve exposure to progesterone had no effect (11).

In an editorial published in 1979, Albright suggested that bupivacaine and etidocaine may be more cardiotoxic than the less potent agents such as lidocaine and mepivacaine (12). This idea was based on six cases of sudden cardiovascular collapse which happened shortly after intravascular injection of large doses of bupivacaine (and etidocaine in one instance)

65

T.H. Stanley and P.G. Schafer (eds.), Pediatric and Obstetrical Anesthesia, 65-67.
© 1995 *Kluwer Academic Publishers.*

intended for epidural anesthesia. Over 50 such cases have become known to date; in approximately 30 of them, resuscitation was unsuccessful.

Since cardiac arrests occurred predominantly in parturients, the question arose as to whether the pregnant patient is more sensitive to the cardiotoxic effects of local anesthetics or, more simply, whether the widespread use of bupivacaine for obstetric anesthesia was responsible for the number of cases reported in pregnant women. In our study, the CNS and cardiovascular toxicity of bupivacaine was compared in pregnant and nonpregnant ewes during continuous intravenous infusion of the drug (13). The mean dose of the drug resulting in cardiovascular collapse was significantly lower in pregnant ewes than in nonpregnant animals. Similarly, bupivacaine blood concentrations at circulatory collapse were lower in the pregnant group. In order to ascertain whether pregnancy enhances the toxicity of other local anesthetics as well, similar studies were conducted using mepivacaine, lidocaine, or ropivacaine (14-16). None of these drugs appeared to be more toxic to pregnant than nonpregnant sheep.

The reasons for the altered toxicity of bupivacaine during pregnancy have not been fully elucidated. A recent study has shown that pretreating rabbits with progesterone increases the in vitro effects of bupivacaine, but not of lidocaine or ropivacaine, on transmembrane action potential parameters in Purkinje fibers and ventricular muscle cells (17,18). Data from our laboratory suggest that the gestational decrease in the protein binding of bupivacaine may be the cause of increased cardiotoxicity of the drug (14). Protein binding of bupivacaine was also lower in parturients than in nonpregnant volunteers (19).

In summary, pregnancy is associated with altered sensitivity of biological membranes to some local anesthetics, resulting in enhanced neural blockade and cardiotoxicity.

REFERENCES

1. Bromage PR: Continuous lumbar epidural analgesia for obstetrics. Can Med Assoc J 85:1136-1140, 1961
2. Hehre FW, Moyes AZ, Senfield RM et al: Continuous lumbar peridural anesthesia in obstetrics. II. Use of minimal amounts of local anesthetics during labor. Anesth Analg 44:89-93, 1965
3. Marx GF, Orkin R: Physiology of obstetric anesthesia. Springfield: Charles C. Thomas, 1969
4. Marx GF: Regional anesthesia in obstetrics. Anaesthesist 21:84-91, 1972

5. Datta S, Hurley RJ, Naulty JS et al: Plasma and cerebrospinal fluid progesterone concentrations in pregnant and nonpregnant women. Anesth Analg 65:950-954, 1986

6. Fagraeus L, Urban BJ, Bromage PR: Spread of epidural analgesia in early pregnancy. Anesthesiology 58:184-187, 1983

7. Buttersworth JF, Walker FO, Lysak SZ: Pregnancy increases median nerve susceptibility to lidocaine. Anesthesiology 72:962-965, 1990

8. Flanagan HL, Datta S, Lambert DH et al: Effect of pregnancy on bupivacaine-induced conduction blockade in the isolated rabbit vagus nerve. Anesth Analg 66:123-126, 1987

9. Datta S, Lambert DH, Gregus J et al: Differential sensitivities of mammalian nerve fibers during pregnancy. Anesth Analg 62:1070-1072, 1983

10. Flanagan HL, Datta S, Moller RA et al: Effect of exogenously administered progesterone on susceptibility of rabbit vagus nerves to progesterone. Anesthesiology 69:A676, 1988

11. Bader AM, Datta S, Moller RA et al: Acute progesterone treatment has no effect on bupivacaine-induced conduction blockade in the isolated rabbit vagus nerve. Anesth Analg 71:545-548, 1990

12. Albright GA: Cardiac arrest following regional anesthesia with etidocaine or bupivacaine (editorial). Anesthesiology 51:285-287, 1979

13. Morishima HO, Pedersen H, Finster M et al: Bupivacaine toxicity in pregnant and nonpregnant ewes. Anesthesiology 63:134-139, 1985

14. Santos AC, Pedersen H, Harmon TW et al: Does pregnancy alter the systemic toxicity of local anesthetics? Anesthesiology 70:991-995, 1989

15. Morishima HO, Finster M, Arthur GR et al: Pregnancy does not alter lidocaine toxicity. Am J Obstet Gynecol 162:1320-1324, 1990

16. Santos AC, Arthur GR, Pedersen H et al: Systemic toxicity of ropivacaine during ovine pregnancy. Anesthesiology 75:137-141, 1991

17. Moller RA, Datta S, Fox J et al: Effects of progesterone on the cardiac electrophysiologic action of bupivacaine and lidocaine. Anesthesiology 76:604-608, 1992

18. Moller RA, Covino BG: Effect of progesterone on cardiac electrophysiological alteration produced by ropivacaine and bupivacaine (suppl). Reg Anesth 17:46, 1992

19. Wulf H, Münstedt P, Maier C: Plasma protein binding of bupivacaine in pregnant women at term. Acta Anaesthesiol Scand 35:129-133, 1991

OBSTETRIC EMERGENCIES

C. P. Gibbs

BREECH PRESENTATION

The incidence of breech presentation is approximately 4%. However, because nearly two-thirds of all breech presentations are able to be changed to vertex presentations by external version, the resulting practical incidence is closer to 1.5%.

The problem with breech presentations is that the largest part of the infant delivers last. Therefore, the obstetrician does not know if the pelvis will be adequate until after committing to vaginal delivery and, in fact, until after the head is delivered. For the term breech, the problem arises when the aftercoming head is too large for the bony pelvis. With the premature breech, the disparity between the dilating wedge and the head is greater than with the term breech. Thus the problem is different, in that it is unlikely that the small premature head will not pass through the bony pelvis; rather, the considerably smaller presenting part will not dilate the cervix adequately. Therefore, the head will not be able to pass through the undilated cervix. In both instances (i.e., the term and premature breech), the obstetrician will allow the breech to deliver spontaneously at least up to the umbilicus to ensure as much cervical dilation as possible.

Risks associated with breech presentation include prematurity (16-33%), major anomalies (6-18%), birth trauma (13 x normal risk), cord prolapse (5-20 x normal risk), intrapartum asphyxia (3-8 x normal risk), spinal cord and deflexion injuries (21%), hyperextension of head (5%), and arrest of aftercoming head (8.8%) (1).

There are several different types of breech presentations. Those most commonly encountered include the frank breech, which occurs approximately 60% of the time. In this instance, the lower extremities are flexed at the hips but extended at the knees. The complete breech (10% of the time) has the lower extremities flexed at both hips and knees, while the footling or incomplete breech (30% of the time) has one or both lower

69

T.H. Stanley and P.G. Schafer (eds.), Pediatric and Obstetrical Anesthesia, 69-78.
© 1995 Kluwer Academic Publishers.

extremities extended at the hip (i.e., the lower extremities are not flexed and one or both feet present).

The type of breech presentation is important because the type determines the effectiveness of the dilating wedge. For example, the frank breech presents a better dilating wedge than does the complete breech, and the complete breech presents a better dilating wedge than do one or 2 feet. Also, the incidence of prolapsed cord is significantly greater when the presenting part does not fill the entire cervical opening. Thus the incidence of prolapsed cord is approximately 15-18% for a footling breech, 4-6% for a complete breech, and .5% for a frank breech. Similarly, the success of vaginal delivery is considerably greater for the frank breech and the complete breech than it is for the footling breech (2).

Pertinent to this discussion, the obstetric management of breech presentation begins before labor and usually at about 37 weeks, when most obstetricians will attempt to turn the breech into a vertex presentation with the help of tocolysis. Thirty-seven weeks is chosen because at that point the breech is unlikely to turn to vertex on its own and, if it is successful, will likely not revert to the breech position. Finally, if fetal distress is caused by the maneuver, the infant will be mature enough to survive should delivery be necessary. External version enjoys a success rate of 60-75% (3).

THE DELIVERY

Probably 50-60% of all breech deliveries will be accomplished by cesarean section. This is so because several earlier studies have indicated that the outcome for the breech baby delivered by cesarean section is better than when delivered vaginally (4,5). Certainly, most footling breeches will be delivered by cesarean section; and most premature breeches will be delivered by cesarean section because of the risk of delivery through an undilated cervix and the trauma of the delivery process itself to the small, more fragile premature infant. When vaginal delivery is attempted, there are several methods:

1. Spontaneous breech delivery. Delivery proceeds without the aid of forceps or extraction by the obstetrician.
2. Assisted breech delivery. The infant delivers spontaneously to the umbilicus, and then the process is assisted by the obstetrician. Delivery to the umbilicus without assistance helps to ensure that the cervix will be as

maximally dilated as possible before birth of the aftercoming head.

3. Assisted breech with piper forceps to the aftercoming head. This is perhaps the most frequently employed method of delivering breeches vaginally. In the process, the procedure is accomplished as above, but piper forceps are applied to the aftercoming head and the head is gently lifted out of the pelvis. Most believe that this is less traumatic to the fetus than without application of forceps.

4. Total breech extraction. In this instance, the obstetrician will not wait for spontaneous delivery of the infant to the umbilicus but rather will attempt to extract the entire body of the infant by way of vaginal and perhaps intrauterine manipulation (this is very rare).

5. Breech decomposition and extraction. In this instance, the obstetrician will attempt to convert the breech presentation to a vertex presentation by intrauterine manipulation (this is very rare).

THE HUNG-UP BREECH

The hung-up breech is a true emergency that may require general anesthesia for satisfactory resolution *if regional anesthesia is not in place.* Because it is not known until the last moment whether or not the delivery can be successfully completed if the head becomes stuck in the pelvis, or if the cervix is not fully dilated, the obstetrician will need the patient to be as cooperative as possible to perform the necessary manipulations to complete the delivery. General anesthesia may very well be necessary and should be provided if requested. The anesthesiologist should also respect the wishes of the obstetrician if s/he requests that the anesthesiologist be present at breech deliveries "just in case." If regional anesthesia is in place, nearly all breech deliveries should be able to be accomplished. Perhaps the most important aspect of the vaginal delivery of a breech infant is that the patient be cooperative and at least not fighting the process. For the patient to be cooperative, she must be as pain free as possible. In most instances, regional anesthesia can provide this requirement. General anesthesia will at least ensure that the patient is not uncooperative and actively resisting. General anesthesia is provided in a manner similar to that for cesarean section.

TWINS

The incidence of twin presentations is approximately 1%. As with breech presentations, the type of presentation is important, and the presentation of the second twin is particularly critical. Twin A is vertex and Twin B is vertex in 42.5% of instances. Twin A is vertex and Twin B is nonvertex (usually breech) in 38.4%, while Twin A is nonvertex (usually breech) in 19.1% (4).

Obstetric management is mostly dependent on presentation and, as above, it is the second twin that presents the biggest challenge (5). If the first twin is a breech, most obstetricians will opt for cesarean section because many twin infants are premature and thus at risk for the complications associated with the breech delivery of a premature infant. If the first twin is vertex, then that delivery can proceed as would a normal vaginal delivery.

When the second twin is a breech presentation, the obstetrician will usually try to allow spontaneous delivery to take place after the first infant is delivered. If contractions do not begin in a reasonable length of time, oxytocin may be initiated to begin contractions. However, some obstetricians will merely reach up and grab the presenting feet and extract the second twin expeditiously. Certainly, this will be the method of choice should fetal distress occur between delivery of the first and second twin. Incidentally, it is always important to monitor the heart rate of the second twin following birth of the first infant so that, if fetal distress occurs secondary to abruption or prolapsed cord, the distress can be identified early. If the second twin is a vertex, then once again, most obstetricians will allow a period of time to pass until the uterus begins contracting spontaneously. If the uterus does not contract spontaneously, then once again, oxytocin will usually be used to initiate labor. If this does not work or if fetal distress ensues, the obstetrician will either elect to do an immediate cesarean section, will try to deliver the infant with the use of vacuum suction, or will attempt to turn the infant from a vertex to a breech presentation and then accomplish delivery by breech extraction. In the latter instance, it will be necessary to provide considerable anesthesia because the manipulations required are painful. It is doubtful if regional anesthesia alone will suffice because the uterus must be relaxed. Uterine relaxation can be accomplished with potent inhalation anesthetic agents— ritodrine or terbutaline, or perhaps even small doses of nitroglycerin (6,7). Recently, it has been described that 50-100 µg boluses of nitroglycerin will provide uterine relaxation without seriously compromising maternal blood pressure (6,7). Thus again, as with the breech presentation, it is reasonable that the obstetrician ask that you be present in case general anesthesia is required. If so, the anesthetic is administered in a manner very similar to that for cesarean section—with the possible addition of halothane or isoflurane should uterine relaxation be required.

SHOULDER DYSTOCIA

Like the hung-up breech, shoulder dystocia can become an extreme emergency (8). In this instance, the head delivers, but the shoulders do not. Again, the obstetrician will need a cooperative and relaxed patient to accomplish the maneuvers necessary to deliver the child in an expeditious manner. If regional anesthesia is in place, it should be adequate. If not, general anesthesia will be required.

SEVERE ACUTE FETAL DISTRESS

In some instances, obstetricians will opt to deliver a patient with severe acute fetal distress vaginally and with the aid of forceps. If so, the application of forceps may once again require that the patient be cooperative and relaxed. General anesthesia can provide these conditions if regional anesthesia is not in place. Some would prefer to institute regional anesthesia in preference to general anesthesia (9). This is a judgment call. If true severe acute fetal distress is present, I would probably choose general anesthesia. What is probably most important is a discussion between the anesthesiologist and obstetrician to determine just how soon the delivery must be accomplished. Once that critical point is determined, the anesthesiologist can make an appropriate decision as to type of anesthesia. Of course, many obstetricians nowadays will simply opt for cesarean section in the presence of severe acute fetal distress. If so, the same discussion regarding degree of acuteness and distress needs to take place.

CARDIAC ARREST AND POSTMORTEM CESAREAN SECTION

Cardiac arrest in the pregnant patient is an obstetric emergency that requires special consideration by the anesthesiologist. Table 1 details 188 instances of perimortem cesarean section performed for maternal cardiac arrest in which the infant survived (10). The role of anesthesia is clear.

Table 1. Reported cases of postmortem cesarean deliveries with surviving infants. In Katz VL et al (10).

Years	Causes of Maternal Death	Cases	Percent
1879-1956	Hypertensive disease	44	39
	Infection	42	37
	Unknown	13	11
	Trauma	5	4
	Aortic aneurysm	3	3
	ANESTHESIA	3	3
	Cardiac	3	3
	Malignancy	1	1
	Subtotal	114	100
1956-1970	Hypertensive disease	10	23
	ANESTHESIA	8	18
	Embolism (pulmonary, amniotic fluid)	8	18
	Cardiac	7	16
	Cerebrovascular accident	3	7
	Malignancy	2	5
	Asthma	2	5
	Subtotal	44	100
1971-1985	Unspecified*	10	33
	ANESTHESIA	9	30
	Embolism (pulmonary, amniotic fluid)	3	10
	Trauma	2	7
	Malignancy	2	7
	Cerebrovascular accident	1	3
	Asthma	1	3
	Infection (meningitis)	1	3
	Cardiac	1	3
	Subtotal	30	100
	TOTAL	**188**	

When cardiac arrest occurs in the pregnant patient, considerations regarding both mother and infant are critical. If the mother cannot be resuscitated adequately, it is obvious that she will suffer. However, when the mother suffers, the fetus is also likely to suffer.

Features of the pregnancy that cause resuscitation difficulty are: aortocaval compression, increased oxygen consumption, and decreased functional residual capacity (11-15). Also, during apnea, PaO_2 falls more rapidly in the pregnant patient (16). In the supine position, cardiac output may be reduced by 30% (17). Katz and colleagues recommend that cesarean section be started after 4 minutes of unsuccessful resuscitation, and that the infant be delivered within 1 minute after cesarean section begins (10). They offer the information in Table 2 to support their recommendation. Although the data indicates that 5 minutes is optimal, it certainly does not indicate that cesarean section should be abandoned if more than 5 minutes have passed. Seven out of 8 and 6 out of 7 infants had normal outcomes when delivered 6-10 minutes and 11-15 minutes, respectively, after the need for resuscitation.

Table 2   Postmortem cesarean deliveries with surviving infants: time from maternal death until delivery (1900-1985). In Katz VL et al (10).

Cases	No. Patients		Percent Normal
0-5 min	42	(normal infants)	100
6-10 min	7	(normal infants)	86
	1	(mild neurologic sequelae)	
11-15 min	6	(normal infants)	83
	1	(severe neurologic sequelae)	
16+ min	1	(severe neurologic sequelae)	25
TOTAL	61		

Regarding the mother, time is also important, as emphasized by Marx (18). She reported a series of 5 patients who arrested during induction of epidural anesthesia. Resuscitation was begun immediately and, in 3 patients, cesarean section was also begun immediately. In 2 others, the operation was delayed for several minutes after arrest. The 3 former patients did well; the latter 2 had irreversible brain damage (19).

Thus resuscitative efforts should not be prolonged. If there is not clear indication of improvement, cesarean section should be instituted after 3-4 minutes of resuscitation. Some have suggested it be accomplished in the labor room, if necessary (10). I'm not so sure about that. A controlled environment would seem desirable.

One of the important, if not *the* most important, features of success during resuscitation in the late pregnant patient is uterine displacement. This *may* be accomplished with a wedge or with table tilt. However, these maneuvers may diminish the effectiveness of cardiac compression. Therefore, *manual* displacement of the uterus to the left may be required, while maintaining the patient in the supine position. In fact, this approach is probably the optimal approach from the beginning. Animal studies clearly demonstrate that inferior vena caval occlusion impairs effective resuscitation (20). Human case reports are confirmatory. Prompt cesarean section will help the fetus by removing it from a progressively more harmful environment while, at the same time, helping the mother by allowing for more effective resuscitation (5,10,19).

CARDIAC ARREST

1. Intubate and ventilate
2. Chest compression
3. Appropriate drugs
4. Shock, if necessary
5. LUD—if resuscitation not okay
6. Manual displacement—if not successful
7. Cesarean section

AMNIOTIC FLUID EMBOLISM

Amniotic fluid embolism (AFE) is a rare but catastrophic obstetric event. The classic picture consists of the sudden onset of hypoxia, hypotension, and DIC. Mortality may be as high as 86% (21) and early death (1-2 hours) runs at perhaps 50% (22). Most occur during labor, but AFE has occurred at the time of cesarean section, at the time of abortion, and as many as 32 hours postpartum (23-25).

Diagnosis is via clinical suspicion and demonstrating fetal squames in the central circulation, even though it has recently been demonstrated that fetal squames are present in normal patients (26,27). X-rays are positive in 70% (22).

The pathophysiology of AFE is becoming clearer. In the past, the process was believed to be sudden pulmonary hypertension followed by right heart failure. Recent central hemodynamic monitoring data indicates that the process may begin with pulmonary hypertension, but in those surviving at least 1-2 hours, the problem becomes one of left-sided heart failure (28). Confirmation of this proposal is supported by echocardiographic data (29). Also, there is frequently a component of non-cardiogenic pulmonary edema or ARDS (22). Apparently, amniotic fluid contains vasoactive substances that, upon entering the pulmonary circulation, cause hypoxia, hypotension, pulmonary hypertension, cor pulmonale, and subsequent left ventricular injury. Left ventricular failure follows and is frequently accompanied by adult respiratory distress syndrome and a consumptive coagulopathy (28,22).

The DIC usually occurs in those surviving the early stages and may be caused by a thromboplastin-like activity of amniotic fluid. Also, amniotic fluid may contain a factor X activating substance (15). Treatment is supportive and guided by central monitoring to determine the phase of the process.

REFERENCES

1. Myers SA, Gleicher N: Breech delivery: Why the dilemma? AJOG 156:6, 1987
2. Collea JV et al: The randomized management of term frank breech presentation: Vaginal delivery vs. cesarean section. AJOG 131:186, 1978
3. Morrison JC et al: External cephalic version of the breech presentation under tocolysis. AJOG 154:900, 1986
4. Chervenak FA et al: Intrapartum management of twin gestation. OB/GYN 65:119, 1985
5. Rabinovici J et al: Randomized management of the second nonvertex twin: Vaginal delivery or cesarean section. AJOG 156:52, 1987
6. DeSimone CA et al: Intravenous nitroglycerin aids manual extraction of a retained placenta. Anesthesiology 73:787, 1990
7. Rolbin SH et al: Uterine relaxation can be life saving. Can J Anaes 39:939-940, 1990
8. Acker DB et al: Risk factors for shoulder dystocia. OB/GYN 66:762, 1985
9. Marx GF et al: Fetal-neonatal status following caesarean section for fetal distress. Br J Anaesth 56:1009, 1984
10. Katz VL et al: Perimortem cesarean delivery. OB/GYN 68:571, 1986
11. Kerr MG et al: Studies of the inferior vena cava in late pregnancy. Br Med J 1:532, 1964
12. Bieniarz J et al: Aortocaval compression by the uterus in late human pregnancy. AJOG 100:203, 1968
13. Cugell DW et al: Pulmonary function in pregnancy. Am Rev Tuberc 67:568, 1953
14. Baldwin GR et al: New lung functions and pregnancy. AJOG 127:235, 1977
15. Pernoll ML et al: Oxygen consumption at rest and during exercise in pregnancy. Resp Physiol 25:285, 1975
16. Archer GW et al: Arterial oxygen tension during apnoea in parturient women. Br J Anaesthesia 46:358, 1974
17. Ueland K et al: Maternal cardiovascular dynamics IV: The influence of gestational age on the maternal cardiovascular response to posture and exercise. Am J Obstet Gynecol 104:856, 1969

18. Marx GF: Cardiopulmonary resuscitation of the late pregnant woman. Anesthesiology 56:156, 1982
19. DePace NL et al: 'Postmortem' cesarean section with recovery of both mother and offspring. JAMA 248:971, 1982
20. Kasten GW, Martin ST: Resuscitation from bupivacaine-induced cardiovascular toxicity during partial inferior vena cava occlusion. Anesth Analg 65:341-344, 1986
21. Morgan M: Amniotic fluid embolism. Anesthesia 34:29, 1979
22. Clark SL: Amniotic fluid embolism. Crit Care Clinics 7:877-882, 1991
23. Watananukul P et al: Amniotic fluid embolism: Report of five cases. Southeast Asian J Trop Med Public Health 10:424, 1979
24. Anderson DG: Amniotic fluid embolism. A re-evaluation. Am J Obstet Gynecol 98:336, 1967.
25. Duff P: Defusing the dangers of amniotic fluid embolism. Contempt Obstet Gynecol 127, 1984
26. Clark SL et al: Squamous cells in the maternal pulmonary artery circulation. Am J Obstet Gynecol 154:104, 1986
27. Cotton DB et al: Squamous and trophoblastic cells in the maternal pulmonary circulation identified by invasive hemodynamic monitoring during the peripartum period. Am J Obstet Gynecol 155:999, 1986
28. Clark SL et al: Central hemodynamic alterations in amniotic fluid embolism. Am J Obstet Gynecol 158:1124-1126, 1988
29. Girard P et al: Left heart failure in amniotic fluid embolism. Anesthesiology 64:262-265, 1986

GENERAL REFERENCES

1. Clark SL, ed. Critical care clinics: Obstetric emergencies. Philadelphia, PA, W. B. Saunders Company, Vol 7, 1991
2. Clark SL, ed. Critical care obstetrics. Oradell, NJ, Medical Economics Books, 1987

ANESTHESIA FOR SURGERY IN THE PREGNANT SURGICAL PATIENT[1]

A. M. Malinow with J. W. Ostheimer (ed.)

INTRODUCTION

Anesthetic management of the pregnant surgical patient must address the well-being of both mother and fetus. The patient's surgical condition, pregnancy-induced physiologic changes, and possible adverse effects (both direct and indirect) of anesthesia all have a bearing on anesthetic management. Attention must be paid to the duration of the planned surgical procedure, the possible sequelae from anesthesia and surgical intervention, the condition of the pregnancy, and the gestational age and viability of the fetus.

Non-obstetric surgery is required in about 1% of pregnancies (1-4). Surgery may be directly related to pregnancy (e.g., cerclage procedures), associated with pregnancy e.g., torsion of an ovarian pedicle), or incidental to pregnancy (e.g., trauma or appendicitis) (5). The consultant anesthesiologist must be patient and understanding in answering difficult questions from both patient and surgeon about "what is best." Decreasing the psychologic stress of both patient and surgeon will help optimize operating room conditions.

FETAL CONSIDERATIONS

TERATOGENICITY

Teratogenic susceptibility/resistance differs among species, making any correlation between animal data and humans difficult. Retrospective epidemiologic studies of anesthetic exposure provide the only human data available; direct control of the experimental conditions has been lost. For

---

[1]A. M. Malinow: Anesthetic management of the pregnant surgical patient G.W. Ostheimer, ed. *Manual of Obstetric Anesthesia*, 2nd edition. Churchill-Livingstone, New York, 1992, Reproduced with permission.

T.H. Stanley and P.G. Schafer (eds.), Pediatric and Obstetrical Anesthesia, 79-87.
© 1995 *Kluwer Academic Publishers.*

a teratogenic effect to occur, a fetus must be exposed to a teratogenic dose of drug for a particular duration and during a susceptible period of embryonal development. In humans, days 14-56 comprise the susceptible period of organogenesis. Development of the central nervous system and peripheral nervous system continue into the neonatal period. Results of multiple surveys reveal that there is no increase in the incidence of congenital abnormalities in pregnant patients who have undergone surgery during this period (1-4,6,7). These thoughts must be tempered with the fact that there are most probably insufficient numbers of anesthetic exposure during pregnancy reported in the world literature to possibly detect human teratogenesis. Matching of gestational age, duration of anesthetic exposure, dose of drug, and surgical stress can best be accomplished in animal models. The only controlled experimental data are all from animal studies.

INHALATIONAL AGENTS

Halothane, isoflurane, enflurane, and nitrous oxide have not been shown to be associated with congenital malformation in rats repeatedly exposed to anesthetic concentrations of inhaled agent (8).

NITROUS OXIDE (N_2O) CONTROVERSIES

The use of N_2O during early pregnancy presents a difficult problem. Nitrous oxide inhibits methionine synthetase activity through the inactivation of vitamin B_{12}, interfering with thymidine and, therefore, DNA synthesis (9). Twenty-four-hour exposure of pregnant rats to 50% or greater inspired N_2O concentrations will produce teratogenic effects (10).

In humans, only significant exposures (approximately 2 hours or more) to N_2O have resulted in altered enzyme activity (9). Additionally, epidemiologic studies have presented evidence, albeit weak, that early N_2O exposure in clinically administered anesthetic concentrations does not produce teratogenic effects (11). There is some animal data that reports a degree of protection conferred by supplemental (IM) folinic acid (12), although this is controversial (10). Administration of supplemental folinic acid to pregnant surgical patients is routinely practiced at some major obstetric anesthesia centers (13).

EFFECT ON GESTATIONAL VIABILITY

Surgery and/or anesthesia in early pregnancy lead to an increased risk of spontaneous abortion (6). Traditionally, surgical procedures anatomically distant to the pregnant, and therefore irritable, uterus were thought to carry a lower risk of premature labor and possible pregnancy loss. However, recent large epidemiologic surveys present conflicting evidence (6,7). Pregnancy loss is increased particularly when associated with gynecologic procedures (2,6) and general anesthesia for non-abdominal procedures (6). More low birthweight infants (due to both prematurity and intrauterine growth retardation) are born to mothers that have had surgery and anesthesia during pregnancy (7). This increased incidence was not associated with a specific type of anesthesia or surgery. While the results of these studies are statistically significant, the authors admit that the causative factors are still unknown (6,7). Nitrous oxide has been associated with increased reproductive loss in the pregnant rat model (8,10). Interestingly, the use of low-concentration isoflurane in combination with 50% N_2O has adverse reproductive effects similar to unexposed rats (14).

INDIRECT EFFECTS

Volatile inhalational agents in concentrations of greater than 0.5 MAC will decrease uterine tone. Up to 1 MAC, inhalational agents will produce uterine artery vasodilation and increased blood flow; above 1 MAC, the decrease in maternal cardiac output will offset this vasodilation, decreasing uterine artery flow (15).

DIRECT AND INDIRECT EFFECTS OF OTHER AGENTS

The maternal administration of 100% oxygen will not raise the fetal oxygen much above 60 mm Hg (16) and will not predispose the fetus to the adverse effects of hyperoxia. Maternal hyperventilation may decrease fetal oxygen levels, due to effects on uterine blood flow (17) and a left-shift of the maternal oxyhemoglobin dissociation curve.

Certain narcotics (morphine, meperidine, and hydromorphone) have been associated with animal fetal abnormalities (18), though never in humans. Fentanyl, alfentanil, and sufentanil have been shown not to be teratogenic (19). Fentanyl has shown no deleterious effects on uterine blood flow.

Barbiturates in a single dose have not been shown to be teratogenic. However, barbiturates may further decrease uterine blood flow in an already hypoperfused placenta.

Diazepam has been associated with different fetal abnormalities, notably cleft lip (20), although this relationship is controversial (21). The fetal half-life of diazepam is about 30 hours, which might cause delayed neurobehavioral effects in the fetus if premature delivery is necessary.

Antisialagogues seem to have little, if any, effect on the fetus.

Muscle relaxants do not readily cross the placenta, yet can be measured in the fetal circulation after very large maternal doses. This may necessitate the need for ventilatory support in infants delivered in the perioperative period.

Ketamine in doses greater than 1.5 mg/kg will increase uterine tone and, therefore, decrease uterine blood flow. This tonic effect is seen throughout the second and third trimesters of pregnancy (22).

Vasopressors have predominantly indirect fetal effects on uterine blood flow. Predominantly beta adrenergic agonists are preferred (23), but there may be a place for alpha adrenergic agents in severely hypotensive patients (24).

Drugs used for prophylaxis against acid aspiration (e.g., H2 antagonists) have not been shown to have significant fetal effect in the dosage regimens commonly employed.

Local anesthetics have well-known indirect effects on the fetus. Although presumably cytotoxic, they have not been shown to be teratogenic (25).

Sodium nitroprusside (SNP) has caused fetal cyanide toxicity in laboratory animals when doses far exceeding safe clinical anesthetic practice have been administered (26). SNP has been used without harm for induced hypotension (27,28).

Nitroglycerin and trimethaphan are used often during the management of preeclampsia and have proven human safety records.

Mannitol will cause bulk flow of water from the fetus across the placenta but has been used without apparent harm in low doses (29).

Chronic administration of beta adrenergic blocking agents has been associated with intrauterine growth retardation, as well as expected fetal beta adrenergic blockade. Acute intravenous administration of labetalol in the gravid ewe model has produced insignificant fetal beta adrenergic blockade (30). Clinical observation of infants born to mothers chronically treated with oral labetalol do not demonstrate significant adrenergic blockade (31). Acute intravenous administration of esmolol in non-hypertensive gravid ewes has produced fetal hypoxemia (32).

MATERNAL CONSIDERATIONS

Safeguarding the pregnant patient during surgery requires knowledge of the anesthetic implications of the altered physiology of pregnancy.

HEMATOLOGIC SYSTEM

Hematocrit values less than 35% are considered abnormal, although many pregnant women with a lower hematocrit carry to term and deliver without adverse outcome. Intraoperative blood loss should be replaced, keeping this level in mind. Pregnancy is a hypercoagulable state. Early ambulation or the use of minidose heparin should be considered when appropriate in patients who are confined to bed for extended periods of recovery.

CARDIOVASCULAR SYSTEM

Cardiac output is 40% above prepregnant values by the early third trimester. Increased plasma volume, increased venous capacitance, and cardiac output keep systemic arterial and central venous pressures at essentially nonpregnant values. Aortocaval compression will decrease cardiac output or uterine blood flow, or both. Uterine displacement is required at all times during the second half of pregnancy.

RESPIRATORY SYSTEM

Renal excretion of bicarbonate offsets the respiratory alkalosis produced by normal maternal hyperventilation (pCO_2 = 32 mm Hg). Pregnancy-associated increase in minute ventilation, as well as decrease in dead space, significantly decreases the arterial-to-alveolar carbon dioxide gradient towards zero (33). End-tidal capnography is, therefore, additionally helpful in intraoperative monitoring. Pulse oximetry is invaluable. Increased oxygen demand, increased cardiac output, and decreased functional residual capacity lower apneic blood oxygen tensions faster in the gravida. Denitrogenation before induction, along with facile laryngoscopy and intubation of the trachea, is obligatory. The possible anatomically difficult airway in the gravida requires extra attention to be given to pre-induction positioning of the patient. Immediate availability of endotracheal tubes in a wide selection of internal diameters, as well as a short-handled laryngoscope, is prudent. Vascular, friable nasopharyngeal mucosa may make passage of gastric tubes a bloody mess. Gentle insertion of well-lubricated gastric tubes is necessary. If the gastric tube is used only during the operative procedure, oral placement is an easier and safer choice. Finally, mucosal vasoconstrictors may have negative effects on uterine blood flow (34).

RENAL SYSTEM

Blood urea nitrogen and serum creatinine are decreased to 5-10 mg/dl and 0.5 mg/dl, respectively. These values should be considered when interpreting laboratory data. The possibility of urinary stasis due to ureteral compression by the gravid uterus makes meticulous fluid management necessary in an attempt to minimize the need for bladder catheterization.

GASTROINTESTINAL SYSTEM

Pharmacologic means to alter gastric acidity and volume should be an integral part of acid aspiration prophylaxis. When appropriate, regional anesthesia is preferable (with intact airway reflexes) to general anesthesia. If general anesthesia is selected, then rapid-sequence induction of general anesthesia is routinely advised. If the surgical condition warrants a more deliberate induction of general anesthesia (e.g., severely increased intracranial pressure), then experienced personnel should be available to maintain cricoid pressure and otherwise assist the anesthesiologist from induction of anesthesia through endotracheal intubation.

CENTRAL NERVOUS SYSTEM

The minimum alveolar concentration (MAC) of inhalational agents decreases (35). This is especially important if inhalational analgesia is contemplated. Loss of protective airway reflexes in a possibly anesthetized patient demands careful titration of agent to effect, and then only in the most experienced hands. A fasting pregnant patient presenting electively for surgery in the first trimester would possibly (but rarely) be a candidate for inhalational analgesia. The gravida presenting for surgery in the second trimester and beyond should be treated with the same precautions as the non-fasting patient presenting emergently for surgery. Neural sensitivity to local anesthetics increases during pregnancy (36). The induction of surgical epidural or spinal anesthesia will require less anesthetic in the pregnant patient. Use of continuous epidural or spinal catheters allows the anesthesiologist to titrate the dose of local anesthetic to desired effect.

GENERAL RECOMMENDATIONS

FIRST TRIMESTER

Possible teratogenic effects should be kept in mind but there is no reason to avoid general anesthesia if it is appropriate for the planned surgical procedure or requested by the patient. The use of N_2O in the first trimester, as well as in the entire pregnancy, is controversial. Maintenance of general anesthesia can easily be accomplished while avoiding the use of N_2O.

SECOND AND THIRD TRIMESTERS

Support of uteroplacental perfusion is of prime importance. Uterine displacement is essential in the supine gravida, especially after 20 weeks gestation. Intermittent comparison of brachial blood pressure to blood pressure distal to the uterus (e.g., popliteal area) is helpful in detecting occult supine hypotension. Fetal heart rate should be monitored throughout the perioperative period by personnel familiar with its interpretation in all pregnancies that are thought to be viable. Obstetric consultation should be readily available to evaluate fetal well-being before, during, and after the procedure, and to treat obstetric complications such as premature labor. Gastrointestinal changes demand acid aspiration prophylaxis. Rapid-sequence induction of general anesthesia is indicated.

SUMMARY

Communication among obstetrician, surgeon, neonatologist, and anesthesiologist is obligatory. Viability of the pregnancy is of prime concern if premature labor cannot be arrested and delivery becomes imminent. Effective preoperative communication with the patient and her family about a jointly conceived perioperative plan of management will decrease stress on everyone, including the patient.

Remember: Meticulous care of the mother will help ensure fetal well-being.

REFERENCES

1. Smith BE: Fetal prognosis after anesthesia during gestation. Anesth Analg 42:521, 1963
2. Shnider SM, Webster GM: Maternal and fetal hazards of surgery during pregnancy. Am J Obstet Gynecol 92:891, 1965
3. Brodsky JB, Cohen EN, Brown BW et al: Surgery during pregnancy and fetal outcome. Am J Obstet Gynecol 138:1165, 1980
4. Konieczko KM, Chapk JC, Nunn JF: Fetotoxic potential of general anesthesia in relation to pregnancy. Brit J Anaesth 59:449, 1987
5. Weingold AB, ed: Surgical diseases in pregnancy. Clin Obstet Gynecol 24(4):793, 1983
6. Duncan PG, Pope WDB, Cohen MM et al: Fetal risk of anesthesia and surgery during pregnancy. Anesthesiology 64:790, 1986
7. Mazze RI, Kallen B: Reproductive outcome after anesthesia and operation during pregnancy: A registry study of 5405 cases. Am J Obstet Gynecol 161:1178, 1989
8. Mazze RI, Fujinaga M, Rice SA et al: Reproductive and teratogenic effect of nitrous oxide, halothane, isoflurane and enflurance in Sprague-Dawley rats. Anesthesiology 64:339, 1986
9. Nunn JF: Clinical aspects of the interaction between nitrous oxide and vitamin B12. Brit J Anaesth 59:3, 1987
10. Fujinaga M, Mazze RI, Baden JM: Reconsiderations of the mechanisms of nitrous oxide teratogenicity. Anesthesiology 69:A658, 1988
11. Crawford JS, Lewis M: Nitrous oxide in early human pregnancy. Anaesthesia 41:900, 1986
12. Keeling PA, Rocke DA, Nunn JF et al: Folinic acid as protection against nitrous oxide teratogenicity in the rat. Brit J Anaesth 58:528, 1986
13. Marx GF: The N_2O dilemma. Obstet Anesth Dig 5:126, 1985
14. Fujinaga M, Baden JM, Yhap EO et al: Reproductive and teratogenic effects of nitrous oxide, isoflurane, and their combination in Sprague-Dawley rats. Anesthesiology 67:960, 1987
15. Biehl DR, Yarnell R, Wide JG et al: The uptake of isoflurane by the foetal lamb in utero: Effect on regional blood flow. Can Anaesth Soc J 30:581, 1983
16. Baraka A: Correlation between maternal and foetal PO_2 and PCO_2 during cesarean delivery. Brit J Anaesth 42:434, 1972
17. Levinsohn GL, Shnider SM, deLorimier AA et al: Effects of maternal hyperventilation on uterine blood flow and fetal oxygenation and acid-base status. Anesthesiology 40:340, 1974

18. Geber WF, Schramm LC: Congenital malformations of the central nervous system produced by narcotic analgesics in the hamster. Am J Obstet Gynecol 123:705, 1975

19. Fujinaga M, Mazze RI, Jackson EC et al: Reproductive and teratogenic effects of sufentanil and alfentanil in Sprague-Dawley rats. Anesthesiology 67:166, 1988

20. Safra MJ, Oakley GP: Association between cleft lip with and without cleft palate and prenatal exposure to diazepam. Lancet ii:478, 1975

21. Rosenberg L, Mitchell AA, Parsells JL et al: Lack of relation of oral clefts to diazepam use during pregnancy. N Engl J Med 309:1282, 1983

22. Galloon S: Ketamine for obstetric delivery. Anesthesiology 44:522, 1976

23. Ralston DH, Shnider SM, deLorimier AA: Effects of equipotent metaraminol, mephenteramine and methoxamine on uterine blood flow in the pregnant ewe. Anesthesiology 40:354, 1974

24. Ramanathan S, Friedman S, Moss P et al: Phenylephrine for the treatment of maternal hypotension due to epidural anesthesia. Anesth Analg 63(5):262, 1984

25. Fujinaga M, Mazze RI: Reproductive and teratogenic effects of lidocaine in Sprague Dawley rats. Anesthesiology 65:626, 1986

26. Naulty JS, Cefalo RC, Lewis PE: Fetal toxicity of nitroprusside in the pregnant ewe. Am J Obstet Gynecol 139:708, 1981

27. Kofke WA, Wuest HP, McGinnis CA: Cesarean section following ruptured cerebral aneurysm and neuroresuscitation. Anesthesiology 60:242, 1984

28. Rigg D, McDonogh A: Use of sodium nitroprusside for deliberate hypotension during pregnancy. Brit J Anaesth 53:985, 1981

29. Neuman B, Lam AM: Induced hypotension for clipping of a cerebral aneurysm during pregnancy: A case report and brief review. Anesth Analg 65:675, 1986

30. Eisenach JC: Maternally administered labetalol produces less adrenergic blockade in fetus than in mother. Anesthesiology 71:A915, 1989

31. MacPherson M, Broughton Pipkin F, Rutter N: The effect of maternal labetalol in the newborn infant. Br J Obstet Gynecol 93:539, 1986

32. Eisenach JC, Castro MI: Maternally administered esmolol produces fetal beta adrenergic blockade and hypoxemia. Anesthesiology 71:718, 1989

33. Shankar KB, Moseley H, Kumar Y et al: Arterial to end-tidal carbon dioxide tension difference during Caesarean section. Anaesthesia 41:698, 1986

34. Woods JR, Plessinger MA, Clark KE: Effect of cocaine on uterine blood flow and fetal oxygenation. JAMA 257:957, 1987

35. Palahniuk RJ, Shnider SM, Eger EL II: Pregnancy decreases the requirements of inhaled anesthetic agents. Anesthesiology 41:82, 1974

36. Datta S, Lambert DH, Gregus J et al: Differential sensitivity of mammalian nerve fibers during pregnancy. Anesth Analg 62:1070, 1983

FETAL CONSIDERATIONS IN THE CRITICALLY
ILL OBSTETRIC PATIENT

J. P. Phelan with S. L. Clark (ed).[*]

Unlike any other medical or surgical specialty, obstetrics deals with the simultaneous management of two individuals—and sometimes more. In all circumstances, the obstetrician must delicately balance the effect of each treatment decision on both the pregnant woman and her fetus, seeking always to minimize the risks of harm to each. The goal of this chapter is to highlight, especially for the nonobstetric clinician, the important clinical fetal considerations encountered when caring for high-risk mothers and will review: 1) current techniques for assessing fetal well-being, 2) fetal considerations in several maternal medical and surgical conditions, and 3) the role of post-mortem cesarean delivery in modern obstetrics.

DETECTION OF FETAL DISTRESS IN THE CRITICALLY
ILL OBSTETRIC PATIENT

More than two decades ago, Hon and Quilligan demonstrated the relationship between certain fetal heart rate (FHR) patterns and fetal condition by using continuous electronic FHR monitoring (1). Since then, continuous electronic FHR monitoring has remained a universally accepted method of assessing fetal well-being (2,3). The use of continuous electronic FHR monitoring permits the clinician to promptly identify fetuses at a greater likelihood of asphyxia and fetal death, and to intervene when an FHR abnormality is present.

Although the presence of a normal FHR tracing is associated with a favorable fetal outcome, an abnormal tracing is not always predictive of an adverse fetal outcome. The next few pages present an overview of FHR patterns pertinent to the critically ill patient. For a more detailed

---

[*]Clark SL: Structural cardiac disease in pregrancy. *Critical Care Obstetrics*, II ed. Chpt. 32. SL Clark, DB Cotton, GD Hankins and JP Phelan, eds. Blackwell Scientific Publications, Boston, MA, U.S.A., 1991. Reproduced with permission.

T.H. Stanley and P.G. Schafer (eds.), Pediatric and Obstetrical Anesthesia, 89-115.
© 1995 *Kluwer Academic Publishers.*

description of antepartum and intrapartum FHR tracings, see the classic descriptions by Hon (4).

BASELINE FETAL HEART RATE (FHR) CHANGES

BRADYCARDIA

Bradycardia is defined as an FHR of less than 120 beats per minute (bpm) and is subclassified as mild (100-120 bpm) and marked (<100 bpm). The most common etiology for a sudden FHR bradycardia is acute fetal hypoxia. In the critically ill obstetrical patient with hypertension, pre-eclampsia, or trauma, a common cause of acute fetal hypoxia is abruption of the placenta. Intrapartum, an abrupt FHR bradycardia may be associated with fetal conditions that cause umbilical cord compression, such as cord prolapse, nuchal cord, oligohydramnios, or uterine hypertonus. Investigators have also described the presence of an FHR bradycardia in association with the lowering of maternal blood pressure with antihypertensive agents (5). Of great importance in dealing with the critically ill obstetrical patient is that acute FHR bradycardia may herald, or may be associated with, amniotic fluid embolus syndrome, acute respiratory insufficiency, or an eclamptic seizure (6).

Less commonly, a persistent FHR bradycardia may be associated with an underlying congenital fetal abnormality. For instance, congenital bradyarrhythmias involving fetal heart block may be related to a prior maternal infection, a structural defect of the fetal heart, or systemic lupus erythematosus (7). Moreover, FHR bradycardia has been described in patients undergoing cardiopulmonary bypass. It is believed that this pattern is the result of inadequate maternal flow rates during the bypass procedure, and that it may be alleviated by high flow (8). In addition, fetuses whose mothers are undergoing neurosurgical procedures with hypothermia may exhibit FHR bradycardia (9).

Not all FHR bradycardias are pathologic. However, in the absence of a fetal congenital heart block, the persistence of a fetal heart rate <100 bpm for an extended period of time could constitute an obstetric emergency and require either prompt correction of the precipitating cause or immediate delivery.

TACHYCARDIA

Fetal tachycardia is defined as a baseline FHR of 160 bpm or greater and is subclassified as mild (160-180 bpm) and marked (>180 bpm). Most commonly, this type of baseline FHR abnormality is associated with maternal pyrexia or chorioamnionitis (Figure 1). In addition, betamimetic administration, hyperthyroidism, or fetal cardiac arrhythmias may produce FHR tachycardia. Although an FHR tachycardia may be a normal finding and may not require intervention, one cause for fetal tachycardia is underlying hypoxia, especially in the presence of ominous FHR patterns, such as diminished FHR variability and severely variable or late decelerations.

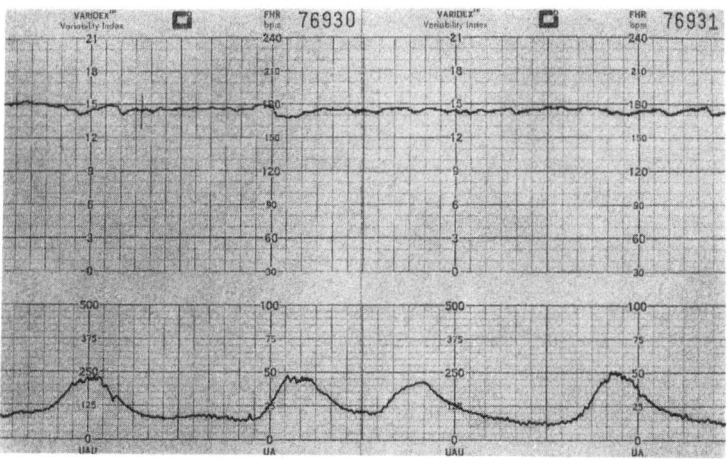

Figure 1.   Baseline fetal heart rate (FHR) tachycardia in a pregnancy complicated by maternal fever resulting from chorioamnionitis.

FETAL HEART RATE VARIABILITY

Short-term variability is defined as the beat-to-beat variation in the FHR resulting from the continuous interaction of the parasympathetic and sympathetic nervous systems on the fetal heart. For clinical purposes, normal FHR variability may be viewed as a beat-to-beat variation of >5 bpm (Figure 2).

In the absence of narcotic administration (10) or magnesium sulfate infusion (11), decreased FHR variability may be indicative of fetal compromise. For example, Paul and associates (12) have shown that when normal rather than diminished FHR variability was present in association with late decelerations of the FHR, the fetal pH was consistently higher. In keeping with that observation, Apgar scores are similarly high in those fetuses who exhibit normal FHR variability. On the other hand, periods of diminished variability are also seen in healthy fetuses.

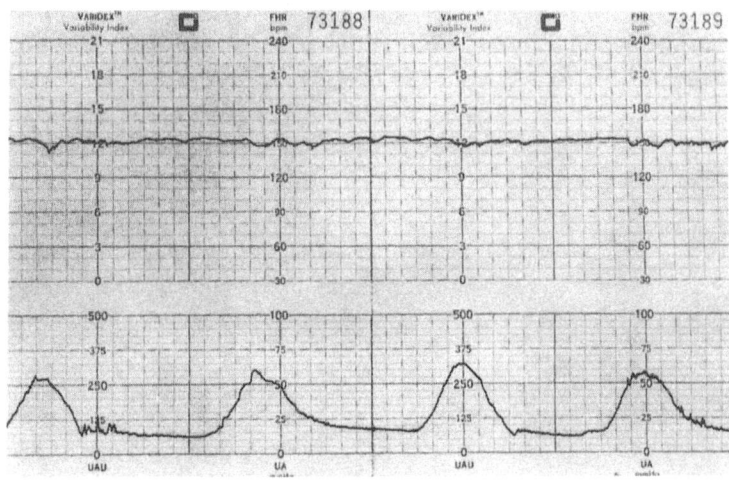

Figure 2. Intrapartum FHR tracing demonstrating diminished FHR variability.

SINUSOIDAL FHR PATTERN

A *sinusoidal FHR pattern* is defined as a regular sine wave variation of the baseline FHR. This sine wave has a frequency of 3-6 cycles per minute (13). The degree of oscillation also correlates with fetal outcome (14). For instance, infants with oscillations of >25 bpm have a significantly greater perinatal mortality rate than do infants whose oscillations are <25 bpm (67% vs. 1%).

The key to managing the sinusoidal FHR pattern is recognition. After the pattern is identified, a search for the underlying cause should be undertaken. One common cause for this FHR abnormality is maternal narcotic administration, such as alphaprodine or meperidine (15,16). When observed in association with FHR accelerations, the sinusoidal FHR pattern is associated with a favorable fetal outcome (16). In the absence of narcotic administration, the presence of this FHR pattern suggests asphyxia or fetal anemia.

Fetal anemia is often associated with placental abruption or previa, fetomaternal hemorrhage, vasa previa, or Rh disease (16). If the sinusoidal FHR pattern is observed in a patient who was involved recently in a motor vehicle accident, for example, the diagnosis of placental abruption should be considered. Abruption may also be suggested by ultrasound demonstration of a retroplacental clot or a positive Kleihaur-Betke test for fetal red blood cells in the maternal circulation. Finally, as suggested by Katz and associates (14), sinusoidal FHR pattern in the absence of accelerations may be associated with fetal hypoxemia. Under such circumstances, either delivery or some form of fetal acid-base assessment should be considered (17)

PERIODIC CHANGES

FHR decelerations associated with head compression ("early" FHR decelerations) are benign and are not included in the following discussion. Instead, the focus is on FHR accelerations, as well as variable and late decelerations.

ACCELERATIONS

An *FHR acceleration* is defined as an abrupt increase in the FHR above baseline, often in relation to uterine activity (Figure 3), fetal body movement (Figure 4), or fetal breathing movements. Criteria for FHR accelerations (i.e., a "reactive" tracing) include a rise in the FHR of at least 15 bpm from baseline that lasts at least 15 seconds from the time it leaves baseline until it returns (18). Whenever spontaneous or induced FHR accelerations are present, significant fetal metabolic acidosis is absent, regardless of other ominous features of the FHR tracing (19-23). The non-stress test (NST) is the primary form of fetal surveillance to assess fetal well-being, and it has a low probability of fetal compromise (18) or death (24). This observation persists, irrespective of the method used to generate the acceleration, whether mechanical (25) or sound stimulation (26,27), scalp sampling (20), or scalp stimulation (21). In contrast, the fetus with a nonreactive FHR pattern has significantly greater probability of an adverse fetal outcome (18), especially if the nonreactivity persists for more than 80 minutes (28).

To assist with immediate assessment of fetal health, acoustic stimulation of the fetus has been introduced (29) and developed into an important clinical tool (26). Its application has permitted prompt and immediate assessment of fetal status (22). A transabdominal vibroacoustic stimulus is applied with an electronic artificial larynx (EAL), a Model 5C (American Telephone Telegraph, New York, U.S.A.), or a Corometrics Acoustic

Stimulator (Wallingford, Connecticut). The EAL emits a fundamental frequency of 80 hertz (Hz) and a sound pressure level averaging 82 decibels (dB) at 1 m through air.

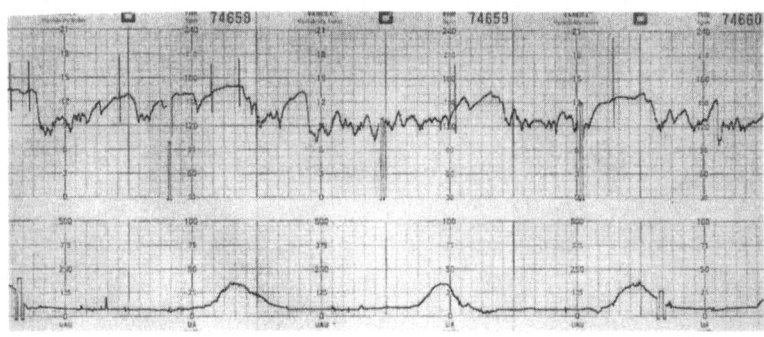

Figure 3. Intrapartum FHR tracing with a normal baseline FHR and FHR accelerations.

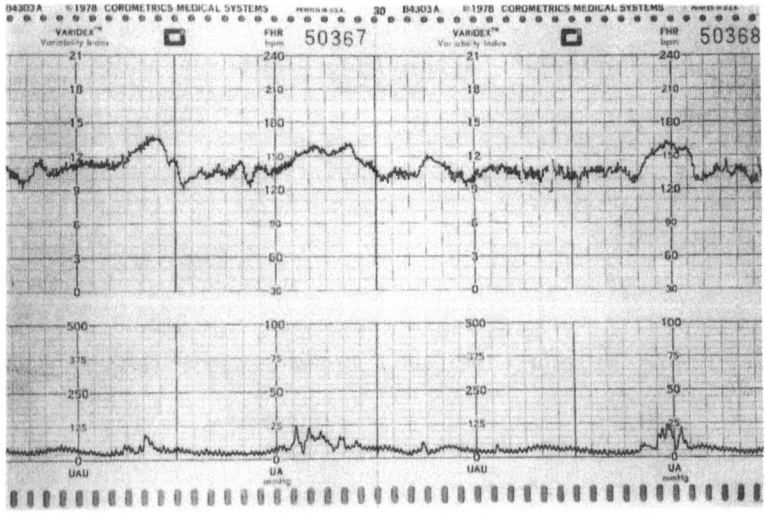

Figure 4. Antepartum nonstress test (NST) with FHR accelerations from fetal movement.

In brief, the clinical approach to fetal assessment with acoustic stimulation begins with monitoring the baseline FHR for 5 minutes. If the test is nonreactive, a sound stimulus is applied for 3 seconds or less. If no response is observed, the stimulus is repeated a maximum of twice more. In a retrospective investigation, this approach reduced the incidence of nonreactive test results by 50% when compared with historical controls (29). In addition, testing time was reduced, and the predictive reliability of a reactive test was unchanged (30). If, after acoustic stimulation, the fetus has a persistent nonreactive pattern, additional assessment with either the contraction stress test (CST) (31) or the fetal biophysical profile (FBP) (32) would be appropriate.

Currently, fetuses with persistent nonreactivity are managed with the FBP (33). The performance of an FBP (see Table 1) requires real-time ultrasound. Recently, the FBP has been modified to include the four-quadrant technique developed by Phelan and associates (34) to determine a normal amniotic fluid volume. Using this approach, the clinician divides the uterus into four quadrants. The linea nigra divides the uterus into right and left halves, while the umbilicus divides it into upper and lower halves. The vertical diameter of the largest pocket in each of these quadrants is determined with the transducer perpendicular to the floor. The summation of these four values provides a single number known as the amniotic fluid index (AFI). From the prior work of Phelan et al (34,35), an AFI ≤ 5.0 cm is considered oligohydramnios. Consequently, if a patient has an AFI ≤ 5.0 cm, her FBP score for that component will be 0. Additional components of the FBP include fetal breathing movements, fetal limb movements, fetal tone, and reactivity on an NST. The patient receives 0 or 2 points, according to the presence or absence of each component.

Table 1. Fetal Biophysical Profile Components

Components	Normal result	Score
Nonstress test (NST)	Reactive	2
Fetal breathing movements	duration ≥ 1 min	2
Fetal movement	≥ 3 movements	2
Fetal tone	Flexion and extension of limb	2
Amniotic fluid volume	Amniotic fluid index > 5.0 cm	2
	Maximum score =	10

Components of the fetal biophysical profile (32), including the modification for determining the amniotic fluid volume using the amniotic fluid index (34,35).

A fetal biophysical profile (FBP) score of 8 or 10 is considered normal (Table 1). Patients with a score of 0, 2, or 4 are evaluated for delivery. Patients with a score of 6 are given a repeat FBP within 12 hours or are evaluated for delivery (33).

VARIABLE DECELERATIONS

As implied by the name, *variable FHR decelerations* have a variable or nonuniform shape and bear no consistent relationship to the uterine contraction. The decline in rate is rapid and is followed by a quick recovery. Umbilical cord compression leading to an increased fetal blood pressure and baroreceptor response is felt to be the most likely etiology. Umbilical cord compression is more likely to occur in circumstances of an abnormal cord position, such as nuchal cords, knots prolapse (36), or a diminished amniotic fluid volume (37). In patients whose pregnancies are complicated by intrauterine growth retardation, as in hypertensive disease or postdatism, variable decelerations frequently occur because of diminished amniotic fluid volume (38,39).

Several investigators have attempted to classify variable decelerations based on the degree of decline in fetal heart rate. Kubli and associates (40) have correlated fetal outcome with mild, moderate, or severe variable decelerations. However, Krebs and associated (41) have advocated a method of interpretation that relies on the characteristics of the variable decelerations rather than the amplitude of the deceleration. These investigators have shown that when atypical variable decelerations are present, there is a greater likelihood of fetal acidosis. These atypical features (Figure 5) include: 1) loss of initial and secondary FHR acceleration, 2) prolonged acceleration, 3) baseline rate continuation at a level lower than that preceding the deceleration, 4) a biphasic deceleration, and 5) delayed return of FHR to baseline. The potential for an adverse fetal outcome associated with one of these types of variable decelerations is significantly higher. Patients with these FHR patterns have both a three-fold greater probability of an Apgar score <7 and a lower mean pH than do patients with "typical" variable decelerations. Consequently, whenever such an FHR abnormality is present and persists in the absence of reassuring signs, strong consideration should be given to fetal acid-base assessment and/or delivery.

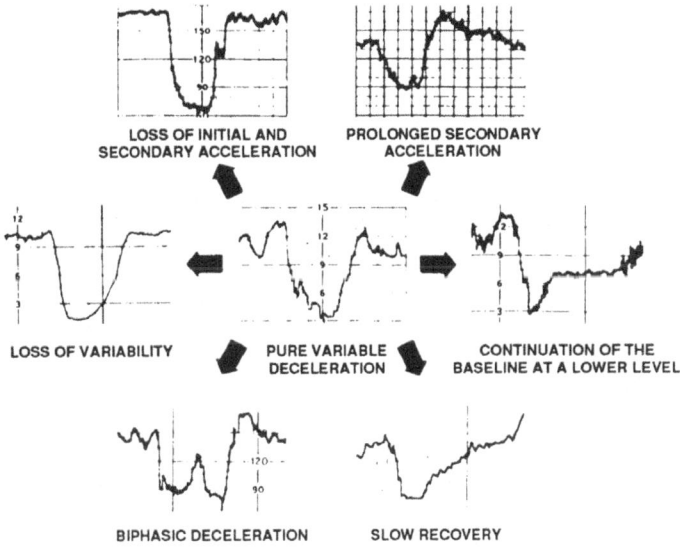

LOSS OF INITIAL AND
SECONDARY ACCELERATION

PROLONGED SECONDARY
ACCELERATION

LOSS OF VARIABILITY

PURE VARIABLE
DECELERATION

CONTINUATION OF THE
BASELINE AT A LOWER LEVEL

BIPHASIC DECELERATION

SLOW RECOVERY

Figure 5.   Atypical variable FHR decelerations. From Krebs HB, Petres RE, Dunn LH:
Intrapartum fetal heart rate monitoring: VII. Atypical variable decelera-
tions. Am J Obstet Gynecol 145:305, 1983. Reproduced with permission from CV
Mosby Co., St Louis, MO.

LATE DECELERATIONS

Late decelerations are uniform deceleration patterns with onset at
or beyond the peak of the uterine contraction, the nadir in heart rate 30-60
seconds after the peak of the uterine contraction, and recovery after the
uterine contraction has terminated (Figure 6). The underlying mechanism for the FHR pattern is fetal hypoxia.

In any patient who presents with the FHR pattern, a search for the
underlying etiology is essential. A review of her history may give some
clue as to the basis of this abnormality. For instance, trauma victims with
placental abruption or patients in hypovolemic shock are likely to manifest repetitive late decelerations on the fetal monitor. In addition, patients
with underlying vascular disease resulting from diabetes mellitus, hypertensive disease, or systemic lupus erythematosus may have fetuses that
manifest the FHR pattern. Whenever late decelerations are observed, the
pregnant woman should be positioned on her left side, oxygen should be
administered, intravenous fluids should be increased, and a search should
be made for a correctable underlying cause (e.g., hypotension). If this

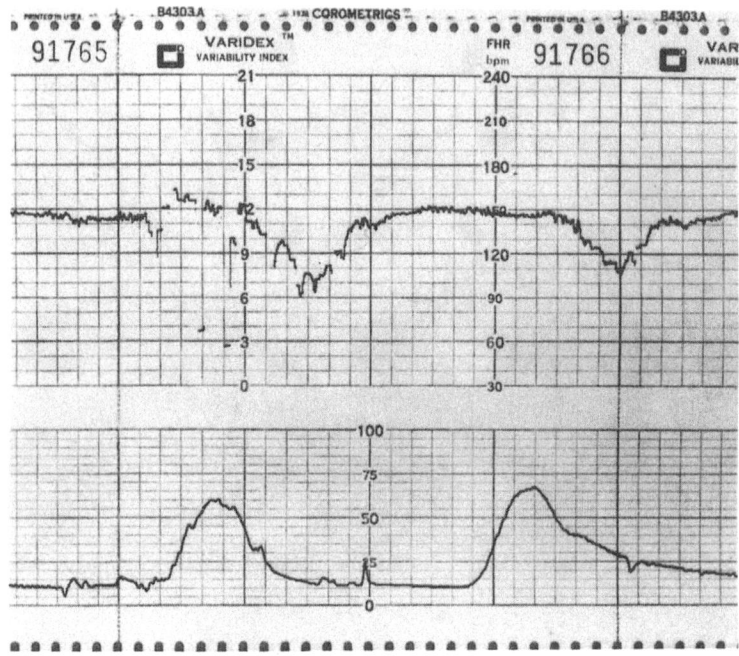

Figure 6. Late decelerations of the fetal heart during labor.

pattern persists in the absence of good variability or FHR accelerations, fetal acid-base status should be assessed or delivery effected (42).

Infrequently, the pregnant diabetic may present in diabetic ketoacidosis with repetitive late decelerations (43,44). With correction of the underlying maternal metabolic abnormality, the FHR abnormality may be resolved, and intervention is often unnecessary. However, persistence of this pattern may suggest an underlying fetal diabetic cardiomyopathy (45) or pre-existing fetal compromise and should lead to some form of fetal acid-base assessment and/or delivery. The fetus of a mother in sickle-cell crisis can also exhibit late decelerations. After the sickle-cell crisis has responded to treatment, this FHR pattern may resolve (46).

FETAL ACID-BASE ASSESSMENT

The criteria indicating a need for assessing acid-base status are illustrated in Table 2. The most common indication is the clinically confusing FHR pattern. This would also include the finding of a persistent nonreactive FHR pattern (28,47).

Table 2. Indications for fetal acid-base assessment or acoustic scalp stimulation.

1.	Repetitive late decelerations
2.	Absent fetal heart rate (FHR) variability
3.	Repetitive severe variable decelerations
4.	Atypical variable decelerations
5.	Sinusoidal patterns
6.	Persistent nonreactive FHR pattern
7.	Clinically confusion FHR pattern

Fetal scalp blood sampling is used in about 3% of all pregnancies (48). The technique was first described by Saling (49), who found that infants with a pH <7.2 were more likely to be delivered physiologically depressed. Conversely, a normal fetal outcome was more likely to be associated with a nonacidotic fetus (pH >7.20) (50).

In many institutions, fetal scalp sampling is technically not feasible because of the lack of readily available equipment. In addition, many clinicians find it cumbersome to use. More importantly, it does require the cervix to be dilated and the membranes ruptured. In the critically ill gravida, this is not always technically feasible. Nevertheless, clinical circumstances may dictate a need to know fetal acid-base status. Alternative techniques that focus on noninvasive approaches to detect fetal acidosis have therefore been developed.

An understanding of noninvasive techniques to assess fetal acid-base status is thus essential in the management of the critically ill obstetric patient. Clark and associates (20) were the first to show a relationship between induced FHR accelerations and normal fetal acid-base status. In that study, the authors reviewed 200 FHR tracings of fetuses who had undergone fetal scalp blood sampling. Of these, 169 had an FHR acceleration in response to fetal scalp blood sampling. All of the 169 had a scalp pH >7.20.

The Clark study formed the basis for a prospective investigation of 100 fetuses with FHR tracings that suggested fetal acidosis (21). These 100 fetuses underwent scalp stimulation with a finger or an Allis clamp, followed by scalp blood sampling. Of the 51 patients who responded with an FHR acceleration to scalp stimulation, 50 (98%) had a normal scalp pH. The single fetus whose pH was <7.20 (pH of 7.19) had a normal outcome. However, in the group that failed to respond with an FHR acceleration, 19 (39%) had evidence of acidosis.

Subsequently, Smith and associates (22) evaluated 64 patients who had abnormal FHR tracings and were judged candidates for fetal acid-base assessment. These patients underwent acoustic stimulation of the fetus, along with acid-base determination. Of these patients, 30 fetuses were found to be reactive, and all had a pH ≥7.25. Of those 34 patients who were nonreactive, 18 (53%) were found to be acidotic. Luz and associates found similar results in their series on fetal auditory evoked responses (51).

Therefore, as part of the management of the critically ill obstetric patient with an abnormal FHR pattern, either scalp or acoustic stimulation of the fetus appears to be a reasonable alternative to scalp blood sampling.

MATERNAL MEDICAL AND SURGICAL CONDITIONS

ANAPHYLAXIS

Anaphylaxis is an acute allergic reaction to food ingestion or drugs. It is generally associated with rapid onset of pruritus and urticaria and may result in respiratory distress, vascular collapse, and shock. Medicines (primarily penicillins), food substances (such as shellfish), exercise, and contrast dyes are common causes of anaphylaxis (52,53).

When an anaphylactic reaction occurs during pregnancy, the accompanying maternal physiologic changes may result in fetal distress. In a case described by Klein and associates (54), a woman at 29 weeks gestation presented with an acute allergic reaction after eating shellfish. On admission, she had evidence of regular uterine contractions and repetitive severe late decelerations. The fetal distress was believed to be the result of maternal hypotension and relative hypovolemia, which accompanied the allergic reaction. Prompt treatment of the patient with intravenous fluids and ephedrine corrected the fetal distress. Subsequently, the patient delivered a healthy male infant at term with normal Apgar scores.

As suggested by these investigators (54) and by Witter and Niebyl (55), acute maternal allergic reactions do pose a threat to the fetus. Treatment directed at the underlying causes should remedy the accompanying fetal distress. Prompt reversal usually will result from the administration of epinephrine and the infusion of intravenous fluids. To give the fetus a wider margin of safety, the maternal systolic blood pressure should be maintained above 90 mm Hg. In addition, oxygen should be administered to correct the maternal and fetal hypoxia (54,55). Maintenance of maternal oxygen tension (PO_2) in excess of 60 mm Hg is essential to ensure adequate fetal oxygenation.

ECLAMPSIA

Maternal seizures are a well-known but fortunately infrequent sequela of preeclampsia. Although the hemodynamic findings of patients with eclampsia are similar to those with severe preeclampsia (56), maternal convulsions require prompt attention and treatment to prevent sequelae to both mother and fetus. During this time, the fetal response usually is manifested as an abrupt FHR bradycardia (6,57). The theoretical underpinnings for the observed FHR changes are illustrated in Figure 7.

According to the work of Paul et al (6), maternal convulsions usually are associated with a sustained uterine contraction. As a result of the contraction and/or pain, the maternal blood pressure rises suddenly. Within 5 minutes of the onset of a seizure, an FHR deceleration is observed. During the seizure, which generally lasts less than 1.5 minutes (6), transient maternal hypoxia and uterine artery vasospasm occur, and they combine to produce a decline in uterine blood flow. In response, spontaneous uterine activity is further increased, resulting in additional compromise of uteroplacental perfusion. Ultimately, fetal hypoxia develops and an FHR deceleration ensues.

Such FHR bradycardia has been reported to last up to 9 minutes (6). Following the seizure and recovery from the FHR bradycardia, a loss of fetal heart rate variability and a compensatory fetal tachycardia are characteristically seen. Fetal response to the maternal convulsion is quite variable and largely depends on the condition of the fetus at the time of the seizure and the severity of the stress.

The cornerstone of patient management during an eclamptic seizure is to maintain adequate maternal oxygenation and to administer appropriate anticonvulsants. After a convulsion occurs, an adequate airway should be maintained and oxygen administered. To optimize uteroplacental perfusion, the mother is repositioned onto her side. Anticonvulsant therapy with intravenous magnesium sulfate (58) to prevent seizure recurrence is recommended. In spite of adequate magnesium

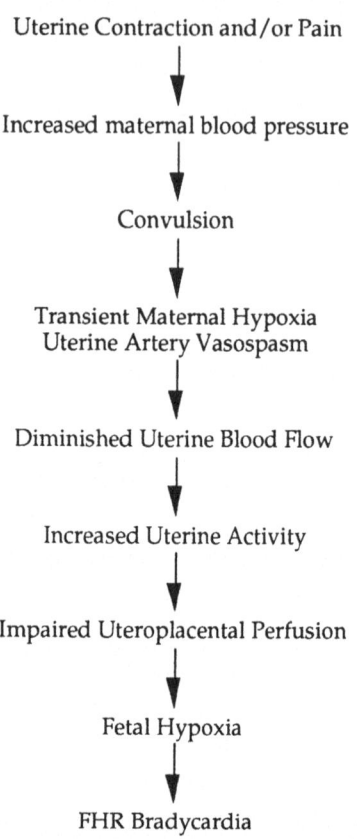

Figure 7.   Theoretical bases for the observed FHR changes associated with
            eclampsia.

sulfate therapy, adjunctive anticonvulsant therapy may be necessary, at
times (6). In addition, intrauterine resuscitation with a betamimetic (59)
or additional magnesium sulfate (60) may be obstetrically necessary for
eclampsia-induced uterine hypertonus.

Continuous electronic fetal monitoring should be used to follow
the fetal condition. After the mother has been stabilized, if the fetus continues to show signs of distress after a reasonable recovery period, assessment of fetal acid-base status (26) and/or delivery would seem prudent.

DISSEMINATED INTRAVASCULAR COAGULOPATHY

Disseminated intravascular coagulopathy (DIC) occurs in a variety
of obstetrical conditions, such as abruptio placenta, the HELLP syndrome,

amniotic fluid embolus, and the dead fetus syndrome. In many instances, DIC is subclinical only.

In other cases, the DIC may be advanced to a clinical level. Laboratory abnormalities are then accompanied by clinical evidence of consumptive coagulopathy. Under the circumstances of fetal distress and a clinically overt maternal coagulopathy, obstetrical management requires prompt replacement of deficient coagulation components before attempting to deliver the distressed fetus. This frequently requires balancing the interests of the pregnant woman and those of her unborn child.

For example, at 33 weeks of gestation, a 34-year-old patient presented to the hospital with the FHR tracing illustrated in Figure 8. Real-time sonography demonstrated asymmetrical intrauterine growth retardation. Oxygen was administered, the patient was repositioned on her left side, appropriate laboratory studies were drawn, and informed consent for a cesarean was obtained. When a Foley catheter was inserted, grossly bloody urine was observed. The previously drawn blood did not clot, and she was observed to be bleeding from the site of her intravenous line. The abnormal FHR pattern persisted.

A clinical decision now had to be made that would protect the well-being of both the mother and her unborn child. But whose interest should the obstetrician protect in this instance? Immediate surgical intervention without blood products would lower the mother's chance of survival. However, if the clinician were to wait for fresh frozen plasma to thaw and/or for platelets to be infused before undertaking surgery, s/he might expose the fetus to a risk of death or brain damage. Ideally, the mother and/or family should participate in such decisions. In reality, though, the often unpredictable nature of such dilemmas and the need for rapid decision making often preclude such family involvement.

In the case illustrated in Figure 8, the decision was made to: 1) place the woman in the operating room, 2) oxygenate her and maintain her in the left lateral recumbent position, 3) prepare to operate with an anesthesiologist, operating room personnel, and surgeons present, and 4) wait for blood replacement products. As soon as the blood was available, she was infused with fresh frozen plasma, platelets, and packed cells, and the cesarean was begun under general anesthesia. Maternal and fetal outcomes were ultimately favorable.

In summary, the cornerstone of managing the patient with full-blown DIC and fetal distress is to correct the maternal clotting abnormality before initiating surgery. While waiting for the blood products for transfusion, the patient should be prepared and ready for immediate cesarean delivery.

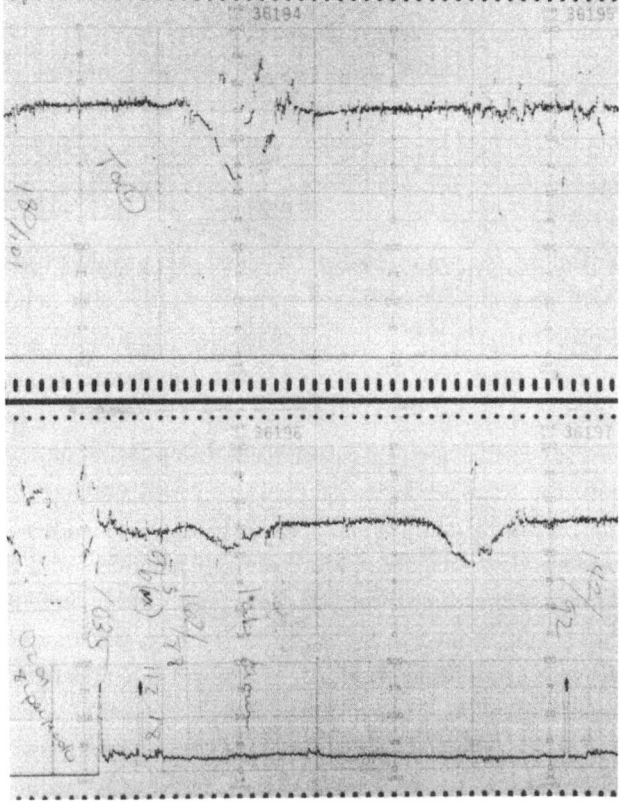

Figure 8.   The FHR pattern from a 33-week fetus whose mother was in clinical disseminated intravascular coagulopathy (DIC).

CARDIAC SURGERY DURING PREGNANCY

Conservative medical management is the current therapeutic mainstay for the pregnant patient with cardiac disease. With the appropriate use of diet, bed rest, prophylactic antibiotics, and cardiovascular drugs, the course of pregnancy in the majority of women is successful. However, when these conservative measures fail, cardiac surgery is an acceptable alternative. A decision in favor of surgical intervention requires an appropriate balancing of the risks and potential complications for the pregnant woman and her fetus. If surgery is undertaken, a team approach, including cardiologist, cardiovascular surgeon, and obstetrician is required (61).

With the recent advances in medical and surgical management of cardiovascular disease, the risk of cardiac surgery to the pregnant woman probably is not increased over that of her nonpregnant counterpart. Paralleling the decline in maternal morbidity and mortality has been a 67% drop in perinatal mortality since 1969 (61). One of the major reasons for the improved fetal outcome has been the use of continuous electronic fetal monitoring during bypass surgery (8). This approach permits the surgical team to continuously monitor fetal condition throughout the surgery and to promptly identify and treat any evident fetal distress (8,62-64).

During bypass surgery, fetal bradycardia, followed by a compensatory tachycardia, is the rule. The theoretical basis for the FHR changes has been suggested to be diminished uteroplacental perfusion. This decline in perfusion is thought to be the result of a lack of pulsatile flow, the opening of uterine arteriovenous shunts, uterine artery spasm, or insufficient flow rates (8,62,65). It appears that there is a direct relationship between flow rates and the FHR (8,62). Intraoperative correction of fetal bradycardia has been achieved simply by increasing flow rates. In instances where the fetal bradycardia has persisted, repositioning the mother to relieve possible compression of the umbilical cord or the inferior vena cava has been suggested (63). If these measures fail and the surgery is to be prolonged, cesarean delivery may be required (66).

Spontaneous uterine activity is increased during and immediately following bypass surgery. Suppression of uterine activity, in the absence of fetal distress, has been suggested during these perioperative periods (62,63).

In summary, to optimize fetal outcome during maternal cardiovascular surgery, continuous electronic fetal monitoring should be used. High-flow, high-pressure, normothermic perfusion appears to be ideal for the fetus. To minimize the risk of diminished uteroplacental perfusion, one should: 1) avoid vasopressors, 2) promptly correct maternal hemorrhage with whole blood or component replacement, 3) increase maternal oxygenation, and 4) infuse glucose to replenish fetal glycogen (63).

MATERNAL BRAIN DEATH

With the advent of artificial life support systems, prolonged viability of the brain-dead pregnant woman is now a reality (67). Consequently, an increasing number of obstetrical patients on artificial life support will be encountered in the medical community. Maternal brain death poses an array of medical, legal, and ethical dilemmas for the obstetrical health care provider (68-70). For instance, should extraordinary care for the brain-dead mother be initiated to preserve the life of her unborn child, and if so, at what gestational age? If artificial life support is elected, how should the pregnancy be managed? When should the fetus be delivered? When should maternal life support be terminated? Is consent required to maintain the pregnancy? If so, from whom should it be obtained? These questions illustrate the complexities of such cases.

It is not within the scope of this chapter to deal with the ethical, moral, and legal issues related to obstetric care of the brain-dead gravida. Rather, the emphasis is on the clinical management of these patients when a decision has been made and consent has been obtained to maintain artificial life support of the brain-dead gravida for the benefit of her unborn child.

To date, three cases of maternal brain death during pregnancy have been reported (Table 3). In one, life support was terminated after a discussion between the patient's physician and family at 19 weeks gestation. However, in the other cases, the pregnancies were maintained for 1 and 9 weeks, respectively (67,70). Infants were delivered by classical cesarean and ultimately had favorable outcomes. For optimal care of such patients and fetuses, a cooperative team of skilled health-care providers is medically necessary. The goal is to maintain maternal somatic survival until fetal viability. To achieve this goal, a number of maternal and fetal considerations are essential (Table 4).

Table 3. Perinatal outcome in reported cases of maternal brain death during pregnancy.

	Gestational age (weeks)		Indication for delivery	Mode of delivery	Apgar scores (5 min)	Weight (g)
	Brain death	Delivery				
Dillon (67)						
Case I	25	36	Fetal distress	Cesarean	8	930
Case II	18	Life support terminated at 19 weeks				
Field (70)	22	31	Growth retardation septicemia	Cesarean	8	1440

Table 4. Medical and obstetrical considerations in providing artificial life support to the brain-dead gravida (70).

Maternal Considerations

Mechanical ventilation

Cardiovascular support

Temperature liability

Hyperalimentation

Panhypopituitarism

Infection surveillance

Prophylactic anticoagulation

Fetal Considerations

Fetal surveillance

Ultrasonography

Steroids

Timing of Delivery

As pointed out by Field and associates (70), maternal medical considerations involve the regulation of most, if not all, maternal bodily functions. For example, the loss of the pneumotaxic center in the pons that is responsible for cyclic respirations and the medullary center responsible for spontaneous respirations makes mechanical ventilation mandatory. Ventilation, under these circumstances, is similar to that of nonpregnant patients. In contrast to the nonpregnant patient, however, the maternal partial pressure of carbon dioxide (pCO_2) should be kept between 28 and 32 mm Hg and the maternal partial pressure of oxygen (PO_2) should be >60 mm Hg to avoid deleterious effects on uteroplacental perfusion. In selected cases, such as the development of adult respiratory distress syndrome, the use of positive end-expiratory pressure (PEEP) also may be necessary.

Maternal hypotension occurs frequently in these patients and is believed to be due to a combination of factors, such as hypothermia, myocardial hypoxia, and panhypopituitarism. Maintenance of maternal blood pressure can be achieved with the infusion of low-dose dopamine and careful central hemodynamic monitoring. Dopamine is effective because it causes vasoconstriction of skeletal muscles and, as a result, elevates the blood pressure without affecting renal or splanchnic blood flow.

With maternal brain death, the thermoregulatory center located in the hypothalamus does not function, and maternal body temperature cannot be normally maintained. As a rule, hypothermia results. Maintenance of maternal euthermia is important and can usually be accomplished through the use of warming blankets and the administration of warm, inspired, humidified air.

Maternal pyrexia suggests an infectious process and the need for a thorough septic workup. If the maternal temperature remains elevated for a protracted period of time, cooling blankets will be necessary to avoid deleterious effects on the fetus (71).

Nutritional support, usually in the form of enteral or parenteral hyperalimentation, is required for maternal maintenance and fetal growth and development. Because of poor gastric motility, parenteral rather than enteral hyperalimentation is preferred (70). The use of hyperalimentation during pregnancy does not appear to have deleterious effects on the fetus (72). As a rule, the amount of hyperalimentation should be in keeping with the caloric requirements of pregnancy.

In such patients, panhypopituitarism frequently occurs. As a result, a variety of hypoendocrinopathies, such as diabetes insipidus, secondary adrenal insufficiency, and hypothyroidism, may develop, each mandating therapy in order to maintain the pregnancy. Treatment of these conditions requires the use of vasopressin, corticosteroids, and thyroid replacement, respectively.

Brain-dead gravidas are also at an increased risk of thromboembolism because, first, pregnancy is a hypercoagulable state, and second, these women are confined to bed and are immobile. Therefore, to minimize the potential for a deep venous thrombosis or pulmonary embolus, heparin prophylaxis (5000 units twice a day) and support stockings would appear prudent (70).

By artificially supporting the maternal system, the intrauterine environment can be maintained to allow for adequate fetal growth and development (Table 4). To optimize fetal outcome, obstetrical management should focus on monitoring fetal growth with serial ultrasonography, antepartum FHR assessment, and, at times, the administration of corticosteroids to enhance fetal lung maturation (70). For stimulation of fetal lung maturity, betamethasone (12 mg) is recommended twice on the first day, at 12-hour intervals. Subsequently, weekly injections of 12 mg are recommended between 28 and 32 weeks.

The timing of delivery is based on either the deterioration of maternal or fetal status, or the presence of fetal lung maturity. If any of these events arises, maternal fraction of inspired air (FiO_2) should be increased to 100% (70). Classical cesarean is the procedure of choice (70) and is the least traumatic procedure to the fetus (73). To ensure immediate cesarean capability, a cesarean pack and neonatal resuscitation equipment should be immediately available.

In summary, maternal brain death during pregnancy does occur. With careful clinical management of these complicated patients, as outlined by Field and associates (70), a favorable fetal outcome can often be achieved.

PERIMORTEM CESAREAN DELIVERY

For centuries, post-mortem cesarean delivery has been recognized as an attempt to preserve the life of the unborn child (74). In 237 BC, Pliny and Elder described the first successful post-mortem cesarean delivery—of Scipio Africanus. Subsequently, in 1280, the Catholic Church at the Council of Cologne decreed that post-mortem cesarean delivery must be performed to permit the unborn child to be baptized and undergo a proper burial. Failure to perform the delivery was considered a punishable offense. This law mandated post-mortem cesarean delivery only in women whose pregnancies were advanced beyond 6 months. To date, there have been 269 cases of post-mortem cesarean delivery reported in the English literature, with 188 (70%) surviving infants (75).

Since Weber's monumental review of the subject in 1971 (74), the causes of maternal death leading to a post-mortem cesarean delivery have not changed substantially (76). These include hypertension, hemorrhage, and sepsis. With unanticipated or sudden death, such as amniotic fluid embolus syndrome, pulmonary embolus, or acute respiratory failure, the timing of cesarean delivery is a critical issue.

If a pregnant woman does sustain a cardiopulmonary arrest, cardiopulmonary resuscitation (CPR) should be initiated immediately. Optimal performance CPR results in a cardiac output of 30-40% of normal in the nonpregnant patient. For best efficiency, the patient should be placed in the supine position. However, in this position, dextrorotation of the uterus may impede venous return and may further reduce maternal cardiac output. Consequently, placental perfusion may become severely compromised. Manual uterine displacement may help to remedy this problem.

If maternal and fetal outcomes area to be optimized, the timing of the cesarean delivery is critical. Katz and associates (76) have suggested that, "cesarean delivery should be begun within 4 minutes, and the baby delivered within 5 minutes of maternal cardiac arrest," to optimize maternal and fetal outcomes. According to the authors, delivery within this tie interval permits restoration of maternal cardiac output and the greatest possibility of maternal and fetal survival. Moreover, care must be taken to continue maternal CPR, not only until the birth of the fetus but also after the delivery. On occasion, a woman has been resuscitated and has lived postcesarean.

As demonstrated in Table 5, fetal survival is linked closely to the interval between maternal arrest and delivery. For optimal fetal results, delivery should be accomplished within 5 minutes of the maternal death, and the fetus should be resuscitated promptly. Although the probability of a surviving, normal infant diminishes the longer the time interval from maternal death, the potential exists for a favorable fetal outcome at more than 20 minutes from maternal cardiac arrest.

Table 5. Perimortem cesarean delivery with the outcome of surviving infants from the time of maternal death until delivery (75).

Time interval (min)	Surviving infants (no)	Normal (%)
0-5	42	100%
6-10	8	88%
11-15	7	86%
16-20	1	0%
21+	3	33%

While the timing of cesarean delivery is a major determinant of subsequent fetal outcome, the gestational age of the fetus is also an important consideration, the probability of survival being related directly to the neonatal birth weight or gestational age (Table 6) (77).

Table 6. Neonatal birth weight and subsequent outcome (77).

Birth weight (g)	Number	Surviving infants	%
≤ 500	27	0	0
501-750	47	20	43
751-1000	49	32	65
1001-1250	49	43	88
1251-1500	79	73	92

At what gestational age should a post-mortem cesarean delivery be considered? Is there a lower limit? It becomes immediately obvious that there are no clear answers to these questions. As a general rule, intervention appears prudent whenever the fetus is potentially viable or is, according to *Roe v. Wade*, "capable of a meaningful existence outside the mother's womb" (78). Therefore, criteria for intervention need to be established and can be formulated with the aid of the institution's current neonatal survival statistics and guidance from its bioethics committee. In light of the continual technological advances in neonatology, care must be taken to periodically review these criteria, because the gestational age and weight criteria may be lowered in the future.

Maternal death is not always an unforeseeable event. For instance, patients hospitalized with terminal cancer, Class IV cardiac disease, pulmonary hypertension, or previous myocardial infarction are at an increased risk of death during pregnancy. Although these cases are infrequent, it seems reasonable to prepare for such an eventuality. One option is to have a cesarean delivery pack and neonatal resuscitation equipment immediately available.

Is informed consent necessary? In the unforeseeable, sudden, unexpected maternal death, consent to deliver the potentially viable fetus does not appear to be required (76). However, when maternal death is foreseeable, maternal consent for cesarean delivery in the event of death would appear reasonable.

REFERENCES

1. Hon EH, Quilligan EJ: Electronic evaluation of the fetal heart rate. Clin Obstet Gynecol 11:145, 1968
2. Paul RH, Gauthier RJ, Quilligan EJ: Clinical fetal monitoring: The usage and relationship to trends in cesarean delivery and perinatal mortality. Acta Obstet Gynaecol Scan 59:289, 1980
3. Shenker L, Post RC, Seiler JS: Routine electronic monitoring of fetal heart rate and uterine activity during labor. Obstet Gynecol 46:185, 1980
4. Hon EH, ed. An atlas of fetal heart rate patterns. New Haven, Conn, Hardy Press, 1968
5. Rigg D, McDonough J: Use of sodium nitroprusside in deliberate hypotension during pregnancy. Br J Anaesth 53:985, 1981
6. Paul RH, Koh KS, Bernstein SG: Changes in fetal heart rate: Uterine contraction patterns associated with eclampsia. Am J Obstet Gynecol 130:165, 1978
7. Lee LA, Weston WL: New findings in neonatal lupus syndrome. Am J Dis Child 138:233, 1984
8. Koh KD, Friesen RM, Livingstone RA et al: Fetal monitoring during maternal cardiac surgery with cardiopulmonary bypass. Can Med Assn J 112:1102, 1983
9. Strange K, Halldin M: Hypothermia in pregnancy. Anesthesiology 58:460, 1983
10. Petrie RH, Yeh SY, Maurata Y et al: Effect of drugs on fetal heart rate variability. Am J Obstet Gynecol 130:294, 1978
11. Babkania A, Niebyl R: The effect of magnesium sulfate on fetal heart rate variability. Obstet Gynecol 51:2, 1978
12. Paul RH, Suidan AK, Yeh SY et al: Clinical fetal monitoring. VII. The evaluation and significance of baseline FHR variability. Am J Obstet Gynecol 123:206, 1975
13. Clark SL: Sinusoidal fetal heart rate pattern associated with massive fetomaternal transfusion. Am J Obstet Gynecol 149:97, 1984
14. Katz M, Meizner I, Shani N et al: Clinical significance of sinusoidal fetal heart rate pattern. Br J Obstet Gynecol 149:97, 1984
15. Epstein H, Waxman A, Feicher N et al: Meperidine-induced sinusoidal fetal heart rate pattern and its reversal with naloxone. Obstet Gynecol (supplement) 59:22, 1982
16. Modanlou HD, Freeman RK: Sinusoidal fetal rate pattern: Its definition and clinical significance. Am J Obstet Gynecol 142:1033, 1982
17. Theard FC, Penny LL, Otterson WN: Sinusoidal fetal heart rate: Ominous or benign? J Reprod Med 29:265, 1984
18. Phelan JP: The non-stress test: A review of 3000 tests. Am J Obstet Gynecol 139:7, 1982
19. Lee CY, DiLoreto RC, O'Lane JM: A study of fetal heart rate acceleration patterns. Obstet Gynecol 45:142, 1975
20. Clark SL, Gimovsky ML, Miller FD: Fetal heart rate response to scalp blood sampling. Am J Gynecol 144:706, 1982

21. Clark SL, Gomovsky ML, Miller FC: The scalp stimulation test: A clinical alternative to fetal scalp blood sampling. Am J Gynecol 148:274, 1984

22. Smith CV, Nguyen HM, Phelan JP et al: Intrapartum assessment of fetal well-being: A comparison of fetal acoustic stimulation with acid-base determination. Am J Gynecol 155:726, 1986

23. Shaw K, Clark SL: Reliability of intrapartum fetal heart rate monitoring in the postterm fetus with meconium passage. Gynecol 72:886-889, 1988

24. Phelan JP, Cromartie AP, Smith CV: The nonstress test: The false negative test. Am J Gynecol 142:293, 1982

25. Druzin ML, Gratacos J, Paul RH et al: Antepartum fetal heart rate testing. XII. The effect of manual manipulation of the fetus on the nonstress test. Am J Gynecol 151:61, 1985

26. Phelan JP, Ahn MO: Fetal acoustic stimulation. In Chervenak FA, Isaacson G, Campbell S, eds. Textbook of ultrasound in obstetrics and gynecology. Boston, Mass, Little Brown (in press)

27. Clark SL, Sabey P, Jolly K: Non-stress testing with acoustic stimulation: 5960 tests without a fetal demise. Am J Gynecol 160:694, 1989

28. Leveno KJ, Williams ML, DePalma RT et al: Perinatal outcome in the absence of antepartum fetal heart rate acceleration. Gynecol 61:347, 1983

29. Smith CV, Phelan JP, Paul RH et al: Fetal acoustic stimulation testing: A retrospective experience with the fetal acoustic stimulation test. Am J Gynecol 153:131, 1985

30. Smith CV, Phelan JP, Platt LD et al: Fetal acoustic stimulation testing (the "FASTEST"). II. A randomized clinical comparison with the nonstress test. Am J Gynecol 155:131, 1986

31. Phelan JP, Smith CV: Antepartum fetal assessment: The contraction stress test. In Hill A and Volpe JJ, eds. Fetal neurology. New York, Raven Press, 1989, pp 75-90

32. Manning FA, Platt LD, Sipos L: Antepartum fetal evaluation: Development of a fetal biophysical profile. Am J Gynecol 136:787, 1980

33. Phelan JP: Antepartum fetal assessment—newer techniques. Semin Perinatol 12:57-65, 1988

34. Phelan JP, Smith CV, Broussard P et al: Amniotic fluid volume assessment using the four-quadrant technique in the pregnancy between 36 and 42 weeks' gestation. J Reprod Med 32:540-542, 1987

35. Phelan JP: The amniotic fluid index. In Chervenak FA, Isaacson G, Campbell S, eds. Textbook of ultrasound in obstetrics and gynecology. Boston, Mass, Little Brown (in press)

36. Phelan JP, Lewis PE: Fetal heart rate decelerations during a nonstress test. Gynecol 57:228, 1981

37. Gabbe SG, Ettinger RB, Freeman RK et al: Umbilical cord compression with amniotomy: Laboratory observations. Am J Gynecol 126:253, 1976

38. Phelan JP: The postdate pregnancy: An overview. Clin Gynecol 32:221-227, 1989
39. Vorherr H: Placental insufficiency in relation to postterm pregnancy and fetal postmaturity. Am J Gynecol 123:67, 1975
40. Kubli FW, Hon EH, Hhazin AF et al: Observations in heart rate and pH in the human fetus during labor. Am J Gynecol 104:1190, 1969
41. Krebs HB, Petres RE, Dunn LH: Intrapartum fetal heart rate monitoring. VII. Atypical variable decelerations. Am J Gynecol 145:297-305, 1983
42. Smith CV: Fetal distress. In Phelan JP and Clark SL, eds. Cesarean delivery. New York, Elsevier Science Publishing, 1988, pp 70-90
43. LoBue C, Goodlin RC: Treatment of fetal distress during diabetic ketoacidosis. J Reprod Med 20:101, 1978
44. Rhodes RW, Ogburn PL: Treatment of severe diabetic ketoacidosis in the early third trimester in a patient with fetal distress. J Reprod Med 29:621, 1984
45. Sheehan PQ, Rowland TW, Shah BL et al: Maternal diabetic control and hypertrophic cardiomyopathy in infants of diabetic mother. Clin Pediatr 25:266, 1986
46. Cruz AC, Spellacy WN, Jarrell M: Fetal heart rate tracing during sickle cell crisis: A cause for transient late decelerations. Gynecol 54:647, 1979
47. Phelan JP, Ahn MO, Sarno A: The fetal admission test. Presented at the 37th annual clinical meeting of the American College of Obstetrics and Gynecology. Atlanta, Georgia, 1989
48. Clark SL, Paul RH: Intrapartum fetal surveillance. The role of fetal scalp sampling. J Gynecol 153:717, 1985
49. Saling E: Technik der endoskopischen microbluentnahme am feten. Geburtshilfe Frauenheilkd 24:464, 1964
50. Saling E, Schneider D: Biochemical supervision of the fetus during labor. J Gynecol Br Cwlth 74:799, 1967
51. Luz NP, Lima CP, Luz SH et al: Auditory evoked responses of human fetus. I. Behavior during progress of labor. Acta Gynecol Scand 59:395, 1980
52. Van Arsdel PP: Drug allergy update. Med Clin North Am 65:1089, 1981
53. Reisman RE: Responding to acute anaphylaxis. Contemp Ob/Gyn 33(April):45-57, 1989
54. Klein VR, Harris AP, Abraham RA et al: Fetal distress during a maternal systemic allergic reaction. Gynecol 64:155, 1984
55. Witter FR, Niebyl JR: Drug intoxication and anaphylactic shock in the obstetric patient. In Berkowitz RL, ed. Critical care of the obstetric patient. New York, Churchill Livingstone, 1983, pp 527-543
56. Clark SL, Divon M, Phelan JP: Preeclampsia/eclampsia: Hemodynamic and neurologic correlations. Gynecol 66:337, 1985
57. Boehm FH, Growdon JH: The effect of eclamptic convulsions of the fetal heart rate. Am J Gynecol 120:851, 1974

58. Prichard JA, Cunningham FG, Pritchard SA: The Parkland Memorial Hospital protocol for treatment of eclampsia: Evaluation of 245 cases. Am J Gynecol 148:951-963, 1984

59. Barrett JM: Fetal resuscitation with terbutaline during eclampsia-induced uterine hypertonus. Am J Gynecol 150:895, 1984

60. Reece E, Chervenak F, Romero R et al: Magnesium sulfate in the management of acute intrapartum fetal distress. Am J Gynecol 148:104-106, 1984

61. Bernal JM, Growdon JH: Cardiac surgery with cardiopulmonary bypass during pregnancy. Am J Gynecol 41:1, 1986

62. Lamp MP, Ross K, Johnstone AM et al: Fetal heart rate monitoring during open heart surgery: Two case reports. Br J Gynaecol 88:669, 1981

63. Werch A, Lamberg HM: Fetal monitoring and maternal open heart surgery. South Med J 70:1024, 1977

64. Levy DL, Warriner RA, Burgess GE: Fetal response to cardiopulmonary bypass. Gynecol 56:112, 1980

65. Meffert WB, Stansel HC: Open heart surgery during pregnancy. Am J Gynecol 102:1116, 1968

66. Martin MC, Pernoll ML, Boruszak AM et al: Cesarean section while on cardiac bypass. Report of a case. Gynecol 57:415, 1981

67. Dillon WP, Lee RV, Tronolone MJ et al: Life support and maternal brain death during pregnancy. JAMA 248:1089, 1982

68. Black PM: Brain death. N Engl J Med 229:338-344, 393-401, 1978

69. Bernat JL, Culver CM, Gert B: On the definition and criterion of death. Ann Intern Med 94:389, 1982

70. Field DR, Gates EA, Creasy RK et al: Maternal brain death during pregnancy: Medical and ethical issues. JAMA 260:816-822, 1988

71. Edwards MJ, Wanner RA: Extremes of temperature. In Wilson JG and Graser FC, eds. Handbook of teratology, Vol 1. New York, Plenum, 1977, p 421

72. Smith CV, Rufleth P, Phelan JP et al: Longterm enteral hyperalimentation in the pregnant woman with insulin dependent diabetes. Am J Gynecol 141:180-183, 1981

73. Phelan JP, Clark SL: Cesarean delivery: Transperitoneal approach. In Phelan JP and Clark SL, eds. Cesarean delivery. New York, Elsevier Science Publishing, 1988, pp 201-218

74. Weber CE: Postmortem cesarean section: Review of the literature and case reports. Am J Gynecol 110:158, 1971

75. Katz VL, Cefalo RC: The history and the evolution of cesarean delivery. In Phelan JP and Clark SL, eds. Cesarean delivery. New York, Elsevier Publishing, 1988, pp 1-18

76. Katz VL, Dotters DJ, Droegemueller W: Perimortem cesarean delivery. Gynecol 68:571, 1986

77. Westgren M, Paul RH: Delivery of the low birth weight infant by cesarean section. Clin Gynecol 28:752, 1985

78. Roe v. Wade, 410 US 113, 93 Sct 705, 35 Led 2d 147, 1973

DOES EPIDURAL ANALGESIA PROLONG LABOR AND INCREASE THE INCIDENCE OF INSTRUMENTAL OR OPERATIVE DELIVERY?

M. Finster

The potential effects of epidural analgesia on the progress of labor and the incidence of operative or instrumental delivery has been a subject of lasting controversy, particularly between obstetricians and anesthesiologists. This controversy is difficult to resolve, since it is almost impossible to devise fully randomized, prospective studies comparing different modes of pain relief during the first stage of labor. There is no lack of retrospective reviews. Most of them indicate that epidural analgesia is associated with longer labors and/or an increased incidence of forceps delivery or cesarean section (1-7). Similar results were reported in a few nonrandomized prospective studies (8-11), particularly when epidural analgesia was started as early as in the latent phase of labor (9). Most authors tend to see a causal relationship even though, without randomization, selection bias cannot be ruled out. Women having a painful and protracted labor (malpresentation, dystocia) are more likely to request epidural analgesia than the less affected "controls." The same patients are also more likely to require an operative or instrumental delivery. Further, obstetricians are more prone to shorten the second stage of labor with the use of forceps or vacuum extractor when epidural analgesia is present. There are several reports indicating that epidural analgesia has no adverse effects on the progress of labor or the woman's ability to deliver vaginally (12-17). Particularly instructive among them are the studies showing that introduction of an "on demand" epidural service did not increase the primary cesarean section rate (14-17).

Uterine activity usually has significant effect on the progress of labor. Early studies showed that induction of caudal or lumbar epidural analgesia resulted in a transient decrease in uterine contractility, lasting 10-30 minutes (18-22). In some of these reports, this was attributed to the addition of epinephrine to the local anesthetic solution (20,22). Interestingly, the rate of cervical dilation was not affected by the temporary

117

T.H. Stanley and P.G. Schafer (eds.), Pediatric and Obstetrical Anesthesia, 117-121.
© 1995 *Kluwer Academic Publishers.*

decrease in uterine activity (18,20). In another study, uterine activity was not altered by induction of epidural analgesia as long as the supine position was avoided (23)—thus preventing aortocaval compression, which is known to reduce uterine contractility (24). Administration of epidural analgesia may also lead to an increase in uterine activity, particularly an elevation of basal tone, and prolonged decelerations of the fetal heart (25).

The most recent investigations have centered on the effects of epidural analgesia on the duration of the second stage of labor and the incidence of instrumental delivery. These were conducted in a prospective, randomized way, since it is not considered unethical to discontinue the analgesia once the uterine cervix has reached full dilatation and the mother is encouraged to "bear down." With the use of bupivacaine 0.25%, given by intermittent "top-up" injections, maintenance of epidural analgesia throughout labor did not prolong the second stage or increase the forceps delivery rate by comparison with patients in whom "top-up" injections were withheld during the second stage of labor (26). Similar results were obtained with a continuous epidural infusion of 0.75% of lidocaine (27). The duration of the second stage of labor and the frequency of operative delivery were similar in women receiving lidocaine throughout labor and in those having normal saline substituted for the local anesthetic after the uterine cervix reached 8 cm dilatation. In contrast, a study by Chestnut et al involving continuous infusion of bupivacaine, 0.125%, to nulliparous women showed that maintaining epidural analgesia beyond 8 cm cervical dilatation resulted in a prolongation of the second stage of labor (124 ± 70 min, vs. 94 ± 54 min in the saline group) and an increased frequency of instrumental delivery (53% vs. 28%) (28). Later on, Chestnut and another group of investigators reported that with the continuous epidural infusion of 0.0625% bupivacaine, with 0.0002% fentanyl, maintenance of analgesia beyond cervical dilatation of 8 cm had no effect on the duration of the second stage of labor or the incidence of instrumental delivery (29). Thus reducing the concentration of bupivacaine, made possible by the addition of fentanyl, had a salutory effect on the woman's ability to achieve spontaneous vaginal delivery. With intermittent epidural injections of bupivacaine 0.125%, the addition of sufentanil 10-30 µg significantly reduced the incidence of instrumental deliveries (from 36% to 24%) (30). The authors attributed this to the prolongation of the block and reduced local anesthetic requirement with the addition of sufentanil.

The only study in which the effects of premature rupture of membranes (PROM) on the incidence of dystocia and instrumental delivery were evaluated showed that these complications were more frequent among nulliparous women with PROM than among those in whom contractions preceded ROM (31). This was independent of the choice of analgesia used during labor, and the authors concluded that any study which aims to examine the effect of epidural analgesia on the outcome of labor should include the PROM as a bias factor.

Very recently published papers indicate that some researchers were able to conduct prospective, randomized studies comparing the effects of epidural conduction blockade with systemic narcotic analgesia (32,33). Analgesia was begun at cervical dilatation of approximately 4 cm. The results of one study are startling. In the epidural group, the incidence of cesarean section for fetal distress was as high as 8.3% and for dystocia 16.7% (32). The corresponding values in the narcotic group were nil and 2.2%. The high incidence of fetal distress in the epidural group contradicts the results obtained in the other study in which fetal heart rate patterns were examined in parturients randomized to receive epidural bupivacaine or intravenous nalbuphine (33). There were no differences between groups in baseline fetal heart rate, long-term variability, or frequency of variable decelerations. No patient had late decelerations.

In summary, the available data indicate that the effects of epidural analgesia may vary, depending on the timing and extent of the block, the position of the patient, the choice and concentration of local anesthetic, and the addition of epinephrine or an opioid. Finally, premature rupture of membranes may be the most important factor affecting the progress of labor.

REFERENCES

1. Johnson WL, Winter WW, Eng M et al: Effect of pudendal, spinal and peridural block anesthesia on the second stage of labor. Am J Obstet Gynecol 113:166-173, 1972
2. Raabe N, Belfrage P: Lumbar epidural analgesia in labor: A clinical analysis. Acta Obstet Gynecol Scand 55:125-129, 1976
3. Willdeck-Lund G, Lindmark G, Nilsson BA: Effect of segmental epidural block on the course of labour and the condition of the infant during the neonatal period. Acta Anaesthesiol Scand 23:301-311, 1979
4. Walton P, Reynolds F: Epidural analgesia and instrumental delivery. Anaesthesia 39:218-223, 1984
5. Cox SM, Bost JE, Faro S et al: Epidural anesthesia during labor and the incidence of forceps delivery. Texas Med 83:45-47, 1987
6. Kaminski HM, Stafl A, Aiman J: The effect of epidural analgesia on the frequency of instrumental obstetric delivery. Obstet Gynecol 69:770-773, 1987

7. Shyken JM, Smeltzer JS, Baxi LV et al: A comparison of the effect of epidural, general, and no anesthesia on funic acid-base values by stage of labor and type of delivery. Am J Obstet Gynecol 163:802-807, 1990

8. Hoult IJ, MacLennan AH, Carrie LES: Lumbar epidural analgesia in labour: relation to fetal malposition and instrumental delivery. Br Med J 1:14-16, 1977

9. Read MD, Hunt LP, Anderton JM et al: Epidural block and the progress and outcome of labour. J Obstet Gynaecol 4:35-39, 1983

10. Diro M, Beydoun SN: Segmental epidural analgesia in labor: a matched control study. J Natl Med Assoc 78:569-573, 1985

11. Thorp JA, Parisi VM, Boylan PC et al: The effect of continuous epidural analgesia on cesarean section for dystocia in nulliparous women. Am J Obstet Gynecol 161:670-675, 1989

12. Friedman EA, Sachtleben MR: Caudal anesthesia: The factors that influence its effect on labor. Obstet Gynecol 13:442-450, 1959

13. Gal D, Choudhry R, Ung KA et al: Segmental epidural analgesia for labor and delivery. Acta Obstet Gynecol Scand 58:429-431, 1979

14. Chandler CJ, Davidson BA: The influence of lumbar epidural analgesia in labor on mode of delivery. Int J Gynaecol Obstet 20:353-356, 1982

15. Gribble RK, Meier PR: Effect of epidural analgesia on the primary cesarean rate. Obstet Gynecol 78:231-234, 1991

16. Robson M, Boylan P, McParland P et al: Epidural analgesia need not influence the spontaneous vaginal delivery rate. Am J Obstet Gynecol 168:A240, 1993

17. Bailey PW, Howard FA: Epidural analgesia and forceps delivery: laying a bogey. Anaesthesia 38:282-285, 1983

18. Vasicka A, Kretchmer H: Effect of conduction and inhalation anesthesia on uterine contractions. Am J Obstet Gynecol 82:600-611, 1961

19. Alexander JA, Franklin RR: Effects of caudal anesthesia on uterine activity. Obstet Gynecol 27:436-441, 1966

20. Craft JB, Epstein BS, Coakley CS: Effect of lidocaine with epinephrine versus lidocaine (plain) on induced labor. Anesth Analg 51:243-246, 1972

21. Lowensohn RI, Paul RH, Fales S et al: Intrapartum epidural anesthesia: An evaluation of effect on uterine activity. Obstet Gynaecol 44:388-393, 1974

22. Matadial L, Cibils LA: The effect of epidural anesthesia on uterine activity and blood pressure. Am J Obstet Gynecol 125:846-854, 1976

23. Schellenberg JC: Uterine activity during lumbar epidural analgesia with bupivacaine. Am J Obstet Gynecol 127:26-31, 1977

24. Caldeyro-Barcia R, Noriega-Guerra L, Cibils LA et al: Effect of position changes on the intensity and frequency of uterine contractions during labor. Am J Obstet Gynecol 80:284-290, 1960

25. Steiger RM, Nageotte MP: Effect of uterine contractility and maternal hypotension on prolonged decelerations after bupivacaine epidural anesthesia. Am J Obstet Gynecol 163:808-812, 1990

26. Phillips KC, Thomas TA: Second stage of labour with or without extradural analgesia. Anaesthesia 38:972-976, 1983
27. Chestnut DH, Bates JN, Choi WW: Continuous infusion epidural analgesia with lidocaine: Efficacy and influence during the second stage of labor. Obstet Gynecol 69:323-327, 1987
28. Chestnut DH, Vandewalker GE, Owen CL et al: The influence of continuous bupivacaine analgesia on the second stage of labor and method of delivery in nulliparous women. Anesthesiology 66:774-780, 1987
29. Chestnut DH, Laszewski LJ, Pollack KL et al: Continuous epidural infusion of 0.0625% bupivacaine -0.0002% fentanyl during the second stage of labor. Anesthesiology 72:613-618, 1990
30. Vertommen JD, Vandermeulen E, Van Aken H et al: The effects of the addition of sufentanil to 0.125% bupivacaine on the quality of analgesia during labor and the incidence of instrumental deliveries. Anesthesiology 74:809-814, 1991
31. Kong AS, Bates SJ, Rizk B: Rupture of membranes before the onset of spontaneous labour increases the likelihood of instrumental delivery. Br J Anaesth 68:252-255, 1992
32. Thorp JA, Hu D, Albin R et al: The effect of intrapartum epidural analgesia on nulliparous labor: A randomized, controlled, prospective trial. Am J Obstet Gynecol 169:851-858, 1993
33. McGrath J, Chestnut D, Debruyn C: The effect of epidural bupivacaine versus intravenous nalbuphine on fetal heart rate during labor. Anesthesiology 77:A984, 1992

ANESTHESIA FOR THE INNER-CITY PARTURIENT

D. J. Birnbach

The "inner-city parturient" can present many challenges to the obstetric anesthesiologist. The unusual and clinically challenging situations that may arise in this patient population may be due to drug abuse, an unstable home environment, poor diet, failure to receive medical treatment during pregnancy, or the presence of untreated co-existing disease. The patient at greatest risk is the unregistered patient—that is, the obstetric patient in labor who arrives at Labor and Delivery never having seen an obstetrician or midwife. Table 1 summarizes some of the problems that can be seen in the unregistered obstetric patient.

Table 1. Problems seen in the unregistered parturient.

Preterm labor
Fetal distress
Abruptio placenta
Preeclampsia/eclampsia
Drug abuse
Hepatitis
Sexually transmitted disease
AIDS
Poor interaction with medical staff

Of all these problems, the use of illicit drugs presents the biggest challenge to the anesthesiologist. An example would be the patient admitted for a stat cesarean section at 30 weeks gestation in preterm labor with fetal bradycardia, massive bleeding due to an abruptio placenta, hypertension, and cardiac arrhythmias due to recent cocaine use.

DRUG ABUSE

The use of illicit drugs has become endemic in our society (1). As a result, anesthesiologists working on Labor and Delivery are now seeing a

123

T.H. Stanley and P.G. Schafer (eds.), Pediatric and Obstetrical Anesthesia, 123-131.
© 1995 *Kluwer Academic Publishers.*

dramatic increase in the number of patients using illicit drugs. Although drug abuse is a major problem in large inner-city hospitals, it is being seen in all classes of patients and hospitals. Drug abuse in pregnancy involves a wide range of substances and clinical presentations. Although there is a strong association between lack of prenatal care and drug abuse (2), identification of the drug abusing patient is a difficult problem. Patients in whom the anesthesiologist should suspect drug abuse include women who: are unregistered at the time of delivery (no prenatal care), exhibit intrauterine growth retardation, exhibit abruptio placenta, or deliver a depressed neonate.

Most pregnant drug abusers deny drug abuse (3) even when confronted with positive toxicology results. Abuse of multiple drugs is the rule rather than the exception. At St. Luke's-Roosevelt Hospital Center in New York City, more than 50% of our unregistered patients have positive toxicology screens, and more than 75% of these patients deny illicit drug use. Use of these drugs may precipitate life-threatening problems (4). These problems, and the anesthetic and obstetric implications of maternal drug abuse, will be discussed.

COCAINE

Cocaine use has now reached epidemic proportions, with more than 30 million Americans having tried cocaine at least once (5). The prevalence of cocaine use in the obstetric population is also increasing, and anesthesiologists, like obstetricians and pediatricians, are now being affected by the abuse of this potentially lethal drug. Positive cocaine toxicology testing has been reported across the United States, crossing geographic, socioeconomic, and cultural boundaries. Because a majority of cocaine-abusing pregnant patients deny drug abuse, the exact extent of perinatal cocaine use is unknown. It has been estimated, however, that greater than 50% of high-risk women cared for at urban teaching hospitals may be using cocaine during their pregnancies (6). Although patients who do not receive prenatal care tend to have the highest rates of cocaine use, registered private patients at suburban hospitals have also been found to be cocaine positive (7,8).

Perinatal cocaine abuse has been linked to many maternal and neonatal complications that may have a profound effect on the patient's response to the administration of anesthesia. The use of cocaine is associated with high morbidity and mortality, especially when the patient is undergoing anesthesia. There is now adequate animal and human data to demonstrate that cocaine use in pregnancy is dangerous to both mother and fetus (9). This danger is exaggerated by the misconception on the part of some patients that cocaine does not cross the placenta and is, therefore, a safe way to achieve a faster and easier childbirth. It has been shown that cocaine causes profound vasoconstriction, which may, in turn, cause profound alterations to uteroplacental blood flow, and eventually cause uteroplacental insufficiency and "fetal distress."

One of the most difficult aspects of medical care for the cocaine-abusing parturient is recognition of her cocaine abuse. A majority of cocaine abusers deny drug use when interviewed by their physicians (6). Physical examination may lead to the suspicion of cocaine abuse when there is unexpected hypertension and tachycardia, but the differential between recent cocaine use and preeclampsia may be difficult (see Table 2).

Table 2. Signs and symptoms of cocaine abuse.

Hypertension	Tremors
Tachycardia	Hyperpyrexia
Convulsions	Metabolic acidosis
Hyperreflexia	Emotional lability

Lack of prenatal care and cigarette smoking have been shown to be of predictive value in recognition of the cocaine abuser (2). Despite a thorough history and physical exam, however, most often the diagnosis of cocaine abuse can only be made via urine toxicology testing. Current laboratory screening methods for cocaine metabolites include gas chromatography, mass spectrometry, and radioimmunoassay. The difficulty with some of these lab tests is the lag time between sending the sample and getting the results. A new instant latex agglutination test for cocaine metabolites (OnTrak Assay®, Roche Diagnostics, Branchburg, NJ) can provide an accurate result within 4 minutes (6). The controversy continues over whether it is reasonable, ethical, or legal to test all or some patients for cocaine use. The best alternatives in today's litigious society include developing a protocol that is approved by the hospital's legal department, testing all patients (so that a patient cannot claim discrimination), and asking the patient for consent.

Cocaine abusers may have a higher incidence of cesarean section for fetal jeopardy than non-abusing patients. Anesthesiologists often meet these patients in an emergency setting while the obstetrician is waiting to begin a stat cesarean section. The choice of anesthetic is occasionally dictated by the hemodynamic sequelae of cocaine, such as the commonly seen scenario of abruptio placenta with massive hemorrhage after cocaine use. Even the strongest supporters of regional anesthesia will select a general endotracheal anesthetic for the hypotensive, hypovolemic parturient. However, in the more controlled situation, the anesthesiologist will have to choose regional vs. general anesthesia based on a comparison of risks and benefits for the individual patient. Epidural or spinal anesthesia, unless contraindicated, is always my first choice when anesthetizing the cocaine-positive patient. Recently presented data on life-threatening events under anesthesia in the cocaine-abusing parturient showed that life-threatening events during cesarean section were far more common with general anesthesia than with regional anesthesia (4). The most frequently encountered problems in patients under general anesthesia were severe hypertension and arrhythmias. Since severe hypertension after laryngoscopy may be expected in these patients, I treat cocaine-induced hypertension prior to initiation of a general anesthetic, in the hopes of avoiding this exaggerated response to laryngoscopy. Propranolol is relatively contraindicated in the cocaine-abusing patient, since beta blockade may cause unopposed alpha adrenergic stimulation and, therefore, worsen the hypertension (10). Labetalol, however, is very effective in treating the hypertension associated with acute cocaine intoxication (11).

The use of regional anesthesia in the cocaine-abusing parturient is also associated with risks. Thrombocytopenia has been associated with cocaine abuse; therefore, these patients may be at risk of developing an epidural hematoma. Profound hypotension may occur, due to a sympathectomy in an intravascularly depleted patient with abnormal compensatory mechanisms. The response to pressor agents is unpredictable. Ephedrine may not be an effective treatment in the cocaine abuser. These patients may have emotional lability and may, therefore, be uncooperative.

Myocardial ischemia is a common manifestation of cocaine intoxication, and the anesthesiologist should be prepared to treat the complications. Table 3 reviews the therapy for cocaine intoxication.

AMPHETAMINES

Amphetamines are still commonly abused drugs, especially in combination with other illicit drugs, such as opioids and cocaine. Acute

Table 3. Therapy for cocaine intoxication.

Symptom	Therapy
Hypertension/tachycardia	Labetalol
Convulsions	Benzodiazepines/secure airway
Tremors	Benzodiazepines
Anginal syndromes	
with hypertension	Labetalol
with EKG changes	Nitroglycerin

ingestion of amphetamines causes a release of catecholamines from adrenergic nerve terminals. Like cocaine, amphetamines inhibit the re-uptake of catecholamines. Signs and symptoms include hypertension, tachycardia, arrhythmias, tremors, hyperreflexia, fever, pulmonary edema, and confusion (12). Hypertension may occur after only small doses of amphetamine and has been reported as causing cerebral hemorrhage and stroke. The combination of hypertension, convulsions, and proteinuria resulting from ingestion of amphetamines by a pregnant patient has been mistaken for eclampsia (13). Acute amphetamine intoxication has also been reported as increasing ICP (14).

ALCOHOL

The alcoholic parturient poses many problems to the anesthesiologist. During the preoperative evaluation, a history of the quantity and type of alcohol consumed, the duration of abuse, the time of last consumption, and the use of other drugs should be elicited by the anesthesiologist. The medical history and review of symptoms should include the neurologic, cardiac, hepatic, and hematologic systems. If the patient appears intoxicated, a blood alcohol level should be obtained. Table 4 reviews some of the anesthetic implications of alcohol abuse.

NARCOTICS

Problems associated with opioid abuse include AIDS, hepatitis, endocarditis, pulmonary emboli, pulmonary edema, anemia, renal disease, cardiac arrhythmias, electrocardiographic abnormalities, and hemodynamic instability (15). A report has also described spinal/epidural abscess and disc infection in these patients (16,17).

Table 4. Symptoms and anesthetic implications of alcohol abuse.

Symptom	Anesthetic Implication
Peripheral neuropathy	Thorough neurologic evaluation prior to initiation of a regional anesthetic
Cardiomyopathy	Avoid cardiodepressant anesthetics
Increased gastric acid	Administer antacids/H-2 blockers, rapid sequence intubation
Coagulation defects	Regional anesthesia relatively contraindicated
Esophageal varices	Caution with nasogastric tubes/esophageal stethoscopes
Decreased albumin	N-M blockade abnormalities
Cirrhosis	Avoid halothane

The anesthetic of choice at this institution for the narcotic-abusing patient is regional anesthesia, thus avoiding the administration of narcotics. If the patient is actively addicted, a maintenance program is arranged, in order to prevent acute withdrawal. If the patient is no longer abusing narcotics, an effort is made to anesthetize the patient without their use. Unfortunately, regional anesthesia may be contraindicated in some opioid-abusing patients, due to coagulopathy, neuropathy, and infection. The use of pure antagonist or mixed agonist-antagonist drugs must be avoided in these patients, as it may cause acute withdrawal (18). The use of epidurally administered agonist-antagonist agents is also contraindicated because of the potential for precipitating acute withdrawal (19).

AIDS

According to the Centers for Disease Control, as of 1992, more than 250,000 cases of AIDS had been reported, with more than 170,000 deaths (20). AIDS is now one of the leading causes of death among women of reproductive age and is the leading case of death among black women of reproductive age in New York (21). It is, therefore, no longer unusual to be asked to provide anesthesia care for the HIV-infected parturient. AIDS, which can be considered as the final stage of the continuum that begins with HIV infection, may take many years to develop. It is thought that the vast majority of seropositive patients will develop AIDS within 10-15 years of infection. HIV infection can affect almost all organ systems, including the pulmonary, cardiac, hematologic, and nervous systems.

Anesthetic implications of HIV infection are outlined in Table 5. There is no evidence that regional anesthesia predisposes the HIV patient to any further neurologic deterioration. Although many HIV-positive patients have some neurologic symptoms, there appears to be no correlation of spinal and epidural anesthesia to new symptoms or acute central nervous system infection (22). Since most HIV seropositive patients have HIV in the cerebrospinal fluid, this is not considered to be a risk of regional anesthesia. The treatment of postdural puncture headache with autologous epidural blood patch is also unlikely to produce new disease. A study of HIV-positive patients receiving epidural blood patch showed no evidence of worsening neurologic status (23).

Table 5. Anesthetic implications of HIV infection.

- Pulmonary disease may cause decreased functional residual capacity.

- Tonsillar and adenoidal hypertrophy may make endotracheal intubation more difficult.

- Cerebral toxoplasmosis may cause increased intracranial pressure.

- Cardiac manifestations, including cardiomyopathy, may predispose to arrhythmias.

- Coagulation disorders may occur and may contraindicate regional anesthesia.

- Neurologic disorders, including neuropathies, meningitis, encephalitis, and dementia, may have an impact on the anesthetic.

THE TEENAGE PARTURIENT

The pregnant teenager in labor may present with problems related both to her medical care and to interaction with Labor and Delivery staff. Problems may include drug abuse, sexually transmitted disease, inability to handle the pain of parturition, hostile behavior of the birthing partner, and the possibility that pregnancy was the result of child abuse. Psychologic problems with pregnant teenagers may be decreased by careful support that is neither condescending nor frightening. Regional anesthesia, although advantageous, will require great patience and support—especially for cesarean section when a young parturient can misinterpret pressure feelings and complain of a failed block. If general anesthesia becomes necessary, the anesthesiologist should use a small endotracheal tube (e.g., 5-7 mm, depending on age and size of patient). Consent for procedures, including epidural analgesia for labor, varies from state to state. In many states, even if the parturient is less than 18, she is considered emancipated and may give valid consent.

REFERENCES

1. Matera C, Warren W, Moomjy M et al: Prevalence of use of cocaine and other substances in an obstetric population. Am J Obstet Gynecol 163:797-801, 1990
2. McCalla S, Minkoff HL, Feldman J et al: Predictors of cocaine use in pregnancy. Obstet Gynecol 79;641-644, 1992
3. Knisely JS, Spear ER, Green DJ et al: Substance abuse patterns in pregnant women. NIDA Res Monogr Ser 108:280-281, 1991
4. Birnbach DJ, Stein DJ, Thomas K et al: Cocaine abuse in the parturient. What are the implications to the anesthesiologist? Anesthesiology 79:A988, 1993
5. Abelson HI, Miller JD: National Inst Drug Abuse Res Monogr Ser 61:35, 1985
6. Birnbach DJ, Stein DJ, Thomas K et al: Instant recognition of the cocaine abusing parturient. Evaluation of a new technique. Anesthesiology 79:A987, 1993
7. Schutzman DL, Frankenfield-Chernicoff M, Clatterbaugh HE et al: Incidence of intrauterine cocaine exposure in a suburban setting. Pediatrics 88:825-827, 1991
8. Streissguth AP, Grant TM, Barr HM et al: Cocaine and the use of alcohol and other drugs during pregnancy. Am J Obstet Gynecol 164:1239-1243, 1991
9. Little BB, Snell LM, Klein VR et al: Cocaine abuse during pregnancy: Maternal and fetal implications. Obstet Gynecol 73:157-160, 1989
10. Ramoska E, Sacchetti A: Propranolol induced hypertension in the treatment of cocaine intoxication. Ann Emerg Med 14:112, 1985
11. Gay GR, Loper KA. The use of labetalol in the management of cocaine crisis. Ann Emerg Med 17: 282-283, 1988
12. Ong BH: Dextroamphetamine poisoning. N Engl J Med 266:1321-1322, 1962
13. Eliot RH, Rees GB: Amphetamine ingestion presenting as eclampsia. Can J Anaesth 37:130-133, 1990
14. Michel R, Adams AP: Acute amphetamine abuse. Anaesthesia 34:1016, 1979
15. Giuffrida JG: Anesthetic management of the drug abuser. Anesth Analg 49:272-278, 1970
16. Gomar C, Luis M, Nalda MA: Sacro-ilitis in a heroin addict. A contraindication to spinal anesthesia. Anaesthesia 39:167, 1984
17. Koppel BS, Tuchman AJ, Mangiardi JR et al: Epidural spinal infection in intravenous drug abusers. Arch Neurol 45:1331-1337, 1988

18. Tornabene VW: Narcotic withdrawal syndrome caused by naltrexone. Ann Intern Med 81: 785-786, 1974

19. Weintraub SJ, Naulty JS: Acute abstinence syndrome after epidural injection of butorphanol. Anesth Analg 64:452-453, 1985

20. HIV Quarterly Surveillance Report. CDC, Atlanta, GA. February 1993

21. Chu S, Buehler JW, Berkelman RL: Impact on human immuno-deficiency virus epidemic on mortality of women of reproductive age, United States. JAMA 264:225-229, 1990

22. Hughes SC, Dailey PA, Landers D et al: The HIV+ parturient and regional anesthesia: Clinical and immunologic response. Anesthesiology 77:A1036, 1992

23. Tom DJ, Gulevich SJ, Shapiro HM et al: Epidural blood patch in the HIV-positive patient: Review of clinical experience. Anesthesiology 76:943-947, 1992

ASPIRATION: ETIOLOGY, PREVENTION, AND TREATMENT

C. P. Gibbs

INCIDENCE

A reliable incidence of aspiration during or surrounding the time of general anesthesia is difficult to determine because not all cases are diagnosed, and those that are diagnosed are often not reported. Olsson and colleagues' report of 185,000 anesthetics (1) found 83 cases of aspiration allowing for an estimated incidence of 4.7 in 10,000 anesthetics, or 1 in 2,131 anesthetics. The incidence at the time of cesarean section was 1:661—an almost fourfold increase over the general population. More recently, Warner and colleagues (2) reviewed 215,488 general anesthetics and reported aspiration to have an incidence of 1 in 3,216 anesthetics. For emergency operations, the incidence was 1 in 895 anesthetics. Many cesarean sections are done as emergency operations.

MORTALITY AND MORBIDITY

Mortality after aspiration of stomach contents ranges from 3% to 70% (3-8). Five percent and 4.6% are the most recent figures and may be the most reliable (1,2). The difference in mortality rates is at least in part due to the different types of material aspirated and the therapy used, both of which will be discussed in later sections of this chapter. Also, comorbid disease seems to play an important role (2).

Morbidity is more difficult to define but consists of a multitude of serious complications, ranging from simple bronchospasm and mild hypoxia to pneumonitis and lung abscess, to myocardial infarction and renal failure secondary to severe hypoxemia (9-11). Olsson et al (1) reported that 17% of patients who aspirated required mechanical ventilation, and an additional 15% required a prolonged hospital stay. Warner et al (2) reported that 19% of patients who aspirated required mechanical ventilation.

T.H. Stanley and P.G. Schafer (eds.), Pediatric and Obstetrical Anesthesia, 133-149.
© 1995 *Kluwer Academic Publishers.*

ASPIRATION AND PREGNANCY

As identified above, aspiration occurs more commonly in pregnant patients than in the general operating room population. Aspiration in pregnant patients is most likely to occur during a difficult intubation (12). Failed and difficult intubations also occur more commonly in pregnant patients than in the general operating room population (13). Thus the pregnant patient is at considerably more risk than others receiving general anesthesia. Why? Reasons can be divided into two categories: 1) those that are intrinsic to pregnancy, and 2) those that are iatrogenic.

The enlarged uterus increases intra-abdominal pressure and thus intragastric pressure (14). However, the enlarged uterus is not necessary to produce the increased pressure, as the pressure is already elevated during the first trimester before the uterus rises out of the pelvis (15). The production of gastrin, the hormone that increases both acidity and volume of gastric contents, is increased during pregnancy, particularly in the placenta, which is probably the site of production (16). Motilin, a hormone that speeds gastric emptying, is depressed during pregnancy (17). Gastric emptying is delayed during labor, and, although the point is somewhat controversial, emptying time may also be delayed throughout pregnancy (18,19). A recent study by Simpson and colleagues provides evidence that emptying time is delayed in the mid-trimester (20). Some have suggested that the gastroesophageal angle is distorted by the encroaching uterus, making it less competent and perhaps explaining the high incidence of heartburn in pregnancy (21,22). Although some have indicated that lower esophageal sphincter pressures are lower, sphincter pressures are actually normal during pregnancy, and the barrier pressure between the stomach and the esophagus is the same as in nonpregnant patients, except for those patients exhibiting heartburn (23-25).

Iatrogenic factors that increase the risk of pulmonary aspiration in the pregnant patient include the use of narcotics and sedatives during labor. These agents retard gastric emptying even more than the delay caused by labor (19). The lithotomy position increases intragastric pressure (14), as does pushing on the uterus to aid delivery of the infant at the time of vaginal delivery. In this latter instance, if general anesthesia were electively used without an endotracheal tube, the stage would be set for an indefensible disaster.

THE PATIENT

Any discussion of aspiration requires a discussion of the term "at risk." A patient is said to be "at risk" when there is more than 25 ml of gastric contents and the pH is less than 2.5 (5,26,27). Whereas considerable support exists regarding the significance of the pH value (27,28), there is none to validate the volume value of 25 ml. Most authors and investigators now believe that the pH is the more critical determinant for degree of lung injury (29-32). However, because the 25-ml value is so well entrenched in the literature and continues to be requoted despite newer data to the contrary, "at risk" to many clinicians will continue to mean pH less than 2.5 and volume greater than 25 ml.

TYPES OF GASTRIC ASPIRATE

It is important to discuss types of gastric aspirate because the character of the aspirate plays a large role in determining the extent of lung injury. For example, partially digested food causes the most severe injury. Historically, aspirates have been classified according to whether they were acid or nonacid liquids. More recently, investigators have described the histologic and physiologic effects of partially digested food particles. Aspiration of large particles or chunks of food produces airway obstruction and, if not relieved, death by asphyxia ensues. In these patients, all efforts are directed toward removing the food particle. Occasionally, bronchoscopy may be necessary. The other types of aspirate are described below.

Acid liquid disperses throughout the lungs within 12-18 seconds and produces isolated areas of patchy atelectasis; and within 3 minutes, there are extensive areas of atelectasis (33). Histologically, there is significant alveolar-capillary breakdown, intense capillary congestion, and interstitial edema and hemorrhage (34). However, necrosis does not usually occur, and lung architecture remains intact. Physiologically, hypoxemia is the earliest, most dramatic, and most consistent response (35-38). Because actual tissue destruction may not always be significant in the early hours after aspiration of acid, findings at this point are likely to reflect reflex responses, destruction of surfactant, alveolar edema, and atelectasis (39). Later, the loss of fluid secondary to the pulmonary burn and resultant pulmonary edema may become so significant that hypotension and hypovolemia occur (35). Pulmonary hypertension also occurs rapidly, mostly as a result of hypoxic vasoconstriction.

Non-acid liquid (pH greater than 2.5) produces few histologic abnormalities. There are occasional, widely scattered, discrete foci of inflammatory changes. Physiologically, nonacid liquid produces an immediate and significant decrease in PaO_2 and an increase in Qsp/Qt (5,35). However, shunt values usually return to baseline within 4-6 hours and PaO_2 within 24 hours (35). Note that even with aspiration of liquids with a relatively neutral pH, a significant fall in PaO_2 can result from reflex bronchospasm and destruction of lung surfactant, which may lead to atelectasis and pulmonary edema (11).

Nonacid food particles produce inflammation that is readily apparent in the bronchioles and lung tissues and varies from scattered to extensive, almost confluent areas. Edema and hemorrhage are frequently present. Later, the reaction changes more to a foreign-body type of reaction. Lymphocytes and macrophages become prominent, and granuloma formation is evident around aspirated food particles. Physiologically, hypoxemia after nonacid food particle aspiration is more severe than that after acid liquid and is nearly as severe as that after acid food particle aspiration (35).

Acid food particle aspiration produces the most severe damage (35). There are more extensive hemorrhagic pulmonary edema and multiple patches of actual alveolar septal necrosis, occasionally even obliterating the structure of the lung tissue. Hypoxemia in this category is likewise the most severe, as are hypercarbia and acidosis. Hypotension is frequent and pulmonary hypertension common. Most importantly, mortality is high and often early. In one study, 50% of experimental animals who aspirated this material and did not receive specific therapy died between 2 and 4 hours after the insult, and all animals died within 24 hours (35). The Table provides blood gas values after various types of aspiration, and the following Figure depicts histologic changes. A review of both Table and Figure should convince even the most skeptical physician that consumption of food during labor is not humane, it is dangerous.

Table. Arterial Blood Gas Tensions and pH of Dogs 30 Minutes after Aspiration of 2 ml/kg of Various Materials.

Aspirate		Response		
Composition	pH	PaO_2 (mmHg)	$PaCO_2$ (mmHg)	pH
Saline	5.9	61	34	7.37
HCl acid	1.8	41	45	7.29
Food particles	5.9	34	51	7.19
Food particles	1.8	23	56	7.13

HCl acid, PaO_2, arterial oxygen pressure, $PaCO_2$, arterial carbon dioxide pressure. (From Gibbs CP, Modell JH. Pulmonary aspiration of gastric contents: Pathophysiology, prevention, and management. In Miller R, ed. Anesthesia, 4th edition. New York, Churchill Livingstone, 1994, pp 1437-1464.)

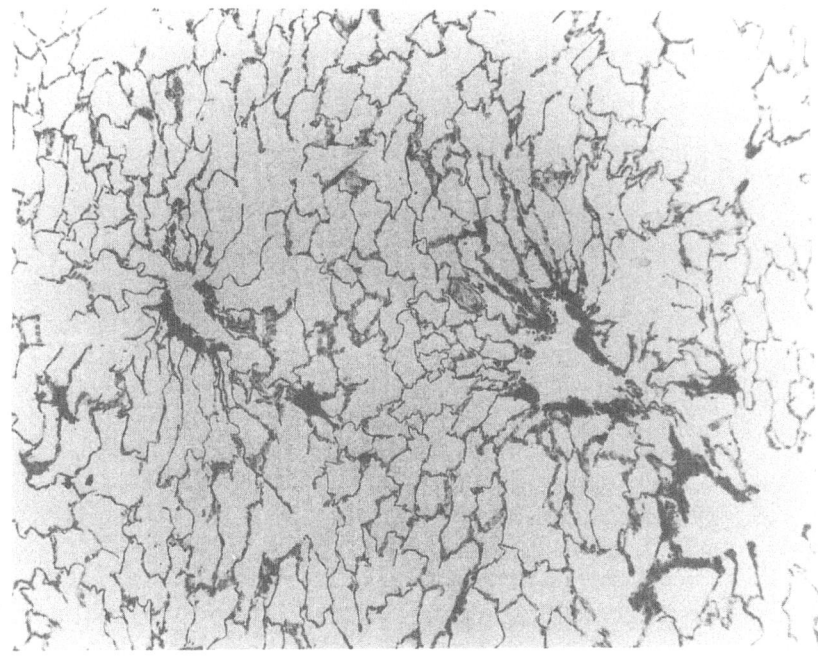

Figure (A,B,C). *Histologic Changes.* **A)** Lung after aspiration of normal saline. Essentially normal lung histology.
(From Gibbs CP, Modell JH. Pulmonary aspiration of gastric contents: Pathophysiology, prevention, and management. In Miller R, ed. Anesthesia, 4th edition. New York, Churchill Livingstone, 1994, pp 1437-1464.)

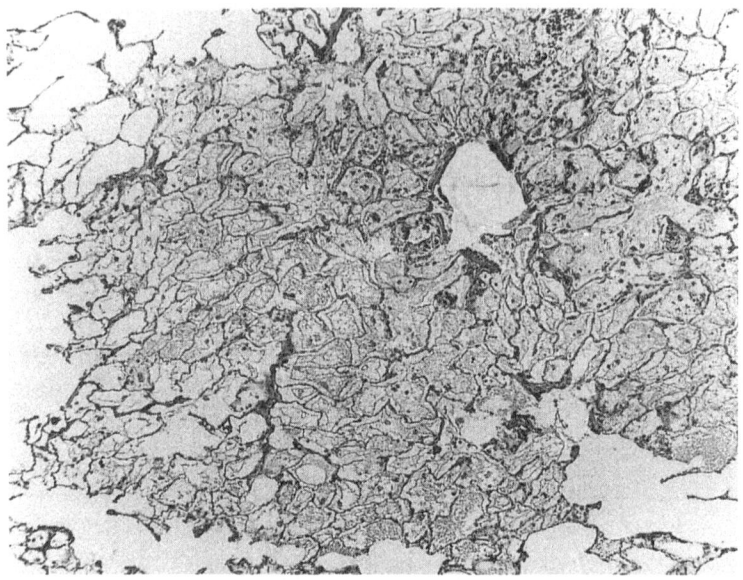

B) Lung after aspiration of liquid acid. Notice hemorrhage (reblood cells) and edema.

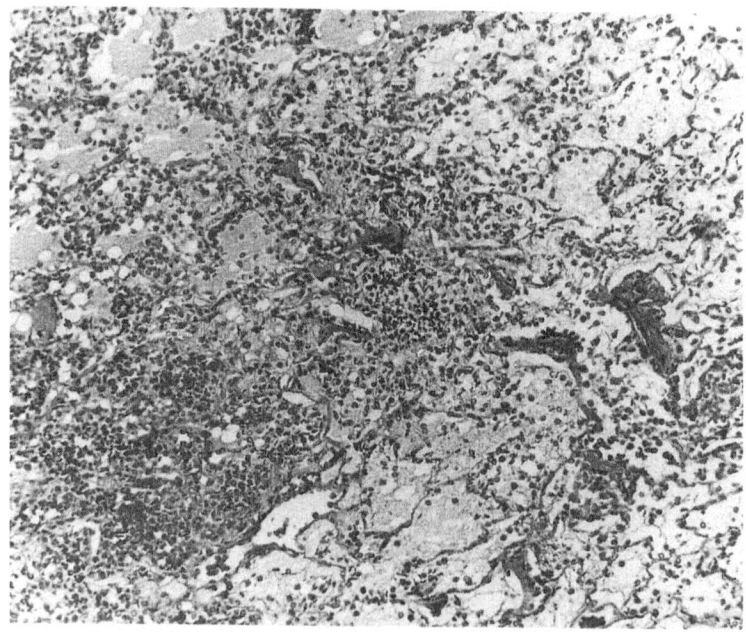

C) Lung after aspiration of acid food particles at pH 1.8. Hemorrhage exudate is more extensive. Actual breakdown of alveolar walls and lung architecture also has occurred.

SIGNS, SYMPTOMS, AND DIAGNOSIS

Aspiration of gastric contents can present dramatically with a full-blown picture that includes gastric contents in the oropharynx, wheezing, coughing, cyanosis, pulmonary edema, shock, hypoxemia, and roentgenographic findings. However, many (or, indeed, all) of these symptoms may be absent (3,19). Often gastric contents are not seen in the oropharynx, particularly when the aspiration is a result of silent regurgitation rather than active vomiting. In this situation, unless stomach contents can be suctioned from the trachea, aspiration of stomach contents is only a presumption, and a positive diagnosis cannot be made.

Some clinicians measure the pH of oral contents to determine if aspiration has occurred. The maneuver is unreliable because the pH of gastric contents is rapidly altered by the more basic oral and tracheal secretions. Radiographic changes, when present, are extremely variable. Small, irregular shadows constitute the most prominent and frequent finding initially. Landay et al (10) found bilateral diffuse infiltrates in approximately 50% and no changes in 15% initially. Distribution is usually bilateral and favors perihilar or basal regions.

The *earliest* and *most reliable* sign of aspiration is hypoxemia, which follows aspiration of even the mildest and most benign aspirate. Even aspirated saline causes a significant degree of hypoxemia (35,36). Therefore, whenever there is any chance that aspiration has occurred, analysis of arterial oxygenation by pulse oximetry or measurement of oxygen tension in arterial blood is indicated. If hypoxemia is present, the patient should be treated.

PREVENTION

Regional anesthesia is the best way to avoid aspiration. However, when general anesthesia is required, the following preventive measures are helpful:
- Nil per os
- Antacids
- Histamine-2 blocking agents
- Metoclopramide
- Head-up position
- Rapid-sequence induction
- Cricoid pressure
- Endotracheal intubation

- Extubation awake

NIL PER OS

Some obstetricians, nurses, and nurse midwives have suggested that physicians liberalize oral intake during labor (37-40). Is nil per os still appropriate? Studies have demonstrated that administration of clear liquids up to 2 hours before elective surgery does not increase gastric volume or acidity in nonpregnant patients, provided those patients do not also consume solid food (41-52). Water, clear liquids, and tea—but not milk—are acceptable oral fluids before elective surgery in nonpregnant patients. However, there are several differences between laboring women and nonpregnant patients undergoing elective surgery, and these differences require a somewhat more cautious approach for the pregnant patient. The interval between the last full meal and the onset of labor varies among patients. Some women are even advised to eat a full meal after the onset of labor and before they present to the Labor and Delivery unit. These advisors are probably well-meaning but ill-informed. Second, many women receive opioids systemically or in the epidural space during labor. Opioids clearly result in delayed gastric emptying. Third, laboring women may require urgent cesarean section at any time. Thus, the interval between the last oral intake and induction of anesthesia may be substantially less than 2 hours for these cesarean section patients.

Guidelines for Perinatal Care, 3rd edition (53), published by the American College of Obstetricians and Gynecologists (ACOG) and the American Academy of Pediatrics, states the following:

> Patients should not ingest anything by mouth during labor except for small sips of water, ice chips, or preparations to moisten the mouth and lips. Hydration and nourishment during a long labor should be provided by means of the intravenous administration of fluids; this measure also minimizes acidemia and electrolyte imbalance.

Thus, it remains appropriate to restrict oral intake during labor. Even a policy that allows ice chips only may not guarantee low volumes of ingested fluid. In our institution, we have observed an oral fluid intake (in the form of ice chips) as low as 22 ml per hour and as high as 120 ml per hour during labor (54). Thus, we encourage judicious ingestion of ice chips and not unlimited consumption. We suggest that oral intake during labor should be limited to 60 ml per hour of water or another clear, nonparticulate liquid. This should represent a reasonable compromise between patient safety and comfort. Food should never be allowed. Not only does it cause severe lung damage if aspirated, it is also more slowly emptied from the stomach (55).

ANTACIDS

An antacid will reduce the acidity of gastric fluid, but it will not reduce gastric volume. Thirty ml of nonparticulate antacid (e.g., 0.3 M sodium citrate, Bicitra, Alka-Seltzer Effervescent) are preferred (56-58). Nonparticulate antacids are recommended over particulate antacids (e.g., magnesium trisilicate) because aspiration of a particulate antacid may cause pulmonary shunting and hypoxemia similar in magnitude to that caused by acid aspiration and greater than that caused by saline (59).

H_2 BLOCKING AGENTS

By blocking histamine receptors on the oxyntic cell, H_2 blockers significantly decrease gastric acid production and decrease volume. Cimetidine (given in doses of 200-400 mg intravenously, intramuscularly, or orally) reduces gastric acidity within 60-90 minutes. The usual regimen is 300 mg orally at bedtime and in the morning (60-63). Intramuscular and intravenous use has few advantages over oral administration unless the patient cannot take anything by mouth. Oral preparations work nearly as fast and are considerably less expensive. The regimen for ranitidine is 150 mg orally at bedtime and in the morning. It is equally effective (64-68).

Omeprazole inhibits the hydrogen ion pump on the gastric surface of the oxyntic cell (69). The decrease in gastric acid production depends not on blood levels of the drug but on the binding of omeprazole to the hydrogen ion pump. Recently, some investigators have evaluated the prophylactic administration of omeprazole before cesarean section (69-74). A two-dose regimen that includes oral administration of 40 mg at bedtime and on the morning of surgery consistently decreases gastric pH (70). Orr et al (73) concluded that a combination of omeprazole and metoclopramide is most effective in reducing both gastric acidity and gastric volume before elective cesarean section.

METOCLOPRAMIDE

This agent is a procainamide derivative that is a cholinergic agonist peripherally and a dopamine receptor antagonist centrally. A 10-mg intravenous dose of metoclopramide increases lower esophageal sphincter tone and reduces gastric volume by increasing gastric peristalsis. Metoclopramide can have a significant effect on gastric volume in as little as 15 minutes (75-77).

HEAD-UP POSITION

For patients subject to passive regurgitation of stomach contents, the head-up position decreases the incidence of actual regurgitation and thereby decreases the risk of pulmonary aspiration. Some clinicians argue in favor of the head-down position, claiming that it decreases the likelihood of pulmonary aspiration if the oropharynx fills with stomach contents. However, the head-up position decreases the likelihood of regurgitation itself.

RAPID-SEQUENCE INDUCTION

If the anesthesiologist feels confident that endotracheal intubation will not present a problem, a rapid-sequence induction is indicated in patients considered at risk for aspiration. During general anesthesia, the most dangerous time in terms of aspiration of gastric contents is the period from loss of consciousness to tracheal intubation with a cuffed endotracheal tube. A rapid-sequence induction permits completion of this process in the shortest possible time. The rapid-sequence induction is not itself without danger and risk. Failure to intubate the trachea once unconsciousness and paralysis are accomplished can result in hypoxia, asphyxia, aspiration, or all three. Results of a survey describing events surrounding 21 cases of aspiration revealed that 14 of 21 cases occurred during the process of a difficult intubation. In one instance, 7 attempts had been made and in another instance 4 attempts had been made (12). As indicated above, the incidence of difficult intubation is 0.04% in all patients and 0.35% in obstetric patients (13).

CRICOID PRESSURE (SELLICK'S MANEUVER)

Sellick's maneuver is the simplest and most effective measure for minimizing the risk of aspiration (78). However, the person applying cricoid pressure must know how to do so properly. Pressure is applied at the cricoid cartilage, not the thyroid cartilage or over the entire larynx. Pressure applied to the thyroid cartilage makes the intubation process more difficult, whereas pressure applied to the cricoid cartilage makes endotracheal intubation easier. Some prefer to place one hand behind the patient's neck while applying pressure at the cricoid cartilage. In addition to ensuring proper placement of pressure, the attendant must not release the pressure until the intubation is complete, the cuff inflated, and correct placement ensured. Although it is not effective 100% of the time, when applied properly, cricoid pressure should prevent nearly all cases of aspiration. The maneuver will withstand an esophageal pressure of at least 100 cm H_2O (78). Thus it should prevent aspiration of gastric contents after either regurgitation or vomiting. Some have suggested that cricoid pressure should be released when vomiting occurs to prevent rupturing of the esophagus (79). Such a consequence is mostly theoretical. Recently, Sellick (80) advocated that cricoid pressure not be released in these instances. When a trachea cannot be intubated and positive-pressure ventilation is required to prevent hypoxia, it is imperative that cricoid pressure be continued until the trachea is successfully intubated.

ENDOTRACHEAL INTUBATION

Intubation of the trachea should be utilized in all patients at risk for aspiration—and obstetric patients are in the at-risk category. If a difficult intubation is anticipated, the process should be accomplished before the administration of anesthesia. Although an awake intubation may be uncomfortable, the morbidity associated with aspiration is considerably more uncomfortable. Further, utilizing appropriate techniques, the process does not have to be brutal.

AWAKE EXTUBATION

When an awake intubation or a rapid-sequence induction is indicated to prevent aspiration, an awake extubation is also indicated. An awake extubation means that the patient is conscious—that is, awake, aware, and responding appropriately to commands. Gagging, coughing, bucking, and indiscriminately reaching for the endotracheal tube are not necessarily signs of consciousness; rather, they may be signs of stage 2 anesthesia, the excitement stage. If the endotracheal tube is removed during this stage, the patient may continue to be vulnerable to aspiration, as well as laryngospasm.

TREATMENT

A thorough discussion of the treatment of aspiration is beyond the scope of this chapter. However, a few points need to be made. First, if a patient is hypoxic, and if aspiration is even suspected, some form of treatment should be instituted. The mainstay of treatment for most patients with aspiration will be mechanical ventilation with positive end-expiratory pressure. Although most patients will require endotracheal intubation, some may be able to be managed with the application of CPAP via a mask. That decision will be determined by the physicians at the bedside. The amount of positive pressure, positive and expiratory pressure, and percentage of oxygen will also be determined at the bedside.

Although pulmonary lavage has been recommended by some as routine treatment for pulmonary aspiration, this technique can decrease pulmonary compliance and PaO_2, and increase intrapulmonary shunting. Because aspirated acidic material reaches the periphery of the lung within 12-18 seconds (81), lavage with bicarbonate solution is not helpful.

Corticosteroids were first recommended for treatment of patients with acid aspiration in 1961 and 1962 (82,83). Since that time, several studies of both animals and humans indicate that corticosteroid therapy may provide some modification of the inflammatory response early after aspiration but does not alter the course of the disease (84-86). They may, however, interfere with normal healing mechanisms (87). For these reasons, corticosteroids are not usually given.

Prophylactic antibiotics have been recommended by some investigators for patients who have suffered pulmonary aspiration of stomach contents (83). However, they should not be used, because they may alter the normal flora of the respiratory tract and thus may render the patient susceptible to secondary infection with more resistant organisms (88). Antibiotics should be reserved for those patients who show signs of clinical pulmonary infection, in which case the antibiotic most effective for the suspected offending organism, identified by Gram stains and cultures, should be used.

Recent animal reports suggest that instilling a surfactant replacement solution into the trachea after acid aspiration may improve pulmonary function (89). At this time, however, such therapy is probably still experimental.

SUMMARY

Aspiration continues to be a serious threat to pregnant patients undergoing general anesthesia. If proper techniques and preventive measures are used, most cases can be prevented or the consequences ameliorated. Because aspiration of partially digested food causes the most severe physiologic and histologic derangements, patients should not eat once labor has begun.

REFERENCES

1. Olsson GL, Hallen B, Hambracus-Jonzon K: Aspiration during anaesthesia: A computer-aided study of 185,358 anaesthetics. Acta Anaesthesiol Scand 30:84-92, 1986
2. Warner MA, Warner ME, Weber JG: Clinical significance of pulmonary aspiration during the perioperative period. Anesthesiology 78:56, 1993
3. Mendelson CL: The aspiration of stomach contents into the lungs during obstetric anesthesia. Am J Obstet Gynecol 52:191, 1946
4. Arms RA, Dines DE, Tinstman TC: Aspiration pneumonia. Chest 65:136, 1974
5. Awe WC, Fletcher WS, Jacob SW: The pathophysiology of aspiration pneumonitis. Surgery 60:232, 1966
6. Cameron JL, Mitchell WH, Zuidema GD: Aspiration pneumonia: Clinical outcome following documented aspiration. Arch Surg 106:49, 1973
7. Dines DE, Titus JL, Sessler AD: Aspiration pneumonitis. Mayo Clin Proc 45:347, 1970
8. Cameron JL, Caldini P, Toung J-K et al: Aspiration pneumonia: Physiologic data following experimental aspiration. Surgery 72:238, 1972
9. LeFrock JL, Clark TS, Davies B et al: Aspiration pneumonia: A ten-year review. Am Surg 45:305, 1979
10. Landay MJ, Christensen EE, Bynum LJ: Pulmonary manifestations of acute aspiration of gastric contents. AJR 131:587, 1978
11. Wynne JW, Hood CI: Hypoxemia in the first hour after aspiration. Chest 78:546, 1980 (abstract)
12. Gibbs CP, Rolbin SH, Norman P: Cause and prevention of maternal aspiration (letter to the editor). Anesthesiology 61:111, 1984
13. Samsoon GLT, Young JRB: Difficult tracheal intubation: A retrospective study. Anaesthesia 42:487, 1987
14. Spence AA, Mori DD, Finlay WEI: Observations on intragastric pressure. Anaesthesia 22:249, 1967

15. Brock-Utne JG, Dow TGB, Dimopoulos GE et al: Gastric and lower oesophageal sphincter (LOS) pressures in early pregnancy. Br J Anaesth 53:381, 1981

16. Attia RR, Ebeid AM, Fischer JE et al: Maternal, fetal and placental gastrin concentrations. Anaesthesia 37:18, 1982

17. Christofides ND, Ghatei MA, Bloom SR et al: Decreased plasma motilin concentrations in pregnancy. Br Med J 285:1453, 1982

18. Davison JS, Davison MC, Hay DM: Gastric emptying time in late pregnancy and labour. Br J Obstet Gynaecol 77:37, 1970

19. Holdsworth JD: Relationship between stomach contents and analgesia in labour. Br J Anaesth 50:1145, 1978

20. Simpson KH, Stakes AF, Miller M: Pregnancy delays paracetamol absorption and gastric emptying in patients undergoing surgery. Br J Anaesth 60:24, 1988

21. Greenan J: The cardio-oesophageal junction. Br J Anaesth 33:432, 1961

22. Williams NH: Variable significance of heartburn. Am J Obstet Gynecol 42:814, 1941

23. Brock-Utne JG, Dow TGB, Dimopoulos GE et al: The effect of metoclopramide on the lower oesophageal sphincter in late pregnancy. Anaesth Intensive Care 6:26, 1978

24. Dow TGB, Brock-Utne JG, Rubin J et al: The effect of atropine on the lower esophageal sphincter in late pregnancy. Obstet Gynecol 51:426, 1978

25. Lind JF, Smith AM, McIver DK et al: Heartburn in pregnancy—a manometric study. Can Med Assoc J 98:571, 1968

26. Roberts RB, Shirley MA: Reducing the risk of acid aspiration during cesarean section. Anesth Analg 53:859, 1974

27. Teabeaut JR II: Aspiration of gastric contents. An experimental study. Am J Pathol 28:51, 1952

28. Awe WC, Fletcher WS, Jacob SW: The pathophysiology of aspiration pneumonitis. Surgery 60:232, 1966

29. James CF, Modell JH, Gibbs CP et al: Pulmonary aspiration: Effects of volume and pH in the rat. Anesth Analg 63:665, 1984

30. Plourde G, Hardy JF: Aspiration pneumonia: Assessing the risk of regurgitation in the cat. Can Anaesth Soc J 33:345, 1986

31. Raidoo DM, Marszalek A, Brock-Utne JG: Acid aspiration in primates. (A surprising experimental result.) Anaesth Intensive Care 16:375, 1988

32. Kennedy TP, Johnson KJ, Kunkel RG: Acute acid aspiration lung injury in the rat: Biphasic pathogenesis. Anesth Analg 69:87, 1989

33. Hamelberg W, Bosomworth PP: Aspiration pneumonitis: Experimental studies and clinical observations. Anesth Analg 43:669, 1964

34. Jones JG, Grossman RF, Berry M et al: Alveolar capillary membrane permeability—correlation with functional, radiographic and postmortem changes after fluid aspiration. Am Rev Respir Dis 120:399, 1979

35. Schwartz DJ, Wynne JW, Gibbs CP et al: The pulmonary consequences of aspiration of gastric contents at pH values greater than 2.5. Am Rev Respir Dis 121:119, 1980

36. Wynne JW, Hood CI: Hypoxemia in the first hour after aspiration. Chest 78:546, 1980 (abstract)

37. McKay S, Mahan C: How can aspiration of vomitus in obstetrics best be prevented? Birth 15:222-235, 1988

38. Elkington KW: At the water's edge: Where obstetrics and anesthesia meet. Obstet Gynecol 77:304-308, 1991

39. Michael S, Reilly CS, Caunt JA: Policies for oral intake during labour: A survey of maternity units in England and Wales. Anaesthesia 46:1071-1073, 1991

40. Chestnut DH, Cohen SE: At the water's edge: Where obstetrics and anesthesia meet (letter in reply). Obstet Gynecol 77:965-967, 1991

41. Agarwal A, Chari P, Singh H: Fluid deprivation before operation: The effect of a small drink. Anaesthesia 44:632-634, 1989

42. Goodwin AP, Rowe WL, Ogg TW et al: Oral fluids prior to day surgery: The effect of shortening the preoperative fluid fast on postoperative morbidity. Anaesthesia 46:1066-1068, 1991

43. Hutchinson A, Maltby JR, Reid CR: Gastric fluid volume and pH in elective inpatients. I. Coffee or orange juice versus overnight fast. Can J Anaesth 35:12-15, 1988

44. Maltby JR, Sutherland AD, Sale JP et al Preoperative oral fluids: Is a five-hour fast justified prior to elective surgery? Anesth Analg 65:1112-1116, 1986

45. Miller M, Wishart HY, Nimmo WS: Gastric contents at induction of anaesthesia: Is a 4-hour fast necessary? Br J Anaesth 55:1185-1188, 1983

46. Scarr M, Maltby JR, Jani K et al: Volume and acidity of residual gastric fluid after oral fluid ingestion before elective ambulatory surgery. Can Med Assoc J 141:1151-1154, 1989

47. Strunin L: How long should patients fast before surgery? Time for new guidelines (editorial). Br J Anaesth 70:1-3, 1993

48. Schreiner MS, Triebwasser A, Keon TP: Ingestion of liquids compared with preoperative fasting in pediatric outpatients. Anesthesiology 72:593-597, 1990

49. Splinter WM, Schaefer JD: Ingestion of clear fluids is safe for adolescents up to 3 h before anaesthesia. Br J Anaesth 66:45-52, 1991

50. Splinter WM, Schaefer JD: Unlimited clear fluid ingestion two hours before surgery in children does not affect volume or pH of stomach contents. Anaesth Intensive Care 18:522-526, 1990

51. Van der Walt JH, Carter JA: The effect of different pre-operative feeding regimens on plasma glucose and gastric volume and pH in infancy. Anaes Intensive Care 14:352-359, 1986

52. Van der Walt JH, Foate JA, Murrell D et al: A study of preoperative fasting in infants aged less than three months. Anaesth Intensive Care 18:527-531, 1990

53. Freeman RK, Poland RL, eds: Guidelines for perinatal care, 3rd edition. American Academy of Pediatrics and American College of Obstetricians and Gynecologists, 76:1992

54. Guyton TS, Gibbs CP: Ice chip consumption during labor. Unpublished data, 1993

55. Hinder RA, Kelly KA: Canine gastric emptying of solids and liquids. Am J Physiol 233:335, 1977

56. Gibbs CP, Spohr L, Schmidt D: The effectiveness of sodium citrate as an antacid. Anesthesiology 57:44-46, 1982

57. Viegas OJ, Ravindran RS, Shumacker CA: Gastric fluid pH in patients receiving sodium citrate. Anesth Analg 60:521-523, 1981

58. Chen CT, Toung TJ, Haupt HM et al: Evaluation of the efficacy of Alka-Seltzer Effervescent in gastric acid neutralization. Anesth Analg 63:325-329, 1984

59. Gibbs CP, Schwartz DJ, Wynne JW et al: Antacid pulmonary aspiration in the dog. Anesthesiology 51:380-385, 1979

60. Coombs DW, Hooper D, Colton T: Acid-aspiration prophylaxis by use of preoperative oral administration of cimetidine. Anesthesiology 51:352-356, 1979

61. Johnston JR, McCaughey W, Moore J et al: Cimetidine as an oral antacid before elective caesarean section. Anaesthesia 37:26-32, 1982

62. Manchikanti L, Kraus JW, Edds SP: Cimetidine and related drugs in anesthesia. Anesth Analg 61:595-608, 1982

63. Williams JG, Strunin L: Pre-operative intramuscular ranitidine and cimetidine: Double blind comparative trial, effect on gastric pH and volume. Anaesthesia 40:242-245, 1985

64. Dammann HG, Muller P, Simon B: Parenteral ranitidine: Onset and duration of action. Br J Anaesth 54:1235-1236, 1982

65. Francis RN, Kwik RS: Oral ranitidine for prophylaxis against Mendelson's syndrome. Anesth Analg 61:130-132, 1982

66. Maile CJ, Francis RN: Pre-operative ranitidine: effect of a single intravenous dose on pH and volume of gastric aspirate. Anaesthesia 38:324-326, 1983

67. Brock-Utne JG, Downing JW, Humphrey D: Effect of ranitidine given before atropine sulphate on lower oesophageal sphincter tone. Anaesth Intensive Care 12:140-142, 1984

68. Rout CC, Rock DA, Gouws E: Intravenous ranitidine reduces the risk of acid aspiration of gastric contents at emergency cesarean section. Anesth Analg 76:156-161, 1993

69. Massoomi F, Savage J, Destache CJ: Omeprazole: A comprehensive review. Pharmacotherapy 13:46-59, 1993

70. Yau G, Kan AF, Gin T et al: A comparison of omeprazole and ranitidine for prophylaxis against aspiration pneumonitis in emergency caesarean section. Anaesthesia 47:101-104, 1992

71. Moore J, Flynn RJ, Sampaio M et al: Effect of single-dose omeprazole on intragastric acidity and volume during obstetric anaesthesia. Anaesthesia 44:559-562, 1989

72. Ching MS, Morgan DJ, Mihaly GW et al: Placental transfer of omeprazole in maternal and fetal sheep. Dev Pharmacol Ther 9:323-331, 1986

73. Orr DA, Bill KM, Gillon KR et al: Effects of omeprazole, with and without metoclopramide, in elective obstetric anaesthesia. Anaesthesia 48:114-119, 1993

74. Ewart MC, Yau G, Gin T et al: A comparison of the effects of omeprazole and ranitidine on gastric secretion in women undergoing elective caesarean section. Anaesthesia 45:527-530, 1990

75. Wyner J, Cohen SE: Gastric volume in early pregnancy: Effect of metoclopramide. Anesthesiology 57:209-212, 1982

76. Olsson GL, Hallen B. Pharmacological evacuation of the stomach with metoclopramide. Acta Anaesthesiol Scand 26:417-420, 1982

77. Brock-Utne JG, Dow TG, Welman S et al: The effect of metoclopramide on the lower oesophageal sphincter in late pregnancy. Anaesth Intensive Care 6:26-29, 1978

78. Sellick BA: Cricoid pressure to control regurgitation of stomach contents during induction of anesthesia. Lancet 2:404, 1961

79. Notcutt WG: Rupture of the oesophagus following cricoid pressure? Anaesthesia 36:911, 1981

80. Sellick BA: Rupture of the oesophagus following cricoid pressure? Anaesthesia 37:213, 1982

81. Hamelberg W, Bosomworth PP: Aspiration pneumonitis: Experimental studies and clinical observations. Anesth Analg 43:669, 1964

82. Bannister WK, Sattilaro AJ, Otis RD: Therapeutic aspects of aspiration pneumonitis in experimental animals. Anesthesiology 22:440, 1961

83. Bannister WK, Sattilaro AJ: Vomiting and aspiration during anesthesia. Anesthesiology 23:251, 1962

84. Downs JB, Chapman RL Jr., Modell JH et al: An evaluation of steroid therapy in aspiration pneumonitis. Anesthesiology 40:129, 1974

85. Chapman RL Jr., Downs JB, Modell JH et al: The ineffectiveness of steroid therapy in treating aspiration of hydrochloric acid. Arch Surg 108:858, 1974

86. Chapman RL Jr., Modell JH, Ruiz BC et al: Effect of continuous positive-pressure ventilation and steroids on aspiration of hydrochloric acid (pH 1.8) in dogs. Anesth Analg 53:556, 1974

87. Wynne JW, Reynolds JC, Hood CI et al: Steroid therapy for pneumonitis induced in rabbits by aspiration of foodstuff. Anesthesiology 51:11, 1979

88. Wynne JW, Modell JH: Respiratory aspiration of stomach contents. Ann Intern Med 87:466, 1977

89. Eijking EP, Gommers D, Vergear M et al: Surfactant treatment of respiratory failure induced by hydrochloric acid aspiration in rats. Anesthesiology 78:1145, 1993

COMBINED SPINAL-EPIDURAL ANESTHESIA (CSE)
FOR LABOR AND DELIVERY

D. J. Birnbach

Combined spinal-epidural anesthesia (CSE) was first described by Brownridge in 1981 (1) as a method that could be used to provide anesthesia for cesarean sections when an alternative to "one-shot" spinal or epidural anesthesia was necessary. This technique allowed for renewability of an epidural while allowing the fast onset and dense block of a spinal. In the past 2 years, particularly due to the introduction and increased availability of atraumatic spinal needles (such as the Sprotte, Whitacre, and Gertie Marx needles), this technique has become more popular as a method of providing analgesia and anesthesia for the parturient.

HISTORY OF CSE

The first report of CSE (1) described placing an epidural catheter at one interspace and subsequently initiating a spinal anesthetic at a second interspace. This technique provided the fast onset and optimum operative conditions associated with a one-shot spinal but also offered the flexibility of an epidural catheter for extending the duration of the block and providing postoperative analgesia. The disadvantage of this technique was that it necessitated two separate anesthetics at two different interspaces.

The evolution of CSE has been in the direction of a sequential technique, accomplished via a needle-through-needle technique. Responding to Brownridge's initial report, Coates described his experience using a needle-through-needle technique (2). This single-level approach offered less patient discomfort and less trauma than the two-level approach. In addition, the needle-through-needle approach had the theoretical advantage of decreased morbidity, since one skin penetration is performed instead of two. Figure 1 demonstrates the needle-through-needle approach.

T.H. Stanley and P.G. Schafer (eds.), Pediatric and Obstetrical Anesthesia, 151-157.

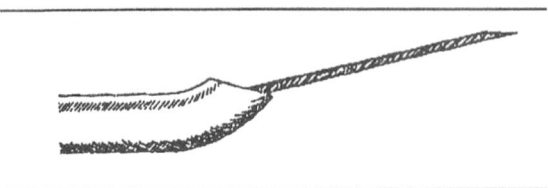

Figure 1. The needle-through-needle technique (2).

A potential hazard of CSE, which many authors addressed early on, was the possibility of passage of the epidural catheter through the newly made hole in the dura. Even without subarachnoid migration of the catheter, there was concern that medications given epidurally could leak through the dural hole and produce subarachnoid effects. In an effort to decrease the risk of the catheter being threaded through the dural hole, several investigators have suggested that the epidural needle be rotated 180 degrees after spinal injection and prior to the placement of the epidural catheter (3,4). Other authors, however, do not agree with the practice of rotating the epidural needle, due to recent evidence that rotation of epidural needles places the patient at a higher risk of dural perforation (5). Clinically, the subarachnoid passage of the epidural catheter has not been found to be a problem; most series looking at CSE have not seen subarachnoid migration. Even without modification of technique, it is unlikely that the 20-gauge epidural catheter will freely thread through the dural puncture made with a 24-26g spinal needle. A test of 3 cc of lidocaine 1.5% should rule out subarachnoid placement of the catheter but will not guarantee proper epidural placement and function of the epidural catheter.

DESCRIPTION OF CSE

An epidural anesthetic is initiated in the usual manner, using a standard or modified epidural needle. When the epidural space is reached, a long (optimally 12-15 mm longer than the epidural needle), atraumatic spinal needle is introduced through the epidural needle. The spinal needle is advanced until the classic pop of dural penetration is felt and its proper position within the subarachnoid space is verified by the appearance of CSF. After injection of the spinal drug (which will vary depending on the clinical setting—cesarean section vs. labor analgesia), the spinal needle is gently removed and an epidural catheter introduced.

A newer, and perhaps improved, method of preventing inadvertent subarachnoid penetration by the catheter has been made possible by the design of a new generation of epidural needles. These needles (such as the Braun "Espocan" pictured in Figure 2) allow the spinal needle to pass in a straight line through a back eye of the epidural needle while the epidural catheter, which is too large to enter the back eye, follows the curved path of the modified Tuohy needle. In a recent study, Joshi and colleagues evaluated two different techniques for combined spinal epidural and concluded that an improved needle set would include a modified Tuohy needle with an aperture at the back and a spinal needle protruding more than 13 mm beyond the Tuohy needle (6).

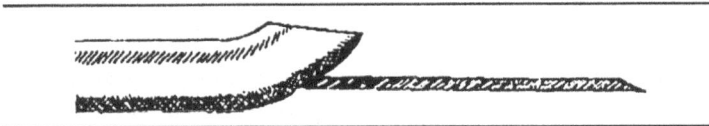

Figure 2. The Braun "Espocan."

Another recent advance in CSE technology is the E-SP® needle (Neurodelivery technology, Lebanon, NH), which allows the anesthesiologist to, first, place the epidural catheter and then, after the epidural catheter placement has been verified, perform the spinal. Although the needle is cumbersome, it does have the advantage of allowing placement of the epidural first (see Figure 3).

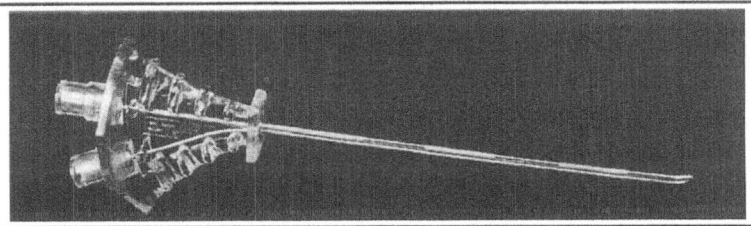

Figure 3. The E-SP® needle.

CSE FOR CESAREAN SECTION

CSE for cesarean delivery offers all the benefits of spinal anesthesia (fast onset, solid block) along with the benefits of epidural anesthesia (catheter allows extending the time of the block, should surgery be prolonged). It is most useful when there is a possibility of a longer duration of surgery, such as in the patient with an abnormal placenta or a repeat cesarean section. The catheter can also be used for postoperative pain management.

Although the procedure can be done in many different positions, I prefer to initiate the CSE for cesarean section with the patient in the right lateral position. Then, after completion of the procedure (at which time there may be a predominantly right-sided block), the patient can be turned to the left lateral position using a right wedge, thus achieving a bilateral block. Using this patient position, even when teaching residents who have not previously performed CSE, we have had no failures. The alternative position, with the patient sitting during placement of the epidural, may prove problematic if the procedure is done slowly because the block may begin to set. This problem is not insurmountable, however, since the catheter can be used to extend the level to the T4 interspace.

Although CSE has been used for patients with morbid obesity, as well as patients with "difficult airways," a modification of the standard CSE technique should be considered in such patients, so that the catheter can be tested for proper placement at time of insertion. The time to discover that the epidural catheter is not functioning is not just as the obstetrician is screaming, "Stat section," nor is it during a long cesarean section in the patient with a difficult airway! In cases where a "difficult airway" exists, if CSE is going to be used, it may be prudent to give a lesser dose of spinal medication and to use the epidural catheter to bring up the level to T4. In this way, the epidural catheter has been tested prior to the start of surgery.

Thoren and colleagues (7) have recently reported on a comparison of sequential spinal/epidural block versus spinal block for cesarean section. They found that both spinal and CSE block provided good surgical analgesia for cesarean section. Although maternal hypotension was a risk in both groups, it occurred earlier in the spinal group. These authors further found that there was no difference in neonatal outcome between spinal and CSE groups, provided that maternal hypotension is promptly treated.

CSE FOR LABOR

CSE can be safely used to provide analgesia in any patient who is to receive an epidural. There are, however, some patients who will greatly benefit from this technique. This group includes patients in very early, or very late, labor. The beauty of CSE for early labor is that the patient can be made comfortable with spinal narcotics (sufentanil or fentanyl), which will last for approximately 2-3 hours, during which time the patient will not have a motor block and can actually ambulate. By the time the spinal narcotic wears off, the patient is usually in the active phase of labor, when many obstetricians feel more comfortable with the use of epidural analgesia. The advantage of CSE over a one-shot spinal injection of narcotic for labor is that the epidural catheter is in place. In the event of a cesarean section, a level can be achieved quickly, thus decreasing the likelihood of general anesthesia. The spinal opioid will produce profound pain relief within minutes, and in the event that the labor continues for more than 2 hours (the approximate duration of spinal narcotics), the catheter can be used to administer local anesthetic solution. Recently, CSE has been described as a method of providing labor analgesia; this allows patients to ambulate and has been termed the "walking epidural" (8).

DRUGS USED IN CSE FOR LABOR

The following drugs can be used to produce labor analgesia using CSE (9-12):

1. Sufentanil 10 µg
2. Fentanyl 10-25 µg
3. Morphine 0.2 mg
4. Morphine 0.25 mg plus fentanyl 25 µg
5. Meperidine 10-20 mg

Recently, Camann et al (13) described the use of sufentanil plus bupivacaine for parturients who are in advanced stages of labor. They found that the addition of dilute bupivacaine to the spinal sufentanil produced prolonged duration of analgesia and achievement of a higher sensory level.

Although the administration of subarachnoid morphine provides the longest period of analgesia, it also provides the longest duration of side effects. Many clinicians believe that the risk of producing 24 hours of nausea, pruritus, and respiratory depression outweigh the advantage of prolonged analgesia, especially since in many cases the labor will not last long enough to warrant the longer-lasting analgesia afforded by morphine.

POTENTIAL SIDE EFFECTS OF INTRATHECAL OPIOIDS FOR LABOR

1. Pruritus
2. Nausea/vomiting

3. Hypotension
4. Urinary retention

POTENTIAL PROBLEMS OF CSE

1. Inability to locate the spinal space after placing the epidural needle in the epidural space.
   There are 3 possible explanations for this:
   - Spinal needle is not long enough. Advancing the epidural needle will resolve this.
   - Epidural needle is off midline and spinal needle is therefore missing dura.
   - The epidural needle is not where you think it is!
2. Inadequate analgesia
   This may occur when the drug is not injected into the spinal space, for example, as occurs when the spinal needle is moved during injection. The solution to this problem is to use the epidural catheter to supplement the level.
3. Postdural puncture headache
   The risks of PDPH may be decreased by the use of atraumatic spinal needles.
4. Migration of the epidural catheter into the spinal space
   The risk of accidental subarachnoid migration of the epidural catheter after CSE can be minimized either by turning the epidural needle 180 degrees after injection of the spinal, or by using an epidural needle with a "back hole." Onset of a solid motor block after administration of an epidural test dose through the catheter should alert the anesthesiologist to a subarachnoid catheter.
5. Cauda equina syndrome
   Cases of cauda equina syndrome have been generally reported as occurring after use of a spinal microcatheter. There have been no reported cases of cauda equina syndrome occurring after the use of CSE. Since almost all cases occurred after the use of hyperbaric 5% lidocaine, to decrease the risk 1 cauda equina syndrome (if the catheter is subarachnoid), the anesthesiologist can either use a different drug (bupivacaine or isobaric 2% lidocaine) or dilute the 5% lidocaine.

REFERENCES

1. Brownridge P: Epidural and subarachnoid analgesia for elective caesarean section. Anaesthesia 36:70, 1981
2. Coates MB: Combined subarachnoid and epidural techniques. Anaesthesia 37:89-90, 1982
3. Rawal N: Single segment combined subarachnoid and epidural block for caesarean section. Can J Anaesth 33:254-255, 1986
4. Hughes JA, Oldroyd GJ: A technique to avoid dural puncture by the epidural catheter. Anaesthesia 46:802, 1991
5. Meiklejohn BH: The effect of rotation of an epidural needle. Anaesthesia 2:1180-1182, 1984
6. Joshi GP, McCarroll SM: Evaluation of combined spinal-epidural anesthesia using two different techniques. Reg Anesth 19:169-174, 1994
7. Thoren T, Holmstrom B, Rawal N et al: Sequential combined spinal epidural block versus spinal block for cesarean section: Effects on maternal hypotension and neurobehavioral function of the newborn. Anesth Analg 78:1087-1092, 1994
8. Collis RE, Baxandall ML, Srikantharajah ID et al: Combined spinal epidural analgesia with ability to walk throughout labour. Lancet 341:767-768, 1993
9. Zakowski MI, Goldstein MJ, Ramanathan S et al: Intrathecal fentanyl for labor analgesia. Anesthesiology 75:A840, 1991
10. Honet JE, Arkoosh VA, Norris MC et al: Comparison among intrathecal fentanyl, meperidine and sufentanil for labor analgesia. Anesth Analg 75:734-739, 1992
11. Leighton BL, DeSimone CA, Norris MC et al: Intrathecal narcotics for labor revisited: The combination of fentanyl and morphine intrathecally provides rapid onset of profound, prolonged analgesia. Anesth Analg 69:122-125, 1989
12. Swayze CR, Sholte FG, Walker EB et al: Efficacy of intrathecal meperidine for labor analgesia. Anesth Analg 72:287, 1991
13. Campbell DC, Camann WR, Datta S: Combined spinal-epidural for labor analgesia: Comparison of intrathecal sufentanil vs. bupivicaine vs. sufentanil plus bupivicaine. Abstracts of the Society for Obstetric Anesthesia and Perinatology Annual Meeting. Vol 41. 1994

RESUSCITATION OF THE NEWBORN

G. W. Ostheimer

Birth is a time of physiologic stress and change for the fetus. Usually, the asphyxial stress of birth is mild-to-moderate, and the neonate is able to compensate for it. When the neonate's compensatory ability is decreased or the asphyxial stress is excessive, resuscitative intervention is necessary to assist in the conversion from fetal to neonatal physiology.

Who should assume responsibility for resuscitation of the depressed neonate? Guideline VII of the American Society of Anesthesiologists (ASA) *Guidelines for Regional Anesthesia in Obstetrics* states: "Qualified personnel, other than the anesthesiologist attending the mother, should be immediately available to assume responsibility for resuscitation of the newborn." (The primary responsibility of the anesthesiologist is to provide care to the mother. If the anesthesiologist is also requested to provide brief assistance in the care of the newborn, the benefit to the child must be compared to the risk to the mother).

The first minutes of life may determine the quality of that life. The need for a prompt, organized, and skilled response to immediate neonatal emergencies requires written policies delineating responsibility for immediate newborn care, resuscitation, selection and maintenance of necessary equipment, and training of personnel in proper techniques.

ROUTINE CARE

The delivery physician or nurse-midwife is responsible for providing immediate postdelivery care of the newborn, and for ascertaining that the newborn adaptations to extrauterine life are proceeding normally, unless the care has been transferred. The hospital rules and regulations should include protocols for the transfer of medical care of the neonate in both routine and emergency circumstances. Routine care of the healthy newborn may be

159

T.H. Stanley and P.G. Schafer (eds.), Pediatric and Obstetrical Anesthesia, 159-186.
© 1995 *Kluwer Academic Publishers.*

delegated to appropriately trained nurses, or transferred to a family physician or pediatrician.

Information to be transmitted to the physician caring for the infant after delivery includes both the infant's and the mother's names and medical record numbers; the mother's blood type, serology result, rubella status, hepatitis B screen result, diabetes screen, exposure to group B streptococci, and record of substance abuse; and the presence of fetal anomalies.

At least one person skilled in initiating resuscitation should be present at every delivery. The skills and responsibilities of that individual should be defined at the institutional level.

RESUSCITATION

Recognition and immediate resuscitation of a distressed neonate requires an organized plan of action and the immediate availability of qualified personnel and equipment, as described in the American Academy of Pediatrics and the American Heart Association *Textbook of Neonatal Resuscitation*. Responsibility for identification and resuscitation of a distressed neonate should be assigned to a qualified individual, who may be a physician or an appropriately trained nurse-midwife, Labor and Delivery nurse, nurse-anesthetist, nursery nurse, or respiratory therapist. The provision of services and equipment for resuscitation should be planned jointly by the directors of the departments of obstetrics, anesthesia, and pediatrics, with the approval of the medical staff. A physician should be designated to assume primary responsibility for initiating, supervising, and reviewing the plan for management of depressed neonates in the delivery room. The following factors should be considered in this plan:

1. A list of maternal and fetal complications that require presence in the delivery room of someone specifically qualified in all aspects of newborn resuscitation should be developed.

2. Individuals qualified to perform neonatal resuscitation should demonstrate the following capabilities:

   - Skills in rapid and accurate evaluation of the newborn condition, including Apgar scoring.
   - Knowledge of the pathogenesis and causes of a low Apgar score (e.g., hypoxia, drugs, hypovolemia, trauma,

anomalies, infections, and prematurity), as well as specific indications for resuscitation.

- Skills in airway management (e.g., laryngoscopy, endotracheal intubation, suctioning of the airway), artificial ventilation, cardiac massage, emergency administration of drugs and fluids, and maintenance of thermal stability. The ability to recognize and decompress tension pneumothorax by needle aspiration is also a desirable skill.

3. Procedures should be developed to ensure the readiness of equipment and personnel, and to provide for intermittent review and evaluation of the system's effectiveness.

4. Contingency plans should be established for multiple births and other unusual circumstances.

5. A physician for the neonate need not be present at a delivery, provided that no complications are anticipated and another skilled individual is present to care for the neonate.

6. The resuscitation steps should be documented in the records (1).

However, it would seem that these guidelines are not necessarily followed. Gibbs et al (2) found that in small units in the Unites States, with less than 500 deliveries per year, personnel other than an anesthesiologist, nurse-anesthetist, pediatrician, or obstetrician perform neonatal resuscitation after vaginal delivery almost 50% of the time and, for cesarean delivery, 25% of the time.

CARDIOVASCULAR PHYSIOLOGY (FETUS TO NEONATE)

The fetal circulation operates in parallel, in contrast to the adult circulation, which operates in series (3,4). In the fetus, oxygenated blood returns from the placenta via the umbilical vein, largely passing the liver through the ductus venosus. Owing to a streaming effect, this blood is preferentially shunted from the right atrium through the foramen ovale to the left atrium and via the left ventricle into the systemic circulation. This streaming of ductus venosus blood to the left side of the circulation enhances the oxygen content of the blood, perfusing the organs of highest oxygen consumption—the heart and the brain.

Desaturated blood returns from the upper part of the body via the superior vena cava and streams into the right ventricle. Right ventricular output encounters high pulmonary vascular resistance due to arteriolar vasoconstriction. About 90% of the right-sided output passes through the ductus arteriosus and enters the aorta distal to the branches of the aortic arch; thus, less well oxygenated blood perfuses the lower body, which has a lower oxygen consumption (Figure 1).

At birth, two primary events initiate the conversion from fetal to adult circulatory patterns (5). First, cessation of the umbilical artery flow (by clamping the cord or exposing the cord to air) increases systemic vascular resistance and aortic pressure, and the clamping of the umbilical vein decreases venous return and right atrial pressure. This effects a decrease in the right-to-left shunts, both at the foramen ovale from the right atrium to the left and the ductus arteriosus from the pulmonary artery to the aorta. Second, the expansion of the lungs at birth stimulates pulmonary vasodilation, with resulting falls in pulmonary vascular resistance and pulmonary arterial pressure, which helps to reduce further the right-to-left flow through the patent ductus arteriosus. Pulmonary blood flow increases, oxygenation improves, and left atrial pressure rises, further decreasing the shunt across the foramen ovale (Figures 2,3).

The hallmarks of conversion to adult circulation are a rise in systemic arterial pressure, accomplished mainly by cord clamping, and a rise in pulmonary blood flow, accomplished by filling the lungs with air. Therefore, the major effect of resuscitation is usually to assist the neonate with the initiation of ventilation. More severely depressed neonates may require additional forms of intervention.

The adult circulatory pattern is established rapidly in the normal, healthy neonate. However, for the first 2 weeks of life (longer in the premature neonate), the circulation can revert to the fetal pattern when the neonate is subjected to certain stresses such as hypoxemia, acidosis, hypercarbia, hypovolemia, shock, and hypothermia (5).

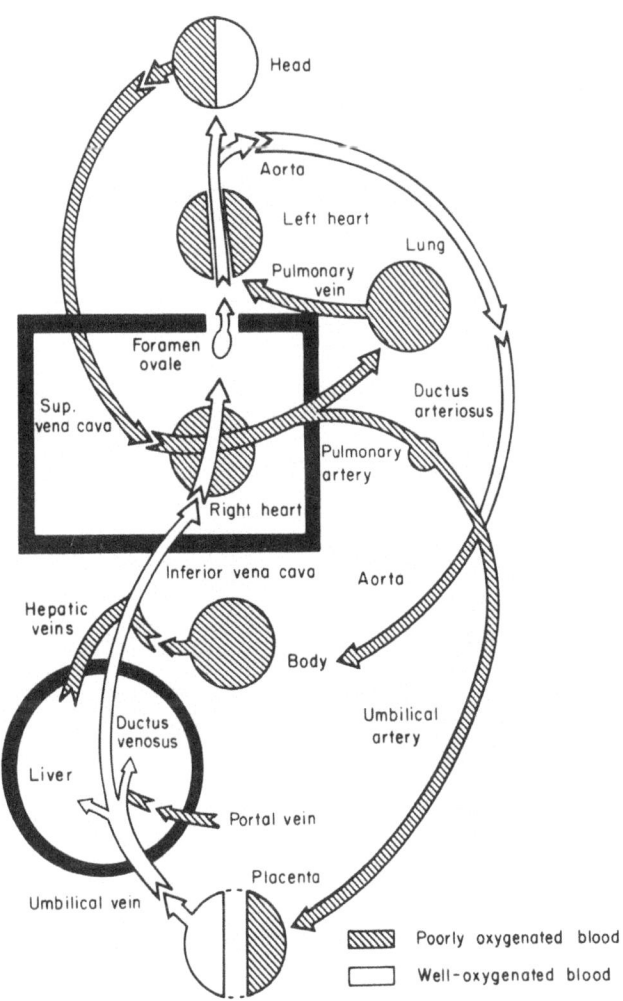

Figure 1. Fetal circulation. Modified from Ostheimer, with permission (29).

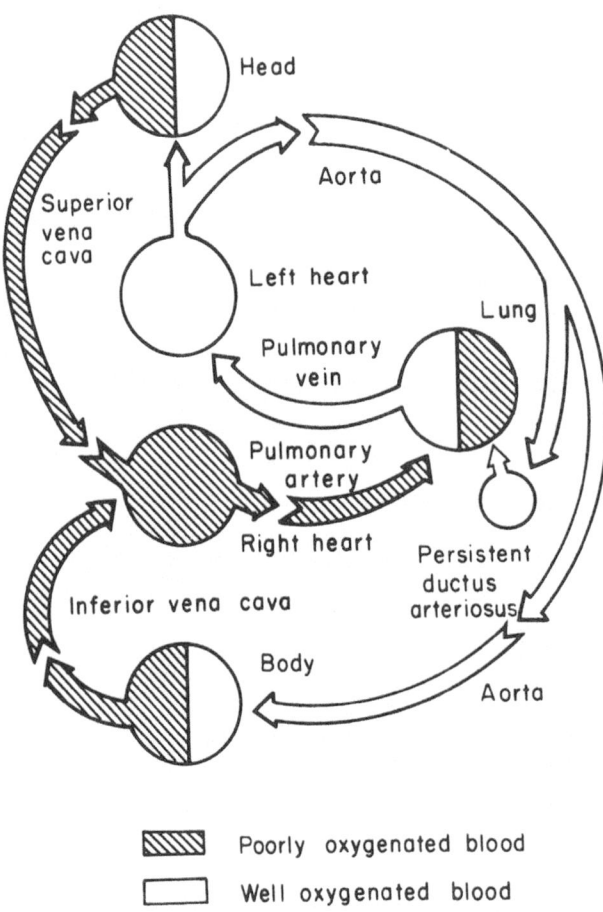

Figure 2.   Postdelivery circulation: intermediate phase. Modified from Ostheimer, with permission (29).

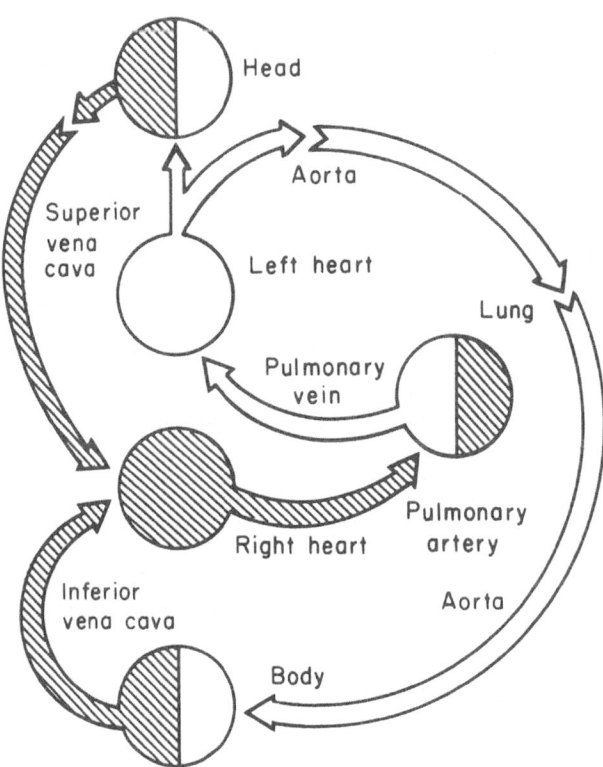

Figure 3.   Normal circulation: final phase. Modified from Ostheimer, with permission (29).

RESPIRATORY SYSTEM

The fetal lung develops by a budding process from the foregut at approximately 24 days of gestation. By 20 weeks, the airways are lined with epithelium, and pulmonary capillaries are developing in the mesenchyme. By 26-28 weeks, the capillaries are close to the developing airways so that oxygen and carbon dioxide exchange can occur, making extrauterine life possible. Surfactant-like material is present in the airway epithelium between 22 and 24 weeks but is not present on the alveolar surface until 26-28 weeks. Steroids administered to the mother facilitate the development of the epithelial cells lining the alveoli and the production of surfactant. The onset of fetal breathing is stimulated by stress (usually hypoxia), and amniotic fluid can be drawn into the lung, as can be demonstrated by meconium aspiration in the stillborn (6,7).

Normal neonates will begin spontaneous respirations within 30-60 seconds. Stimuli to breathe include rebound of the thoracic cage after vaginal birth, mild-to-moderate hypoxia, cord clamping, a cold environment, and tactile stimulation. (Note: only gentle stimulation is needed. Vigorous spanking, cold and hot water baths, and other excessive stimulation have no therapeutic value and may be harmful). The volume of the first breath is 20-75 ml. Subsequent tidal volume is 15-20 ml. When rhythmic breathing is established and the lungs are fully expanded, the normal respiratory rate is 30-40 breaths/min. In the first few hours of life, during the resorption of residual lung fluid, respiratory rates may be as high as 60-90 breaths/min. Central cyanosis should clear by 5 minutes after birth. Some peripheral cyanosis may persist because of peripheral vasoconstriction. During vaginal delivery, the baby's chest is compressed with a pressure of 30-250 cmH$_2$O (8). This "squeeze" expresses much of the fluid from the lungs, but the lungs remain collapsed and are not aerated. In order to expand the lungs against the collapsing forces of alveolar tension and elastic pulmonary recoil, the neonate exerts 40-80 cmH$_2$O negative pressure (9,10). The resuscitator may, therefore, need to use higher than normal pressures when assisting with the initiation of ventilation, as long as the potential for pneumothorax is kept in mind (Figure 4). The neonate will respond to a large rapid inflation of its lungs with a sharp inspiration of its own (Head's paradoxical reflex).

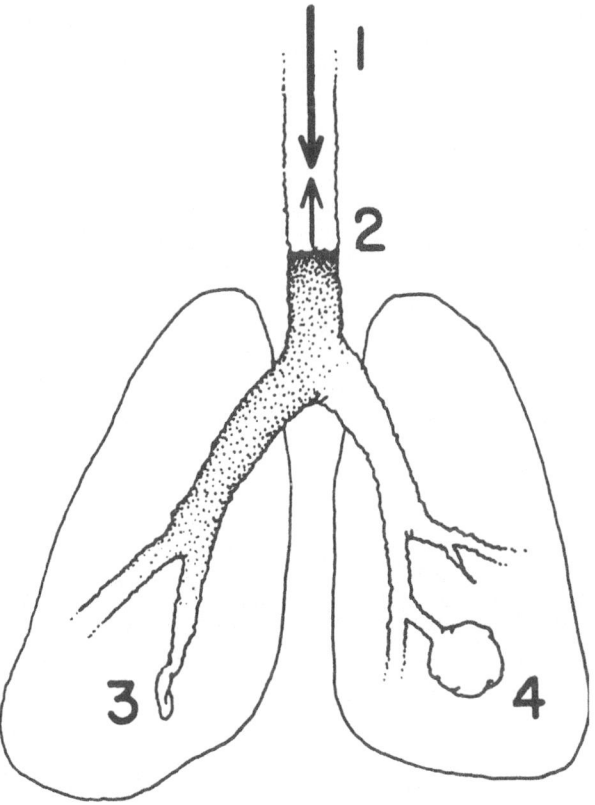

Figure 4.   The lung immediately after delivery. Expansion of the collapsed lung requires higher pressures than those needed to move air into the lung (1) once aerated. Several forces must be overcome; outward flow of fluid in the trachea and bronchi (2); surface tension of the collapsed alveoli (3); and elastic forces of the lung (4). Modified from Ostheimer, with permission (30).

CARDIOVASCULAR SYSTEM

The heart rate may vary from 100 to 200 beats per minute (bpm) during the first 30 minutes of life but should stabilize at 120 ± 20 bpm thereafter. Normal blood pressure varies with birthweight, as shown in Table 1 (11). A systolic pressure less than 50 mmHg in a term neonate is abnormally low and should be treated promptly with intravascular volume expansion. Normal intravascular volume is 85-100 ml/kg in the newborn.

Table 1. Normal neonatal blood pressure (11).

Birthweight (kg)	Pressure (mmHg)	
	Systolic	Diastolic
<1.0	40-60	15-35
1.0-2.0	50-65	20-40
2.0-3.0	50-70	25-45
>3.0	50-80	30-50

THERMOREGULATION

Humans are homeothermic, that is, we increase our heat production to maintain body temperature when exposed to a cold environment. Poikilotherms, such as reptiles, cannot increase their heat production, and their body temperature drifts to that of the environment. There are two methods of increasing heat production: a physical method of muscle contraction (shivering), used by children and adults, and a chemical method used by neonates called nonshivering thermogenesis (Figure 5). When neonates are cold stressed, they increase their oxygen consumption and metabolic activity. Large amounts of norepinephrine are released (in contrast to epinephrine in adults), which activates an adipose tissue lipase to break down brown fat (so called because of its rich vascular supply) into triglycerides and nonesterified fatty acids (NEFAs). The NEFAs may pass out of the cell, are oxidized to carbon dioxide and water in the cell—which is an exothermic (heat-producing) reaction—or are re-esterified with glycerol to form triglycerides. Adipose tissue is not able to phosphorylate the glycerol derived

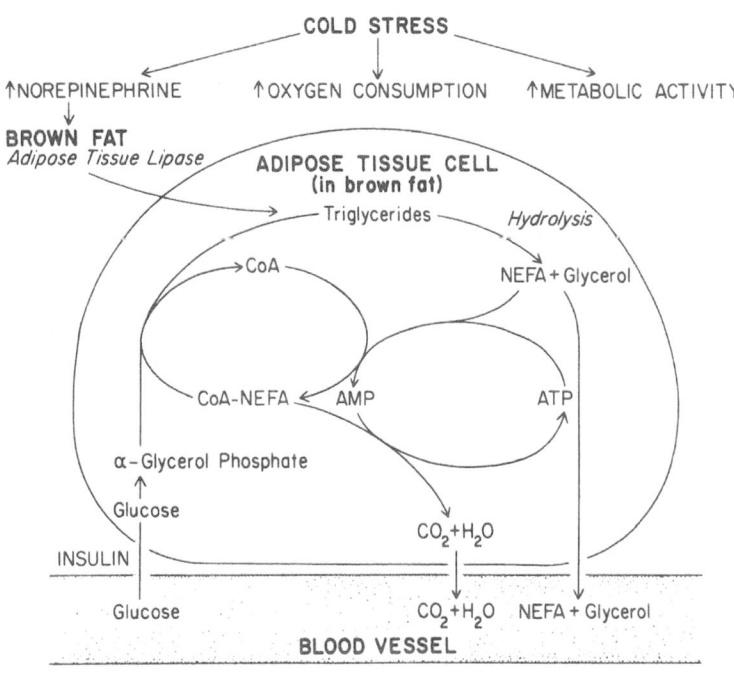

Figure 5. Nonshivering thermogenesis. Modified from Ostheimer, with permission (30).

from the triglycerides; therefore, re-esterification via the coenzyme A-NEFA complex requires a supply of α-glycerol phosphate derived from the glucose that comes from outside the cell. Resynthesis of triglycerides is also an exothermic reaction because of the utilization of adenosine triphosphate (ATP) in the formation of the coenzyme A-NEFA complex.

Nonshivering thermogenesis occurs mainly in the brown fat of the neonate, which is found in an interscapular mass (the "hibernating gland"), muscles and blood vessels entering the thoracic inlet, and the abdominal viscera, especially around the kidneys and adrenal glands. The venous drainage from the interscapular adipose tissue joins the drainage from the muscles of the back to form the external vertebral plexus, which drains to the rich venous plexus around the spinal cord, which in turn enters the jugular

170

or azygous veins, depending on the level, thus supplying heat to the spinal cord and the heart (Figure 6).

We must strive to maintain a neutral thermal environment (32-34°C for neonates), at which metabolism (as reflected by oxygen consumption) is minimal yet sufficient to maintain body temperature. Minimal oxygen consumption occurs when the difference between skin and environmental temperature is less than 1.5°C. The infant, born into the cold environment of the delivery room, suffers an enormous heat loss, initially by evaporation, since the neonate is wet from amniotic fluid and has a large surface area. Once the skin is dried, heat is lost mainly by radiation. Dahm and James (12)

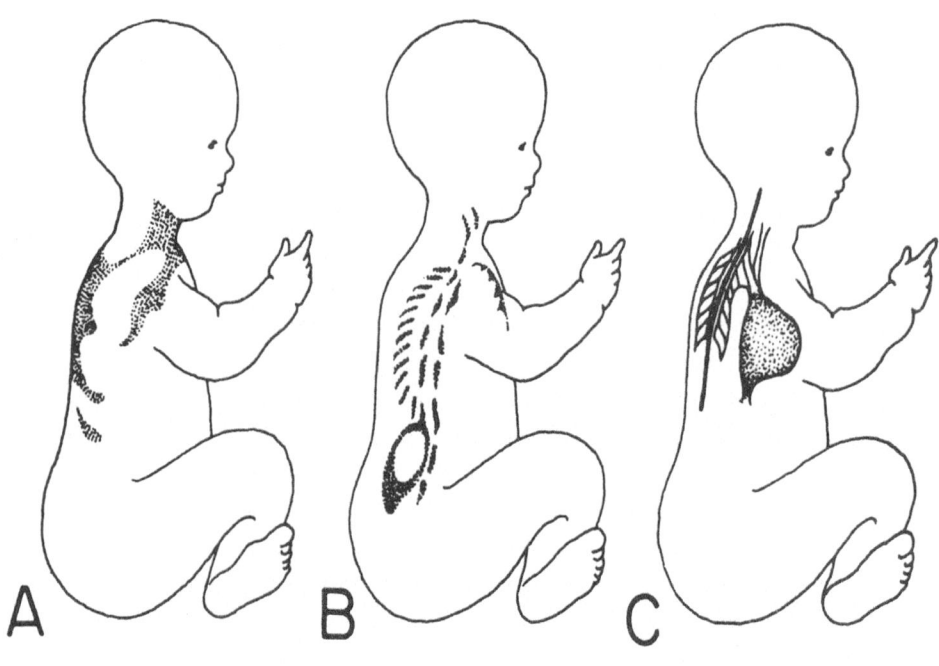

Figure 6. (A&B) Sites of brown fat. (C) Route of venous drainage.

investigated heat loss in the first 30 minutes after delivery and found that wet infants exposed to room air lost nearly 5 times more heat than those who were dried and warmed.

In vigorous infants, promptly drying the skin and wrapping the baby in a warm blanket is almost as effective in decreasing heat loss as placing the baby under a radiant heater. However, in depressed or immature infants who may be asphyxiated or have reduced energy stores, an overhead radiant heater maintains body temperature while allowing access to the patient during resuscitation.

ROUTINE DELIVERY ROOM CARE OF THE NORMAL NEONATE

The following measures are all that is necessary in 85-90% of deliveries:
1. Aspiration of the mouth and nose by bulb syringe
2. Drying the skin and maintaining normal newborn temperature
3. Routine identification procedures
4. Ophthalmic prophylaxis (required by law in most states).

In the remainder, in whom neonatal depression has occurred, further measures will be necessary.

PRINCIPLES OF NEONATAL RESUSCITATION

The principles of newborn resuscitation are the same as those for adult resuscitation:
1. Airway management
2. Breathing
3. Circulation or adequate cardiac output to maintain cerebral oxygenation.

After birth of the baby's head, the oropharynx is suctioned with a bulb syringe before the baby's first breath and while the chest is still compressed in the vaginal canal (vaginal squeeze) to prevent aspiration of mucus and debris into the trachea with the onset of respiration (Figure 7). The baby is then delivered; the umbilical cord is clamped and cut, and the newborn is transferred by the obstetrician to a warmed bassinet that has been placed in a 20-30 degree head-down position to facilitate the gravity drainage of liquid material into the oropharynx. A slight lateral tilt of the newborn concentrates

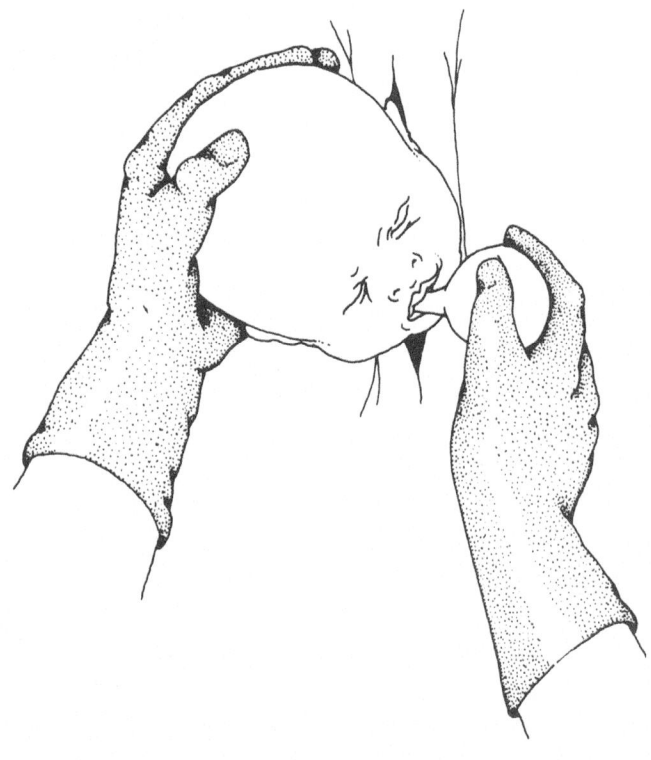

Figure 7.   Pharyngeal suction with the baby's head on the perineum. Modified from
Ostheimer, with permission (30).

the pooling of secretions into one corner of the oropharynx. Management of
the airway is accomplished by gentle suction with a bulb syringe, if possible—
not a plastic or rubber suction catheter. Cordero and Hon (13) investigated the
effect of nasopharyngeal or oropharyngeal stimulation on heart rate and
respiration. In 41 infants who received repeated nasopharyngeal suction with
a bulb syringe, no decrease in heart rate or respiration was noted. However,
in 46 neonates who were suctioned blindly with a catheter through the nose
or mouth, 7 developed severe cardiac arrhythmias and 5 became apneic.

These undesirable responses resulted from stimulation of afferent vagal fibers in the posterior pharynx of already highly vagotonic newborns.

Gentle slapping of the feet is all the stimulation needed for the healthy newborn. Spanking, cold-water showers, jack-knifing, "milking" the trachea, dilation of the anaphincter, alternating hot and cold baths, bed rocking, and excessive rubbing of the back are all condemned as having no therapeutic value and being potentially harmful.

RESUSCITATION EQUIPMENT

Every delivery area should have the following equipment readily available for the resuscitation of the newborn:

1. A source of 100% oxygen.
2. A bag and mask for intermittent positive-pressure ventilation (IPPV). A flow-through system that does not require positive pressure for oxygen delivery should be used, since most neonates will not need positive-pressure ventilation, just oxygen therapy.
3. A bulb syringe for suctioning the nose and oropharynx.
4. A DeLee suction catheter with mucus trap for aspiration of mucus, meconium, blood, and other secretions or stomach contents.
5. Laryngoscopes with size 0 and 1 straight blades.
6. Endotracheal tubes (Cole orotracheal tubes or straight endotracheal tubes with stylets in place in sizes 1.5 mm, 2.0 mm, 2.5 mm, 3.0 mm and 3.5 mm). The Cole tubes are more rigid and do not require a stylet. If the neonate requires long-term ventilation, the oral tube should be changed to a straight nasotracheal tube when the infant's condition is stable.
7. Oral airways, size 00 and 0, are rarely needed but should be available.
8. A radiant heater with servomechanisms.

A neonatal "code cart" should also be available and should contain equipment for vascular access, blood sampling, and intravenous infusion, as well as drugs commonly employed in resuscitation, and charts showing typical doses and dilutions.

With the increasing concern about body fluid being contaminated with hepatitis or human immunodeficiency virus (HIV), personnel participating in newborn resuscitation are using one of several devices that allows

Table 2. The Apgar Scoring System.

Evaluation	Sign	Stimulus	Score		
			0	1	2
appearance	color	visual assessment	blue, pale	body pink, extremities blue	completely pink
pulse	heart rate	count cord pulse or auscultate heart	absent	< 100 bpm	> 100 bpm
grimace	reflex irritability	flick sole of foot	no response	some motion	cry
activity	muscle tone	manipulate extremity	limp flaccid	some flexion of extremities	well-flexed
respiration	respiratory effort	visual assessment	absent	slow, irregular hypoventilation	good strong cry

aspiration of fluids from the mouth, trachea, and stomach of the newborn by vacuum suction (>80 cmH2O). This approach should eliminate the possibility of inhaling contaminants through a mask or gauze covering while aspirating via the endotracheal tube or DeLee suction apparatus.

EVALUATION AND TREATMENT OF THE DEPRESSED NEONATE

APGAR SCORING

It is easy to recognize the vigorous, healthy, normal neonate and the severely depressed neonate needing immediate cardiopulmonary resuscitation. Between these two extremes lie varying degrees of neonatal depression. While the Apgar scoring system was not meant to be used as a guide to resuscitators, it has proven useful as a means of quantifying the degree of depression (Table 2). The 1-minute score (14) is used here as a guide to the intervention required. However, resuscitation should not be delayed awaiting the 1-minute Apgar score. A follow-up score is determined at 5 minutes of life and will indicate the progress of the neonate. Additionally, 10-, 15-, and 20-minute scores may be assigned to document the response of the neonate to resuscitation efforts.

VIGOROUS, CRYING INFANT (APGAR SCORE 7-10)

No therapy is necessary beyond the routine measures mentioned above.

MODERATE DEPRESSION (APGAR 4-6)

1. Administer 100% oxygen by mask (Figure 8).
2. Stimulate by slapping the feet or drying the skin with a soft cloth towel or blanket.
3. If the heart rate is below 100 bpm and/or respirations are inadequate, begin IPPV by bag and mask, and continue it as long as necessary.
4. Monitor the heart rate and spontaneous respiratory efforts. If these deteriorate or fail to improve, treat as a severely depressed neonate.

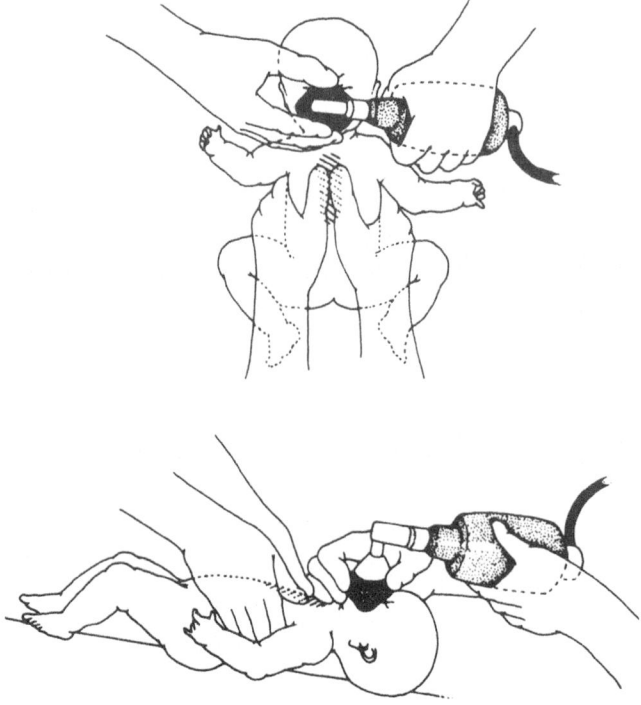

Figure 8.   Technique of ventilation and closed-chest cardiac massage. Modified from
Ostheimer, with permission (30).

SEVERE DEPRESSION (APGAR SCORE 0-3)

1. Administer 100% oxygen by bag and mask as soon as possible.
    2. If there is no response (increased heart rate, respiratory effort) within a few minutes, perform laryngoscopy, suction the oropharynx and/or trachea, and intubate the trachea to facilitate ventilation (Figure 9).
    3. Initiate closed-chest cardiac massage (CCCM) if the heart rate remains below 100 bpm. Place both thumbs over the mid- to lower third of the sternum and the fingers behind the chest.

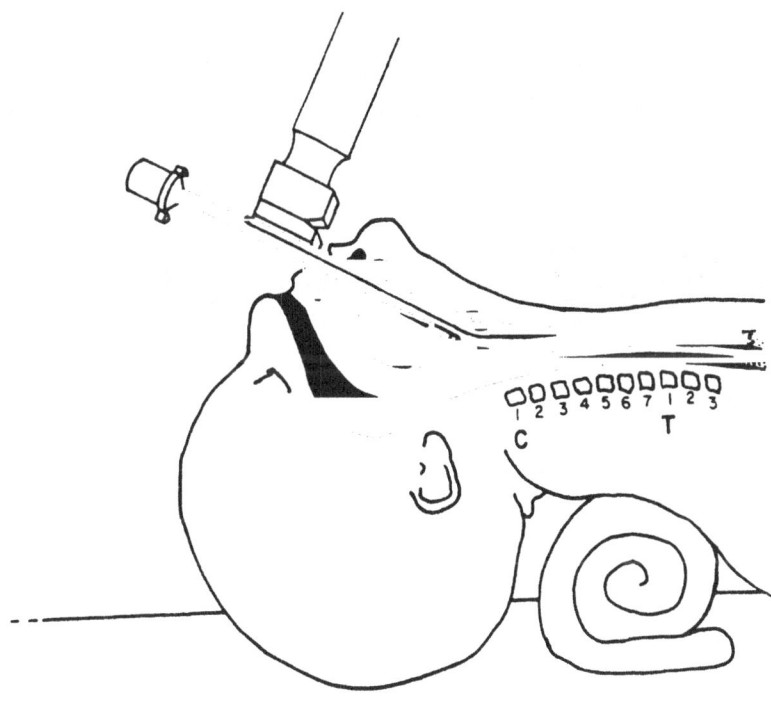

Figure 9. Laryngoscopy and endotracheal intubation with a Cole tube.

Compress the chest at a rate of 120 bpm, depress the sternum two-thirds of the way to the vertebral column (Figure 8).

4. Monitor the adequacy of cardiopulmonary resuscitation. With proper intubation and ventilation, the chest should expand and breath sounds should be heard in both axillae (Figure 10). Auscultate over the abdomen to rule out esophageal intubation. If ventilation and/or intubation are difficult, repositioning of the head may be necessary. Because of the relatively large head of the neonate, as well as the edema fluid (caput) that collects over the occiput during labor, the neck may be flexed enough to compress the trachea when the baby is supine. Placing a small roll under the baby's shoulders will alleviate this problem by extending the neck (Figure 11). However, excessive hyperextension may also compress the soft trachea of the neonate.

5. Gastric aspiration should not be done in the first few minutes of life, in order to avoid causing any arrhythmias from nasopharyngeal or oropharyngeal stimulation—unless there is massive gastric dilatation secondary to IPPV with the bag and mask or a tracheoesophageal fistula is suspected. Cordero and Hon (13) suggest that after 5 minutes of age, the neonate has become physiologically more stable and will tolerate passage of a nasogastric tube.

CONTINUED MODERATE-TO-SEVERE DEPRESSION

The newborn who fails to respond to adequate ventilation with oxygen and circulatory support with CCCM will require further therapy.

PHARMACOLOGIC INTERVENTION

Drugs commonly used in neonatal resuscitation are administered through an umbilical artery or vein catheter, although epinephrine can be given intratracheally if vascular access has not yet been established. A 5 or 8 French catheter can be threaded into the umbilical artery, although intense vasoconstriction of the artery may necessitate use of the umbilical vein in the immediate resuscitative period. In the latter case, the catheter should be threaded no more than 2 cm into the vein to avoid cannulation of a major hepatic vessel.

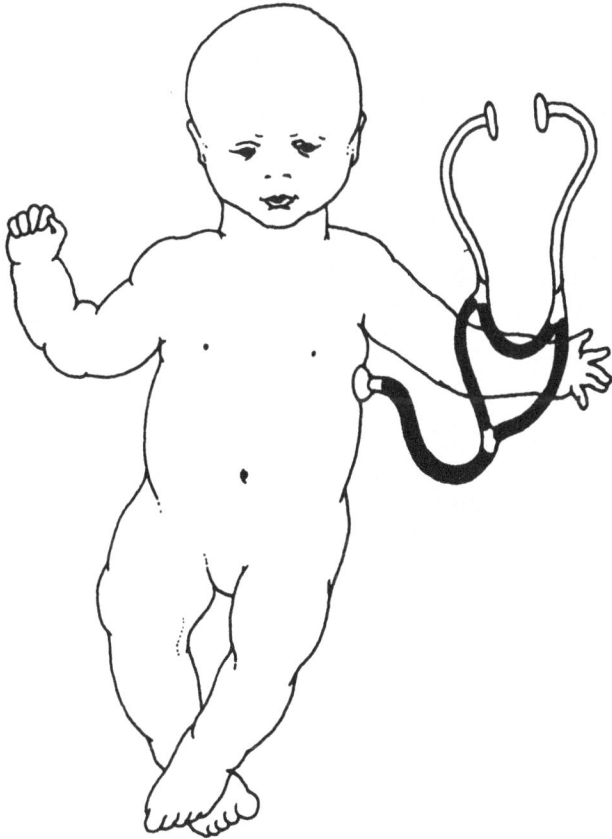

Figure 10.   Evaluation of ventilation by auscultation. Modified from Ostheimer, with permission (30).

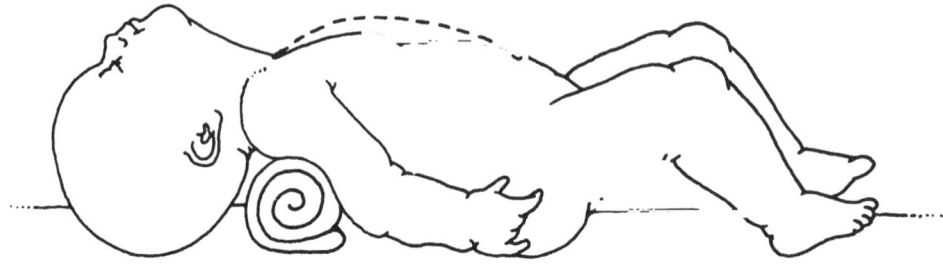

Figure 11. Moderate hyperextension to relieve soft tissue obstruction. Modified from
Ostheimer, with permission (30).

DRUGS USED IN PHARMACOLOGIC RESUSCITATION

SODIUM BICARBONATE (1-2 MEQ/KG)

The neonate suffering from severe birth asphyxia and not responding
well to oxygen and ventilator support probably has a respiratory and
metabolic acidosis. The initial dose of sodium bicarbonate will improve the
acidosis, but further doses should be administered only as indicated by the
infant's pH. A sample of blood (arterial or venous) should be drawn for blood
gas analysis upon insertion of the umbilical artery or vein catheter.
Ventilation must be adequate to reverse the respiratory component of the
acidosis.

Bicarbonate therapy has several potential complications (17-20). It is a
hyperosmolar solution, and its rapid administration in the acidotic and
hypoxic newborn can lead to profound vasodilation and hypotension due to
skeletal muscle vasodilation and venous pooling. Because of its lower
osmolarity, a 0.22 mmol/ml solution is preferred to the 0.45 mmol/ml
solution. It should be given in an intravenous infusion (5-10% dextrose or
0.45% saline) so that the solution can serve as a diluent to decrease the bolus

effect of the sodium bicarbonate. Excessive sodium bicarbonate therapy has been shown to cause hypernatremia, which has been implicated in intracerebral hemorrhage in the sick neonate (20). However, appropriate doses, guided by the infant's pH, appear to be safe in this regard.

DEXTROSE (2 G/KG IV, PUSH, THEN 5-8 MG/KG/MIN)

Severely asphyxiated infants are often hypoglycemic because of their increased catecholamine levels, with initial elevation of glucose and stimulation of insulin secretion in the presence of decreased glycogen reserves and immature gluconeogenetic pathways (5). Neonates born to diabetic mothers are at risk of hypoglycemia, with fetal islet cell hyperplasia and elevated insulin secretion. Those neonates who are small for gestational age or have suffered from uteroplacental insufficiency may also develop hypoglycemia because of depleted glycogen stores. Hypoglycemia in these infants may be of later onset, and they will require longer monitoring of blood glucose levels.

EPINEPHRINE (ADRENALINE) (0.01-0.1 MG/KG)

The hypotensive, bradycardic infant who is still acidotic may require this high dose of epinephrine for cardiac stimulation. In the nonacidotic infant, the usual dose of epinephrine is 0.01 mg/kg.

NALOXONE (0.1 MG/KG IV OR 0.2 MG/KG IM)

Naloxone is used to reverse opioid-related depression only. If the mother has received opioids, the neonate may require naloxone. If this is so, the neonate should be observed for at least 4 hours after naloxone administration for evidence of narcotic depression recurrence.

If the mother has received general anesthesia for delivery, the anesthetic can have a depressant effect on the newborn. Usually, all the baby needs is oxygen, stimulation, and time to "wake up." Naloxone is not necessary in this setting, unless the mother has received opioids as part of the anesthetic.

Other drugs may be needed in prolonged resuscitation. The indications for, and methods of, their use are not discussed here in the context of the acute resuscitative effort, and their use is the prerogative of the attending pediatrician.

SPECIFIC NEONATAL PROBLEMS

MECONIUM STAINING

Passage of meconium by the fetus is thought to occur in response to hypoxic stress in the ante- or peripartum period (21). Meconium staining is present in 8-15% of all pregnancies, with a higher incidence occurring in the post-term pregnancy. Over half of infants born through meconium-stained fluid will have meconium in their tracheas and, if left untreated, many will develop meconium aspiration syndrome (22-24). Since the treatment for meconium aspiration syndrome is only supportive and symptomatic, efforts have been concentrated on the prevention of the syndrome through effective airway suctioning at birth (23-25). Immediately after the delivery of the infant's head, while the chest is still in the birth canal, the oropharynx and nasopharynx should be suctioned thoroughly by the obstetrician, using a bulb syringe or a DeLee apparatus. Immediately after delivery and, if possible, before the infant has taken his/her first breath, laryngoscopy and tracheal suctioning should be performed by the most experienced resuscitator present, regardless of the presence or absence of meconium in the oropharynx and nasopharynx, since the obstetrician may have already completely cleared the upper airways of meconium. Tracheal suctioning should be repeated until no further meconium can be aspirated. An assistant should monitor the baby's heart rate during suctioning, since pharyngeal stimulation can cause bradycardia and other arrhythmias through vagal reflexes (13). If the heart rate slows substantially, oxygen by mask or by clean tracheal tube should be given, with assisted ventilation if necessary. Infants who have aspirated meconium should receive chest physical therapy and postural drainage with suctioning, and should be monitored closely for the occurrence of respiratory distress. This sequence of immediate, thorough pharyngeal and tracheal suctioning has been found to be safe, and its implementation has greatly reduced the incidence and severity of meconium aspiration syndrome and its subsequent mortality (23,24).

How often has the obstetric anesthesiologist heard that if there is thin meconium present in the airway at delivery it is not necessary to aspirate the trachea of the newborn? Chen et al (26) demonstrated that even small amounts of meconium in aspirated amniotic fluid can result in inactivation of surface active material from the alveolar lining of the lungs. Therefore, it behooves us to be very aggressive in the management of the neonate with meconium in the amniotic fluid. However, the occurrence of in utero meconium aspiration is still a devastating problem. If we could eliminate this potentially disastrous occurrence during the later stages of pregnancy or during labor, we would virtually eliminate the meconium aspiration syndrome.

NEONATAL SHOCK

Serious hypovolemia with secondary hypoperfusion and tissue hypoxia can occur as a result of numerous factors. Sequestration of blood in the placenta because of elevation of the infant above the mother at the time of cord clamping, prolapsed umbilical cord, abruptio placentae, placenta previa, and rupture of the umbilical cord can significantly decrease the neonate's circulating blood volume. Low-birthweight infants may have decreased total protein concentrations, with a resultant shift of fluid out of the intravascular space because of low intravascular oncotic pressure. Also, maternal sepsis transmitted to the fetus may present as neonatal shock.

A decreasing blood pressure, tachycardia, pallor, decreased urine output, decreasing hematocrit, and metabolic acidemia all indicate that volume expansion may be needed. The preferred therapy is 20 ml/kg of fresh, uncontaminated heparinized fetal whole blood obtained from the placenta, which may be difficult to obtain. If this is unavailable, fresh whole adult blood or packed red blood cells and fresh-frozen plasma in the same quantity may be used. Five percent albumin (1 g/kg) can also serve as a volume expander. Finally, if no blood products are available, lactated Ringer's solution or 0.45% normal saline may be used. The neonate's blood pressure, pulse, respiration, and temperature should be monitored carefully to detect any deterioration before such a change becomes a crisis.

Constant monitoring of the hypotensive neonate is vital to proper management. Management of the infant's blood pressure should become a routine part of the physiologic evaluation at birth if a problem exists, and all infants should have a screening blood pressure measured on admission to the nursery (Figure 12). The neonate is "recovering" from the asphyxia of

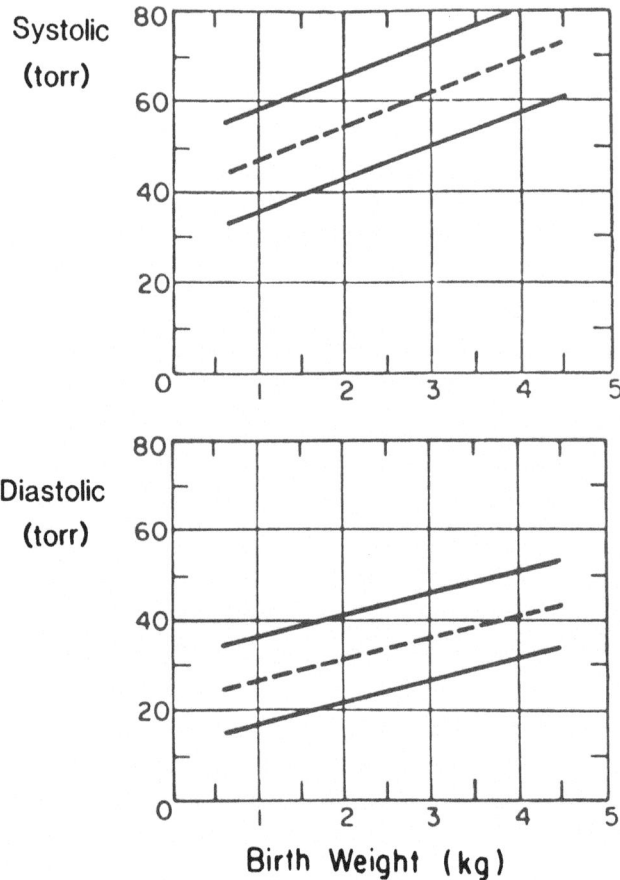

Figure 12. Neonatal systolic and diastolic aortic blood pressure. From Versmold et al, with permission.

delivery and should have the same evaluation as a patient "recovering" from anesthesia and surgery.

SUMMARY

The simple mnemonic ABCDE summarizes the 5 key principles of neonatal resuscitation:
1. Airway
2. Breathing
3. Circulation
4. Drugs
5. Evaluation of concurrent and causative problems and maintenance of a neutral thermal environment.

REFERENCES

1. Freeman RK, Poland RL: Guidelines for perinatal care. 3rd edition. American Academy of Pediatrics and the American College of Obstetricians and Gynecologists, Elk Grove Village, Illinois, 1992
2. Gibbs CP, Krischer J, Peckham BM et al: Obstetric anesthesia: A national survey. Anesthesiology 65:298-306, 1986
3. Behrman RE, Lees MH, Peterson EN et al: Distribution of the circulation in the normal and asphyxiated fetal primate. Am J Obstet Gynecol 108:956-959, 1970
4. Rudolph AM, Heymann MA: Fetal and neonatal circulation and respiration. Ann Rev Physiol 36:187-207, 1974
5. Bowen, FW: Resuscitation and stabilization of the neonate. In Bolognese RJ, ed. Perinatal medicine: Management of the high risk fetus and neonate. Baltimore, Williams & Wilkins, 1982, pp 445-453
6. Brown BL, Gliecher N: Intrauterine meconium aspiration. Obstet Gynecol 57:26-29, 1981
7. Turbeville DF, McCaffress MA, Block MF et al: In uterodistal pulmonary meconium aspiration. South Med J 72:535-553, 1979
8. Karlberg P: The adaptive changes in the immediate post-natal period, with particular reference to respiration. J Pediatr 56:585-586, 1960
9. Vyas H, Milner AD, Hopkin IE: Intrathoracic pressure and volume changes during the spontaneous onset of respiration in babies born by cesarean section and by vaginal delivery. J Pediatr 99:787-791, 1981
10. Milner AD, Vyas H: Lung expansion at birth. J Pediatr 101:879-886, 1972
11. Versmold HT, Ketterman JA, Phibbs RH et al: Aortic blood pressure during the first 12 hours of life in infants with birth weight 610-4220 grams. Pediatrics 67:607-613, 1981

12. Dahm LS, James LS: Newborn temperature and calculated heat loss in the delivery room. Pediatrics 49:504-513, 1972

13. Cordero L, Hon EH: Neonatal bradycardia following nasopharyngeal stimulation. J Pediatr 78:441-447, 1971

14. Apgar V: A proposal for a new method of evaluation of the newborn infant. Curr Res Anesth Analg 32:260-267, 1953

15. Todres ID, Rogers MC: Methods of external cardiac massage in the newborn infant. J Pediatr. 86:781-782, 1975

16. Fiholt DA, Kettrick RG, Wagner HR et al: The heart is under the lower third of the sternum. Am J Dis Child 140:646-649, 1986

17. Simmons MA, Adcock EW, Bard H et al: Hypernatremia and intracranial hemorrhage in neonates. New Engl J Med 291:6-10, 1974

18. Volpe J: Neonatal intracranial hemorrhage-iatrogenic etiology (editorial). New Engl J Med 291:43-45, 1974

19. Cote CJ, Greenhow DE, Marshall BE: The hypotensive response to rapid intravenous administration of hypertonic solutions in man and in the rabbit. Anesthesiology 50:30-35, 1979

20. Wheeler AS, Sadri S, Gutsche BB et al: Intracranial hemorrhage following intravenous administration of sodium bicarbonate or saline solution in the newborn lamb asphyxiated in utero. Anesthesiology 51:517-521, 1979

21. Walker J: Fetal anoxis. J Obstet Gynecol Br Cwlth 60:162-180, 1953

22. Gregory GA, Gooding CA, Phibbs RH et al: Meconium aspiration in infants: Prospective study. J Pediatr 85:848-852, 1974

23. Ting P, Brady JP: Tracheal suction in meconium aspiration. Am J Obstet Gynecol 122:767-771, 1975

24. Carson BS, Losey RW, Bowes WA et al: Combined obstetric and pediatric approach to prevent meconium aspiration syndrome. Am J Obstet Gynecol 126:712-715, 1976

25. Frantz ID, Wang NS, Thach BT: Experimental meconium aspiration: Effects of glucocorticoid treatment. J Pediatr 86:438-441, 1975

26. Chen CT, Toung TJK, Rogers MC: Effect of intra-alveolar meconium on pulmonary surface tension properties. Crit Care Med 13:233, 1983

27. Paxson CL: Collection and use of autologous fetal blood. Am J Obstet Gynecol 134:708-710, 1983

28. Golden SM, O'Brien WF, Metz SA: Anticoagulation of autologous cord blood for neonatal resuscitation. Am J Obstet Gynecol 144:103-104, 1983

29. Ostheimer GW: Resuscitating the depressed neonate. Contemp Obstet Gynecol 15:27, 1980

30. Ostheimer GW: Newborn resuscitation. Wkly Anesth Update, Princeton, NJ, 1978

NEONATAL PHYSIOLOGY OF IMPORTANCE TO THE ANESTHESIOLOGIST

F. A. Berry

Our anesthetic practice is based on, among other things, the physiology of our patient (1). At no other time in life is the physiology as rapidly changing as it is in the neonatal period, when the anesthesiologist is faced with an array of surgical problems. The neonatal period is defined as the first 30 days of life.

TRANSITION AND MATURATION

The initial changes in the physiology of the neonate are due to what is referred to as the adaptation of the fetus to an independent life. It has also been referred to as the transition of the fetus from the fetal state to the newborn, and then the neonatal state. The newborn is defined as an infant in the first 24 hours of life. None of the definitions depend on the conceptual age of the infant.

All of the body and organ systems undergo transition, as well as maturation. Maturation is referred to as the extra-uterine development of the organ systems, whereas transition is primarily a circulatory occurrence where the cardiac output to the various organ systems completely changes and the fluid-filled alveolus becomes air filled. In the fetal state, the amount of circulation to each organ—such as the lung, kidney, and liver—is appropriate to the metabolic needs of a growing and developing organ. There is little organ *function*; therefore, the metabolic demands of organ function, which are great in later life, are not present in the fetus. For that reason, a great deal of the circulation is shunted away from the lungs by the ductus arteriosus, and from the kidneys by a relatively high renal vasculature resistance. Transition occurs in hours, days, and weeks, whereas maturation is a question of weeks, months, and years. Initially they are both going on at the same time.

T.H. Stanley and P.G. Schafer (eds.), Pediatric and Obstetrical Anesthesia, 187-195.
© 1995 *Kluwer Academic Publishers.*

TRANSITION OF THE CIRCULATORY, VENTILATORY, AND RENAL SYSTEMS

This section will primarily focus on the transition of the circulation, the pulmonary system, the renal system, and the liver. The fetus is characterized by three major shunts: 1) the ductus arteriosus, an oxygen sensitive shunt that shunts relatively deoxygenated blood returning from the superior vena cava from the pulmonary artery to the descending aorta; 2) the ductus venosus, which is pressure sensitive, shunts blood through the liver into the inferior vena cava, and essentially bypasses the liver; and 3) the foramen ovale, a pressure-sensitive shunt that shunts the well oxygenated blood from the placenta, via the umbilical vein, from the right atrium to the left atrium and to the left ventricle, where it is then circulated to the brain. The period of the initiation of ventilation and the transition of the circulation occurs at the time of birth. The changes within the cardiorespiratory system work in concert but will be separated for purposes of discussion.

As the infant initiates breathing, the alveoli and the newborn blood become better oxygenated; the ductus arteriosus, which constricts with increasing levels of oxygen, closes. At the same time, as the blood vessels uncoil, the pressures in the left side of the circulation increase, while the pressures within the pulmonary system decrease. This results in the pressure of the left atrium being greater than the right and a functional closure of the foramen ovale. About 10-15% of older children and adults will be found to have at least a probe patent foramen ovale. In addition, the ductus venosus closes as the blood flow from the umbilical vein is decreased, so that the blood will go through the liver. The ductus arteriosus is normally closed by the fourth day, even in premature infants, if they do not have the respiratory distress syndrome (2). Any premature or full-term infant who is hypoxic has the potential for the ductus arteriosus to remain open, since it is oxygen sensitive.

TRANSITION OF THE PULMONARY SYSTEM

At the initiation of ventilation at birth, there is development of the normal tidal ventilation and lung volumes. This occurs because of the presence of surfactant, respiratory muscles, and the ability of the newborn to create negative intrathoracic pressures of 40-50 cm of water, which opens the alveoli and establishes the normal functional residual capacity along with normal tidal ventilation. Usually the blood gases will stabilize at about an hour of life with a PaO_2 of 65 mmHg, a $PaCO_2$ of 38 mmHg, and a pH of 7.35.

PERSISTENT PULMONARY HYPERTENSION

One of the rapidly expanding areas of knowledge is in the pathophysiology of persistent pulmonary hypertension. The causes are either chronic from intrauterine circulatory problems, or post-delivery from hypoxia and acidosis secondary to sepsis, lack of surfactant, and any other causes of hypoxia and acidosis. The pathophysiology of the fetal pulmonary blood vessels from intrauterine hypoxia is that there is an increase in the amount of muscle in the small blood vessels of the distal elements of the respiratory system (3). Therefore, any hypoxia or acidosis will cause pulmonary vasoconstriction, which will result in further hypoxia and respiratory failure. Hypoxia and acidosis occur in association with diaphragmatic hernia. However, in this situation, the major problem is that of hypoplasia of the pulmonary system. The treatment of respiratory failure is primarily through supportive care with intubation and conventional ventilation (4). High-frequency oscillation is being used with increasing frequency in infants who fail conventional ventilation (5). Nitric oxide, which causes smooth muscle relaxation within the pulmonary vascular bed, is the subject of tremendous research in the newborn with persistent pulmonary hypertension from whatever cause (6,7). Nitric oxide can be therapeutic when it relaxes the smooth muscles, which have undergone vasoconstriction. The result is improved oxygenation. It may also be used as a diagnostic tool since, if there is no improvement with nitric oxide, this would suggest that the major problem is not vasoconstriction. In congenital diaphragmatic hernia, it indicates the degree of hypoplasia, which is not correctable by surgery.

THE ANESTHETIC IMPLICATIONS OF PHYSIOLOGY
IN NEONATAL ANESTHESIA

MODULATION OF THE CIRCULATION

One important aspect of the physiology of circulation is the various factors that modulate the circulation in order to meet the challenges of disease, surgery, and the administration of anesthetics. The newborn heart is characterized by a relatively low percentage of the heart weight being contractile mass (30%), as compared to the normal mature heart where 60% of the weight of the heart is contractile mass (1). The result of the relatively low amounts of contractile muscle is that the neonatal heart has relatively low compliance compared to the mature heart. Another factor is that the oxygen consumption of the neonate is in the order of 7-9 ml/kg/min compared to the adult level of 3 ml/kg/min. Due to this high metabolic demand, the cardiac output of the newborn is approximately 200 ml/kg/min compared to the adult level of 70 ml/kg/min. This means that the resting cardiac output of the neonate is very near the maximum cardiac output (8). In addition, the infant, because of the limited contractility, is relatively unable to increase stroke volume, so that cardiac output is primarily dependent upon cardiac rate. The problem is that any decrease in heart rate that is associated with hypoxia, vagal stimulation, and/or anesthesia will reduce the cardiac output.

Bradycardia in the infant indicates a low cardiac output and the need for immediate correction. The definition of bradycardia is age related. The normal neonate has a heart rate of 110-180. The definition of bradycardia in this group is any heart rate below 100. If the heart rate drops from 140 to 110, then atropine is the drug of choice, along with a low threshold for cardiac compressions. Once the heart rate drops below 100, then epinephrine 5-10 µg/kg is the drug of choice. In a normal infant of 1 year of age, the normal heart rates are somewhere between 90 and 110-120. Therefore, in these infants, bradycardia is defined as a heart rate below 80. The treatment for bradycardia, particularly sudden bradycardia, is ventilation with 100% oxygen, epinephrine 5-10 µg/kg, and having a low threshold for chest compression.

SYMPATHETIC NERVOUS SYSTEM AND BARORECEPTORS

The other major factors that assist in the modulation of circulation are the sympathetic nervous system and the baroreceptors, both of which are immature in the newborn. The sympathetic nervous system is immature due to incomplete innervation of the sympathetic nervous system. The baroreceptors are immature and more susceptible to anesthetic drugs than in the mature state (9). The results are twofold. One is that sympathectomy due to epidural or spinal anesthesia results in no appreciable vasodilation and no decrease in blood pressure. This relative lack of sympathetic tone persists up until the age of 2 or 3 years (10). The other is that, with the limited ability to increase cardiac output, blood pressure is a better indicator of blood loss than in the mature state. In other words, with a constant anesthetic concentration, if the blood pressure decreases, it is an indicator of a decrease in blood volume and requires augmentation with volume.

THE RENAL SYSTEM

Glomerulogenesis is complete at 34 weeks conceptual age. Regardless of conceptual age, there is a high renal vascular resistance and low systemic blood pressure during fetal life, resulting in a low renal blood flow and a low glomerular filtration rate. The function of the kidney of the fetus is to produce urine, which adds to amniotic fluid for cushioning of the fetus, as well as normal lung development. Immediately after birth, the renal vascular resistance decreases and systemic vascular pressure increases, leading to an increase in renal blood flow and improvement in the glomerular filtration rate. By 3-4 days of life, there is a moderate increase in renal function; and by 2-3 months of age, renal function is sufficient so that it is not a problem in fluid and electrolyte balance. One of the problems of the first month of life, though, is that the infant is an obligate sodium loser because of immaturity of the distal tubule and an inability to increase the reabsorption of sodium. The result is that all fluids administered to neonates need to contain sodium and, for surgical procedures, the fluid needed is a balanced salt solution.

THE BLOOD-BRAIN BARRIER

The neonatal blood-brain barrier is immature. Consequently, hydrophilic drugs, such as morphine, pass the blood-brain barrier more easily and, therefore, have a greater effect in the neonate than in the mature state. On the other hand, drugs like fentanyl, which are lipophilic, easily cross the blood-brain barrier regardless of its maturation and, therefore, have the same effect in the neonate as in the mature state.

LIVER MATURATION AND THE DUCTUS VENOSUS

Two drugs commonly used in anesthesia, fentanyl and vecuronium, depend on the maturity of the liver enzymes for metabolism. In the neonatal period and for several months thereafter, increasing abdominal pressure will decrease the blood flow to the liver, opening the ductus venosus and resulting in a decrease in the metabolism of fentanyl and vecuronium. Therefore, in the first several months of life, muscle relaxants such as atracurium that do not depend upon the liver for metabolism, are the drugs of choice. If the neonate is to be extubated at the conclusion of surgery or shortly thereafter, narcotics should be given in small doses.

THE RESPIRATORY SYSTEM

The respiratory system of the infant is quite different from that of the adult, based upon the high oxygen consumption of the infant. The tidal ventilation, functional residual capacity, and dead space are all essentially the same in the infant and the adult. However, with an oxygen consumption between 7-9 ml/kg/min compared to the adult of 3 ml/kg/min, the respiratory frequency in breaths-per-minute and alveolar ventilation is 2-3 times that of the adult. The other result of the need for greater alveolar ventilation is that the relative ratio between minute ventilation and functional residual capacity is greater in the infant than in the adult. The ratio in the infant is 5:1, in the adult 1.5:1.

The practical implications are that the neonate, with a higher minute ventilation, goes to sleep more rapidly and awakens more rapidly because the functional residual capacity, which is a buffer to minimize gas changes within the lung, is relatively small compared to minute ventilation. On the other hand, the downside is that, with tracheal obstruction or any other interruption of ventilation, the functional residual capacity represents the oxygen reserve of the lungs. The high oxygen consumption of the infant rapidly depletes the oxygen reserve, leading to the rapid development of hypoxia and cyanosis. In addition, the closing volume of the lung, which is defined as the alveolar closing volume where blood no longer is ventilated and is therefore effectively shunted, is much closer to the normal expiratory reserve volume than in the adult. Another factor is that hypoxia may reopen the ductus arteriosus and cause further problems (11). The result in the infant is that at the end of normal expiration, the closing volumes are achieved in some alveoli and the PaO_2 of the infant will be lower. A slight cough will cause a much more rapid encroachment on closing volumes and a much more rapid development of desaturation in the infant than in the adult.

VARIABILITY IN DRUG RESPONSE

The variability in drug response among neonates is greater than at any other time during life. This applies to muscle relaxants and narcotics, as well as to volatile agents. Also, during the first year there is tremendous variability of drug response. The value for the mean alveolar concentration (MAC) of the volatile anesthetics has great variability from the time of birth to 6-12 months of age and in the mature state. For halothane, MAC in the neonate is 0.8%. In the 6-12-month old, it is 1.2%, and in the 18-year old, 0.8%. The same differences are true for the other volatile anesthetics.

ANESTHETIC TECHNIQUES BASED ON NEONATAL PHYSIOLOGY

The major decision in neonatal anesthesia is the question of whether or not the infant needs postoperative ventilation and/or resuscitation. If the neonate following surgery is going to need continued ventilation and/or resuscitation, then the anesthetic technique is of little importance. Any anesthetic technique can be used, as long as it provides blood pressure control and oxygenation. However, if extubation is anticipated at the end of surgery or shortly thereafter, anesthetic technique is crucial. If extubation is anticipated, a general anesthetic technique plus regional anesthesia will usually result in a neonate who rapidly regains control of his/her reflexes and can be extubated. The regional anesthesia is usually in the form of a caudal that is given in a dose of 2-3 mg/kg of bupivacaine. This is usually administered in a solution of 0.25% bupivacaine with 1 to 200,000 epinephrine. The advantage of regional anesthesia is that it reduces the need for muscle relaxants, reduces the concentration of volatile anesthetics, and reduces or eliminates the need for narcotics. The value is that the infant will be more alert and awake, and able to manage his/her airway at the end of the surgical procedure or shortly thereafter. The regional anesthetic can be continued for postoperative analgesia, or small titrated doses of intravenous narcotics can be administered (12).

SUMMARY

Our anesthetic management depends very critically on the physiology of the infant and the confounding effects of the surgical problem and anesthetic. Appreciation of these factors enables the anesthesiologist to select the anesthetic management that differentiates between the infant who may need continued support and the infant in whom early extubation is anticipated.

REFERENCES

1. Berry FA: Physiology and surgery of the infant. In Anesthetic management of difficult and routine pediatric patients. 2nd edition. New York, Churchill Livingstone, 1990.
2. Reller MD, Rice MJ, McDonald RW: Review of studies evaluating ductal patency in the premature infant. J Pediatr 122:S59-62, 1993
3. Murphy JD, Vawter GF, Reid LM: Pulmonary vascular disease in fetal meconium aspiration. J Pediatr 104:758, 1984
4. Wung J-T, James LS, Kilchevsky E et al: Management of infants with severe respiratory failure and persistence of the fetal circulation, without hyperventilation. Pediatrics 76:488, 1985
5. Clark RH, Yoder BA, Sell MS: Prospective, randomized comparison of high-frequency oscillation and conventional ventilation in candidates for extracorporeal membrane oxygenation. J Pediatr 124:447-454, 1994
6. Johns RA: EDRF/nitric oxide: The endogenous nitrovasodilator and a new cellular messenger. Anesthesiology 75:927-931, 1991

7. Finer NN, Etches PC, Kamstra B et al: Inhaled nitric oxide in infants referred for extracorporeal membrane oxygenation: Dose response. J Pediatr 124:302-308, 1994

8. Friedman WF, George BL: Treatment of congestive heart failure by altering loading conditions of the heart. J Pediatr 106:697, 1985

9. Murat I, Lapeyre G, Saint-Maurice C: Isoflurane attenuates baroreflex control of heart rate in human neonates. Anesthesiology 70:395, 1989

10. Dohi S, Naito H, Takahaski T: Age-related changes in blood pressure and duration of motor block in spinal anesthesia. Anesthesiology 50:319, 1979

11. Moorthy SS, Dierdorf SF, Krishna G: Transient hypoxemia from a transient right-to-left shunt in a child during emergence from anesthesia. Anesthesiology 66:234-235, 1987

12. Woolf CJ, Chong MS: Preemptive analgesia: Treating postoperative pain by preventing the establishment of central sensitization. Anesth Analg 77:362-379, 1993

ANESTHESIA FOR THE NEONATE: EMERGENT AND NON-EMERGENT

J. M. Badgwell

Anesthesia for the neonate (newborn to age 1 month) is usually challenging and exciting, and is almost always rewarding. Notwithstanding the current debate concerning whether only pediatric sub-specialists should anesthetize neonates (1), it is the goal of this presentation to prepare you for the challenge of neonatal anesthesia, and to shift the potential excitement of these cases toward their positive rewards.

PREANESTHETIC ASSESSMENT

Remember that a child with one congenital anomaly may have others. For instance, tracheoesophageal fistula (TEF) is associated with congenital heart defects in about 25% of cases. Nonsurviving infants with TEF have congenital heart defects in 50% of cases. Infants with congenital diaphragmatic hernia (CDH), if born stillborn, are found to have associated anomalies in 95% of cases, whereas liveborn patients with CDH have associated anomalies in 20% of cases.

THE PREANESTHETIC HISTORY

Infants of diabetic mothers may be prone to hypoglycemia or hypocalcemia. Infants with a history of perinatal asphyxia may have impaired autoregulation of the central nervous system and depressed myocardial function.

The preoperative assessment should include a careful calculation of the patient's various "ages." *Gestational age* is the time period from conception to birth. *Postnatal age* is the time period from birth to the present. *Conceptual age* is from conception to the present time. A "term" infant is defined as one with a gestational age of 37-42 weeks, whereas a preterm infant is less than 37 weeks gestational age. Term infants weighing less than 2500 g are defined as small for gestational age (SGA). These infants are prone to aspiration pneumonia and hypoglycemia. Preterm infants,

197

T.H. Stanley and P.G. Schafer (eds.), Pediatric and Obstetrical Anesthesia, 197-213.
© *1995 Kluwer Academic Publishers.*

on the other hand, have a high incidence of hyalin membrane disease and perioperative apnea.

PHYSICAL EXAMINATION

HEAD AND NECK

The head and neck are examined for physical characteristics suggesting difficult intubation: micrognathia (Pierre Robin), cleft palate hemangioma, lymphangioma, and hygroma of the cervical region.

CARDIORESPIRATORY

Newborn infants with respiratory distress syndrome (RDS) exhibit tachypnea, inspiratory retraction, expiratory grunt, and oxygen-hemoglobin denaturation.

Evaluation of the cardiovascular system includes examination of the skin and mucous membrane color, capillary filling time, vital signs, and peripheral pulses. Peripheral pulses are decreased with coarctation of the aorta and markedly increased with patent ductus arteriosus. Hepatomegaly is a cardinal sign of congestive heart failure.

INFANT HEMATOLOGY

The term infant at birth has a hemoglobin of around 18-20 g/dl, whereas in the preterm it may be 13 g/dl. Newborn infants have 75-80% fetal hemoglobin. Fetal hemoglobin has a greater affinity for oxygen (i.e., the oxygen-hemoglobin association curve is shifted to the left, and less oxygen is available for delivery to the tissues). Therefore, a sick newborn needs about 10-12 g/dl hemoglobin before surgery to provide adequate oxygen delivery to tissues.

WHAT AGENTS CAN WE USE?

INHALATION ANESTHETICS

PHARMACOKINETICS

The rate of rise from alveolar-to-inspired partial pressures of inhaled anesthetics is more rapid in neonates than in adults. The rapid wash-in of inhalation agents in neonates is attributed to: 1) greater alveolar ventilation to functional residual capacity ratio (5:1 in the neonate compared to 1.5:1 in the adult), 2) greater fraction of the cardiac output distributed to the vessel rich group, 3) lower tissue/blood and blood/gas solubilities. The blood solubilities of inhaled anesthetics are 18% less in neonates than in adults (2), and tissue solubilities are 50% less (3). These factors speed the rate of rise of alveolar-to-inspired anesthetic partial pressures in neonates compared to adults. This rapid wash-in to brain and heart tissues of neonates may produce exaggerated hemo-dynamic responses early in the induction sequence, especially if a high inspired concentration (the overpressure technique) is used.

PHARMACODYNAMICS: MINIMUM ALVEOLAR CONCENTRATIONS (MAC)

In the pediatric age range, and particularly in neonates, the effect of age on MAC has important clinical implications. Lerman et al found that the MAC of halothane was 25% less in neonates (0.87 ± 0.03%) than it was in infants 1-6 months of age (1.2 ± 0.06%) (4). Lerman also investigated the anesthetic requirements of isoflurane in neonates and found that the MAC for isoflurane is 1.28 ± 0.17% in preterm infants less than 32 weeks gestational age, 1.4 ± 0.18% in neonates 32-37 weeks, and 1.60 ± 0.03% in full-term infants (5).

CIRCULATION: IS ISOFLURANE SAFER THAN HALOTHANE?

In infants and children (as in adults), halothane decreases systolic arterial pressure, decreases heart rate, depresses myocardial contractility, and has minimal effect on vasodilation (6,7). By contrast, isoflurane increases heart rate but depresses myocardial contractility to a lesser extent than halothane, and dilates the peripheral vasculature (6,7). Isoflurane has a similar net effect to halothane on the systolic arterial pressure. It has been suggested that cardiac output is decreased more by halothane than it is by isoflurane (8). Does this mean that isoflurane is a safer anesthetic to use in neonates than halothane? In a recently published paper, it was found that equipotent concentrations of halothane and isoflurane decreased cardiac output, stroke volume, and injection fraction similarly in neonates (9). The cardiovascular depression was found to be dose dependent with decreases of more than 30% in ejection fraction and stroke volume at 1.5 MAC concentrations of either agent. It was observed in a previous study by the same authors that older infants and children anesthetized with isoflurane maintained cardiac output better than those anesthetized with halothane when presented with a fluid challenge (6).

Therefore, there may be some advantage to using isoflurane rather than halothane in critically ill neonates.

ARE NEONATES MORE SENSITIVE THAN OLDER INFANTS?

Heart rate and systolic arterial pressure decrease similarly in neonates and infants 1-6 months of age when compared at equipotent concentrations of halothane (4). These data suggested that neonates are *not* more sensitive to the cardiodepressant effect of volatile agents. There are two recent studies, however, to suggest that hemodynamic depression is greater in neonates compared to older infants and children anesthetized at equivalent age-adjusted MAC concentrations of isoflurane and halothane (9,10). Much has been written in an attempt to explain this relative myocardial depression in neonates. Work in rabbits suggests that the myocardial depression seen in neonates may be attributed to the effects of volatile anesthetics on immature contractile proteins, cell membranes, and the intracellular dynamics of calcium ions (11). The best explanation, however, may be that the hemodynamic depression is due to uptake and redistribution differences and increased anesthetic requirements rather than heightened cardiovascular susceptibility to inhaled anesthetics.

Despite this minor controversy that neonates may be more sensitive to volatile anesthetic agents, the clinical implications are clear. Newborn infants, especially critically ill neonates, may have marked cardiovascular depression secondary to volatile anesthetic agents. Furthermore, there may be no particular "safety" in using isoflurane over halothane. For whatever reasons, neonates may be very sensitive to the cardiodepressant effect of volatile anesthetic agents, especially during controlled ventilation when very high concentrations of anesthetic agents may be rapidly achieved in cardiac tissues.

Although it is generally recommended to administer atropine to neonates to preserve heart rate and cardiac output during volatile anesthesia, recent echocardiographic studies in both neonates and infants suggest that increased heart rate after atropine does not attenuate the myocardial depression as measured by ejection fraction and stroke volume (9). The increase in heart rate after atropine does not compensate for decreased stroke volume and cardiac output (9). Therefore, one may not be able to rely on atropine to counteract the cardiodepressant effects of the volatile anesthetic agents. Lactated Ringer's solution, approximately 10 ml/kg, may be needed to maintain systolic arterial pressure during volatile agent anesthesia.

INTRAVENOUS AGENTS

NARCOTICS

Are Neonates Sensitive to the Respiratory Depressant Effect? The misconception that neonates are "sensitive" to the respiratory depressant effects of narcotics began in 1965 when Way et al published a paper showing that 3-day old infants experienced depressed ventilatory response to inspired carbon dioxide after receiving morphine (0.05 mg/kg) (12). Later, it was erroneously assumed that neonates would be equally sensitive to the respiratory depressant effects of all narcotics. However, we now recognize that this is not the case. Because of its high water solubility, morphine readily crosses the immature blood-brain barrier of the neonate. This high water solubility explains why Cordia et al discovered higher brain concentrations of morphine in younger animals despite plasma concentrations that were similar to older animals (13). In contrast to morphine, fentanyl is highly lipid soluble and crosses equally well the immature blood-brain barrier of the newborn and the mature blood-brain barrier of the adult. Therefore, neonates and older patients are affected equally by the same plasma concentration of fentanyl. There is no reason to believe that neonates are more sensitive to the respiratory depressant effects of fentanyl and related drugs because of blood-brain barrier immaturity. Can increased sensitivity in the neonate be explained by other pharmacokinetic reasons?

Pharmacokinetics of Fentanyl in Neonates. Fentanyl is highly lipid soluble and is rapidly distributed to tissues that are well perfused, such as brain and heart. The effect of a single dose of fentanyl is terminated by redistribution, as is thiopental. Fentanyl is then metabolized by the cytochrome P-450 system in the liver. This system is very immature at birth and does not reach adult capacity until the first 1-2 months of life. Fentanyl elimination is also dependent on hepatic blood flow. Therefore, neonates who undergo abdominal surgery or receive volatile anesthetic agents may have compromised hepatic blood flow and prolonged elimination of fentanyl. Furthermore, after multiple or large doses of fentanyl, prolongation of effect may occur because elimination (not redistribution) will determine the duration of effect. The age relationships of fentanyl pharmacokinetics are presented in Figure 1 (14).

The larger steady state volume of distribution (Vdss) in young patients means that the dose of fentanyl is redistributed to a larger peripheral compartment. Therefore, a single dose of fentanyl will result in a lower plasma concentration in a newborn compared to an adult. The

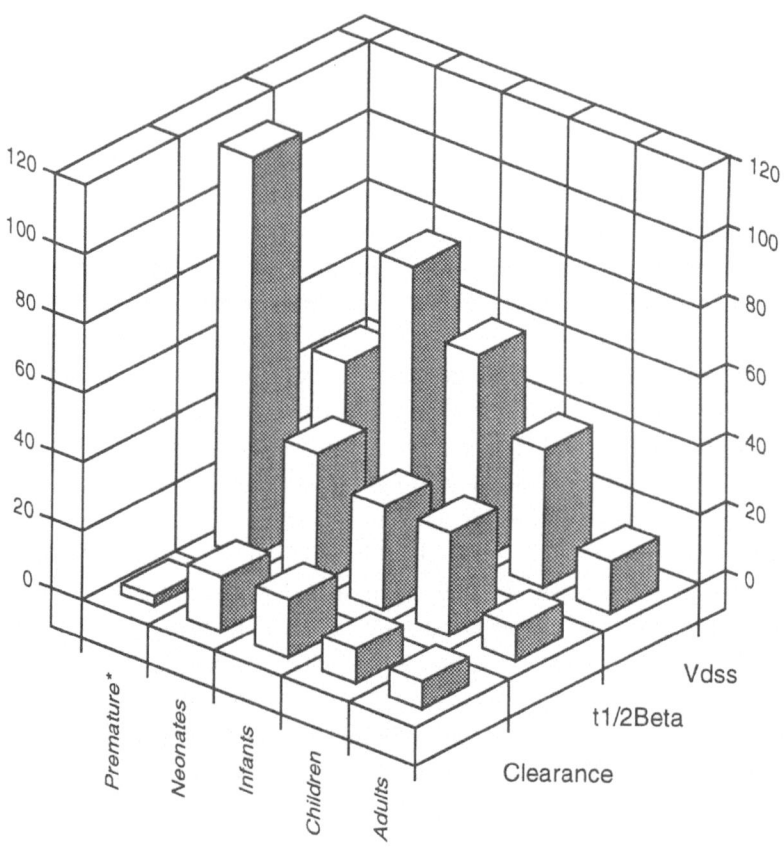

Figure 1.   The relationship of age and fentanyl pharmacokinetics. For the X-axis:
Clearance = X value in ml/kg/min; T1/2 Beta = X value x 10 min; and Vdss = X
value x 0.1 l/kg. Adapted from Johnson (14).

higher clearance (Cl) in the neonate results from a greater hepatic blood
flow per kilogram body weight in the group. Elimination does not vary
with age because of the larger Vdss and higher clearance in younger
patients (T1/2 Beta = 0.093 Vdss/Cl).

The relationship of surgical procedures to fentanyl pharmacokinetics in neonates is shown in Figure 2 (15). This graph demonstrates

the reduced clearance and prolonged elimination of fentanyl in neonates after abdominal surgery, compared to those for patent ductus arteriosus ligation and myelomeningocele repair. These data agree with a reported observation that fentanyl clearance is low, or may even be absent, in neonates having abdominal surgery (15).

Fentanyl Anesthesia for the Neonate—What Dosage? In the past, neonates were often "anesthetized" only with muscle relaxation and oxygen, for fear they were too sick to withstand a real anesthetic. However, in 1981, Robinson and Gregory showed that in neonates undergoing ductus ligation surgery, fentanyl (30-50 µg/kg as the sole agent) maintained very stable hemodynamics and allowed extubation within an hour of the surgery (17). After that report and others (18), the hemodynamic stability associated with fentanyl and sufentanil (18) administration in the neonate have become well known. Hypotension and bradycardia are rare, as long as either pancuronium or atropine is administered concomitantly. However, the safety of fentanyl anesthesia may be compromised when other anesthetic agents (such as volatile agents, barbiturates, benzodiazepines, and nitrous oxide) are administered concomitantly. Also, the effect of intra-abdominal operation, age, and the degree of illness cannot be overemphasized. Fentanyl in doses of 10-12.5 µg/kg produced reliable anesthesia without hemodynamic changes in full-term infants of less than 7 days of age undergoing a variety of thoracic, abdominal, and genitourinary emergency operations (19). These infants were younger (the majority were less than 24 hours old), and probably sicker, than those studied by Robinson and Gregory. Anand and his co-workers have demonstrated that fentanyl anesthesia (10 µg/kg) attenuates the hormonal stress response to surgery in critically ill neonates and prevents the catabolic changes that may worsen outcome (20-25). These investigators noted a decreased incidence of postoperative complications, including intraventricular hemorrhage, in infants anesthetized with a nitrous/narcotic technique independent of postnatal age, type of surgery, and other patient risk factors.

Thiopental. This may be used as an induction agent in neonates. However, there is some uncertainty concerning the dose requirement in neonates. Although Jonmarker observed an increased requirement in infants 1-6 months of age (ED50 = 7 mg/kg) compared to older infants (ED50 = 5 mg/kg), infants less than 1 month of age were not studied (26). It is suggested that these infants may need lower doses of thiopental, similar to what has been reported for the MAC for volatile anesthetics. Despite the uncertainty, it is clear that critically ill neonates (especially if they are

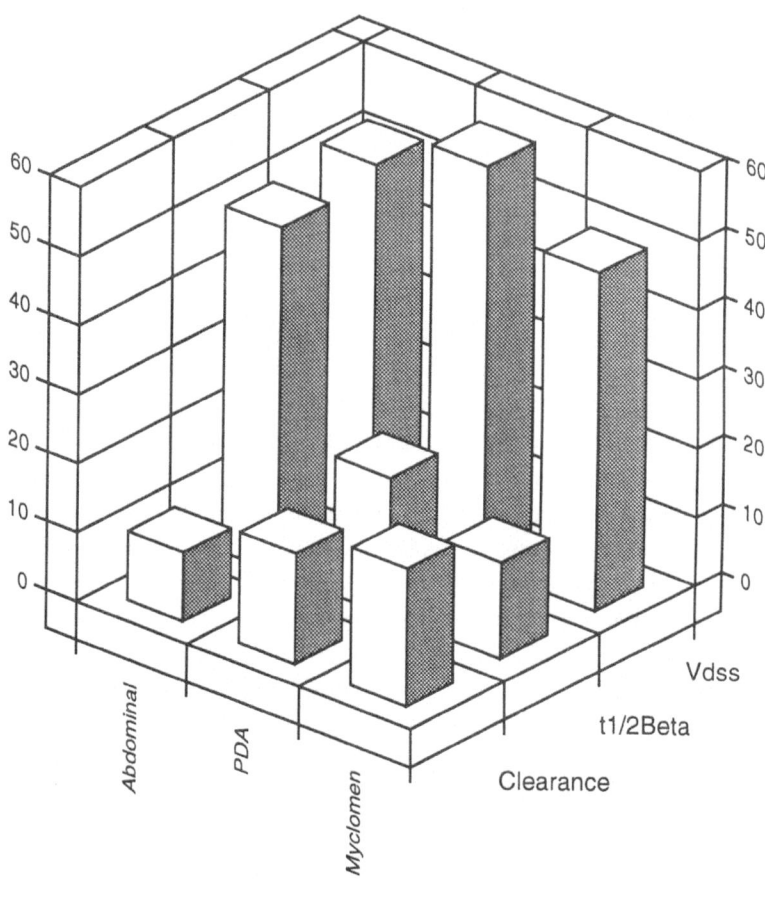

Figure 2.   The relationship of type of surgery and pharmacokinetics. For
the X-axis: Clearance = X value in ml/kg/min; T1/2 Beta = X
value x 10 min; and Vdss = X value x 0.1 l/kg. Adapted from
Koehntop (15).

hypovolemic, acidotic, hypoxic, or have significant cardiopulmonary
disease) may have a reduced requirement for thiopental. In fact, these
infants may not tolerate the cardiac depressant effect of thiopental and
may need either an awake intubation or induction with fentanyl or
ketamine.

Ketamine. This may be a useful induction agent in hypovolemic or
otherwise critically ill infants.   Ketamine may be administered

intravenously or intramuscularly (27). Although there is a wide margin of safe and effective dosage (0.5-8 mg/kg IM or IV), ketamine is known to cause hypotension in catecholamine-depleted older patients. In the absence of data for ketamine in critically ill or hypovolemic neonates, one would be advised to use ketamine cautiously in these patients.

MUSCLE RELAXANTS

Succinylcholine. This remains the neuromuscular-blocking drug with the most rapid onset of action and the shortest duration, and it is the drug of choice to facilitate endotracheal intubation as part of a rapid sequence intubation in the infant with a full stomach, or to treat laryngospasm. Although the ED90 of succinylcholine is 517 µg/kg in neonates (compared to 608 µg/kg in infants and 352 µg/kg in children) (28), the usual dose of this drug in neonates is 2 mg/kg to facilitate endotracheal intubation. Atropine is given prior to the administration of succinylcholine to prevent bradycardia.

There are numerous clinical reports describing masseter muscle rigidity after halothane and succinylcholine, as well as hyperkalemia cardiac arrest after succinylcholine given to children with undiagnosed muscular dystrophy. To the author's knowledge, none of these case reports includes data from neonates. Two years ago, however, we anesthetized a 1-month old infant with halothane who developed total body rigidity after succinylcholine. Endotracheal intubation was accomplished with difficulty. On other occasions, the child was anesthetized using trigger-free agents and had no complications. The case has had an unhappy ending, however, as the child recently died from malignant hyperthermia that developed two hours after a trigger-free anesthetic and completion of surgery. Tissue diagnosis is pending.

Atracurium and Vecuronium. Atracurium (29) and vecuronium (30) are more potent in infants than in children. The ED95 values in µg/kg for atracurium are 217 ± 18 (<1 mon), 234 ± 33 (1-3 mon), 229 ± 22 (3-12 mon), and 310 ± 26 (1-3 yr) (28). For vecuronium, the ED95 values are 48 ± 4 (<1 mon), 44 ± 4 (1-3 mon), 49 ± 3 (3-12 mon), and 57 ± 5 (1-2 yr) (29). Neonates receiving atracurium recover neuromuscular function more rapidly than older infants or children. Therefore, although neonates are more sensitive, they recover more rapidly from the effects of atracurium. Due in part to the age-related difference in potency, neonates are paralyzed significantly more rapidly than older patients. A bolus of 0.5 mg/kg of atracurium depressed 95% twitch height in 0.9 minutes in neonates and 1.4 minutes in children.

In contrast to the rapid recovery from atracurium, the rate of recovery of neuromuscular function after vecuronium is about 50% slower in infants than in children. After 100 µg/kg of vecuronium 90%, neuromuscular blockade persisted for 58 minutes in infants, 18 minutes in children, and 37 minutes in adolescents.

These age-related differences in rate of recovery from vecuronium and atracurium may be due to differences with age, or they may be due to the fact that vecuronium (and not atracurium) requires hepatic metabolism. The same factors that prolong elimination of fentanyl in neonates (see above discussion), such as abdominal surgery and volatile anesthetics, may prolong the elimination of vecuronium.

The reversal of either atracurium or vecuronium may be accomplished with edrophonium (1 mg/kg) preceded by atropine (0.01 mg/kg). Because edrophonium is a very rapid-acting anticholinergic agent that may cause bradycardia, atropine is administered 30 seconds (by the clock) before the administration of edrophonium. It should be noted that atropine may not cause an increase in heart rate in the already tachycardiac infant. Nevertheless, atropine should always precede edrophonium. In the presence of either atracurium or vecuronium, the greater the degree of spontaneous recovery of neuromuscular function at the time of reversal agent administration, the more rapid the recovery of neuromuscular function. Reversal may be accomplished when neuromuscular blockade has returned to 1-2 twitches in a train-of-four. When a reversal agent is administered in the presence of only a slight, single response to train-of-four stimuli, residual paralysis may persist.

Pancuronium. Earlier studies of pancuronium found no significant difference in potency with age, in the range of the first week through 7 years (31). However, a recent study using electromyography has demonstrated increased potency in infants 3-6 months of age (ED95 = 66 µg/kg) compared with children over a year of age (ED95 = 93 µg/kg) (32). Because of its vagolytic action, pancuronium is a useful neuromuscular-blocking agent during fentanyl anesthesia. Its long duration of action may also be helpful in long cases, or when intubation will extend into the postoperative period.

SPECIFIC NEONATAL EMERGENCIES

OMPHALOCELE-GASTROSCHISIS

Omphalocele is herniation of the intestines into the umbilical cord. It differs from gastroschisis in that omphalocele has a peritoneal sac covering the intestines. Twenty-five to thirty percent of omphaloceles occur in infants that are premature or SGA. About two-thirds of these patients with omphalocele have associated anomalies. Infants with omphalocele and Beckwith-Wiedemann syndrome have macroglossia and may be hypoglycemic.

Gastroschisis is a defect of the abdominal wall lateral to the umbilical cord. There is no covering membrane; therefore, the intestines may become edematous or infected and may be the source of large volumes of fluid loss. Adequate volume must be infused perioperatively to maintain hydrational status (7-25 ml/kg/hr).

ANESTHETIC MANAGEMENT

It is important to monitor airway pressure and pulmonary compliance. An arterial line is helpful to monitor blood pressure, arterial blood gases, and serum glucose. A CVP is very useful to monitor volume status. Prior to intubation, the stomach is decompressed. Induction of anesthesia is accomplished with thiopental, atropine, and succinylcholine, and maintained with a balanced technique (avoiding nitrous oxide). Usually, these children can be extubated 24-48 hours after surgery.

TRACHEOESOPHAGEAL FISTULA (TEF) AND ESOPHAGEAL ATRESIA

About 25% of these infants also have congenital heart defects (ventricular septal defect, arterial septal defect, tetralogy of Fallot, atrio-ventricular canal, or coarctation of the aorta). Recent improvements in anesthetic and surgical techniques allow almost 100% survival of these otherwise healthy full-term infants. In premature infants weighing less than 1800 g or with pneumonia, the mortality from TEF ranges from 15% to 60%. The VATER syndrome is an association of V, vertebral defects; A, anal defects; T, TEF; common variation of TEF (90% of cases) is proximal esophageal atresia with a tracheoesophageal fistula between the posterior aspect of the trachea and the distal esophagus. Surgical management may involve a one-stage repair, in which the fistula is ligated and the esophagus is primarily anastomosed. In moderate- or high-risk infants unable to withstand primary repair, a gastrostomy is performed under local or general anesthesia.

ANESTHETIC MANAGEMENT

Awake intubation is usually advocated as the safest approach in infants with TEF. However, anesthesia may be induced with an inhalational agent by allowing the child to spontaneously breathe, or by using very cautious positive pressure ventilation. The endotracheal tube should be advanced gently into the right main stem bronchus and then withdrawn to a position just above the carina. This position is desired because the fistula is usually just proximal to the carina on the posterior aspect of the trachea. Rotation of the endotracheal tube, such that the bevel faces posteriorly, may help to prevent intubation of the fistula itself. In patients with a gastrostomy, proper positioning can be aided by submerging the gastrostomy tube in a beaker of water so that gas bubbles will be evident during ventilation. Even with adequate positioning of the endotracheal tube, ventilation through the fistula may occur. If this happens in patients without a gastrostomy, gastric distention may result and impair ventilation. If this occurs, emergency decompression is necessary with a large bore needle or emergency gastrostomy to permit satisfactory ventilation of the infant. By contrast, a prior gastrostomy may serve as a low-resistance vent through which most of the tidal volume escapes. If this occurs, the gastrostomy tube should be clamped, or a retrograde Fogarty catheter can be inserted. When the airway is secured and ventilation is assured, the child may be paralyzed.

Intraoperative monitoring includes placing the precordial stethoscope in the right axillary line. In high risk infants, an arterial catheter is inserted. Most patients can be extubated after repair of TEF. However, tracheomalacia at the site of the fistula can cause collapse of the airway, requiring reinsertion of the endotracheal tube and prolonged controlled ventilation.

CONGENITAL DIAPHRAGMATIC HERNIA

Gone are the days when these infants were rushed to the operating room on the first day of life for surgical repair. Through the work of Des Bohn (33-36) it is now known that these infants are frequently worse in terms of respiratory mechanics and blood gas values after surgical repair. A system of predicting outcome has been established in these patients. In this system, infants with $PaCO_2$ greater than 40 mm Hg and ventilatory index (mean airway pressure x respiratory rate) greater than 1,500 are predicted to have a very poor outcome. Management of this group of patients involves high-frequency oscillatory ventilation of ECMO and deferred surgical repair. Although many of these infants die before surgery can be performed, surgery does not improve outcome. In those infants whose $PaCO_2$ is less than 40 mm Hg and whose ventilatory index is greater than 1,500, elective repair takes place in the first day of life. In those infants with ventilatory index greater than 1,500 and $PaCO_2$ greater than 40 mm Hg, repair is deferred for greater than 24 hours, and the patients are managed on high-frequency oscillatory ventilation, conventional mechanical ventilation, or ECMO until their medical condition improves.

ANESTHETIC MANAGEMENT

With rare exceptions, these infants are diagnosed in utero and are resuscitated and intubated in the delivery room. Positive pressure ventilation in the operating room is a continuation of the infant's mechanical ventilation preoperatively. Ventilatory rate is usually maintained at relatively high rates (50-100 breaths/min) to achieve adequate oxygenation and hyperventilation. Frequent blood gas determinations, end-tidal CO_2 and pulse oximetry are essential to ensure effective mechanical ventilation. It is very important to correct acidosis, should it occur, and it is equally important to maintain the pH greater than 7.5 by hyperventilation ($PaCO_2$ around 25-35 mm Hg). At least one of the IVs should be in an upper extremity, because the inferior vena cava may become compressed after reduction of the hernia. There is no "magical anesthetic technique" specific to this condition. Usually a balanced technique using fentanyl and muscle relaxants is well tolerated. The use of high-dose narcotics (fentanyl) is also appropriate if tolerated hemodynamically. Continuous narcotic infusion that persists into the postoperative period has an effect on decreasing persistent pulmonary hypertension. Except in infants with small defects and excellent gas exchange, endotracheal intubation, paralysis, and controlled ventilation should be continued postoperatively.

CONGENITAL LOBAR EMPHYSEMA

Congenital lobar emphysema (CLE) is a pathologic accumulation of air in one lobe of the lung, usually an upper lobe or the right middle lobe (37). Although the clinical presentation of CLE is highly variable, it frequently occurs at birth. The pathophysiology of CLE is similar to that of pneumothorax, and the severity of symptoms (severe dyspnea, cyanosis, wheezing, grunting, and coughing) relate to the degree of cardio-pulmonary compromise caused by air accumulation under tension.

Physical examination reveals signs and symptoms similar to hyalin membrane disease (tachypnea, retractions, flaring of the alae nasi, labored breathing, and expiratory wheezing). Lobar distention appears on radiographs as a unilateral radiolucency with marked mediastinal shift away from the affected side and a flattened diaphragm. The presence of bronchial vascular markings differentiate CLE from congenital lung cyst, a disorder that is commonly confused with CLE.

ANESTHETIC MANAGEMENT

Newborns with CLE and severe cardiorespiratory failure demand immediate surgery. An arterial catheter is an essential monitor to allow serial blood gas determinations.

A gentle induction of anesthesia is performed with a volatile anesthetic agent and 100% oxygen. Nitrous oxide and positive pressure ventilation are contraindicated because of the danger of further expanding the emphysematous lobe. The trachea is intubated without the use of muscle relaxants, and spontaneous ventilation is allowed until the chest is opened. If hypotension occurs during the induction or maintenance of anesthesia, the volatile anesthetic agent is decreased or discontinued, and supplemental analgesia is provided with ketamine (1-2 mg/kg IV). Injection of local anesthetic at the incision site will allow lighter levels of general anesthesia. Hypercarbia in these spontaneously breathing infants may exist. If oxygenation is adequate, as reflected by pulse oximetry and arterial PO_2, the transient hypercarbia that results from relative hypoventilation may be ignored. One should not be tempted to hyperventilate the patient with positive pressure ventilation in order to bring the CO_2 down before the chest is opened. After the chest is opened, the emphysematous lobe permeates through the incision, which eliminates intrathoracic compression. Controlled ventilation can then be started, facilitated by muscle relaxants, if desired.

REFERENCES

1. Annual Meeting Summary. Society for Pediatrics Newsletter. Vol 5, No 1. Winter-Spring, 1992
2. Lerman J, Schmitt BI, Willis MM et al: Age and the solubility of volatile anesthetics in blood. Anesthesiology 61:139-143, 1984
3. Lerman J, Schmitt BI, Willis MM et al: Effect of age on the solubility of volatile anesthetics in human tissues. Anesthesiology 65:63-67, 1986
4. Lerman J, Robinson S, Willis MM et al: Anesthetic requirements for halothane in young children 0-1 month and 1-6 months of age. Anesthesiology 59:421-424, 1983
5. LeDez KM, Lerman J: The minimum alveolar concentration (MAC) of isoflurane in pretem neonates. Anesthesiology 67:301-307, 1987
6. Murray D, Vandewalker G, Matherne P et al: Pulsed doppler and two-dimensional echocardiography: Comparison of halothane and isoflurane on cardiac function in infants and small children. Anesthesiology 67:211-217, 1987
7. Wolf WJ, Neal MB, Peterson MD: The hemodynamic and cardiovascular effects of isoflurane and halothane anesthesia in children. Anesthesiology 64:328-333, 1986
8. Lerman J: Inhalation anesthetics in infants and children from anesthesiology clinics of North America. In Lerman J, ed. New developments in pediatric anesthesia. Philadelphia, WB Saunders, p 772
9. Murray DJ, Forbes RB, Mahoney LT: Comparative hemodynamic depression of halothane versus isoflurane in neonates and infants: An echocardiographic study. Anesth Analg 74:329-337, 1992
10. Charlton GA, Friesen RH: Age related cardiovascular sensitivity to halothane. Presented at the 1992 annual spring meeting, American Academy of Pediatrics Anesthesiology Section, New York City. (Resident's research competition award winner)
11. Murat I, Hoester J, Ventura-Cloper R: Developmental changes in effects of halothane and isoflurane on contractile properties of rabbit cardiac skinned fibers. Anesthesiology 73:137-145, 1990
12. Way WL, Costley EC, Way EL: Respiratory sensitivity of the newborn infant to mepreidine and morphine. Clin Pharmcol Ther 6:454-461,1965
13. Kupferberg HJ, Way EL: Pharmacologic basis for the increased sensitivity of the newborn rate to morphine. J Pharmacol Exp Ther 141:105-112, 1963
14. Johson KL, Erickson JP, Holley FO et al: Fentanyl pharmacokinetics in the pediatric population. Anesthesiology 61:A441, 1984
15. Koehntop DE, Rodman JH, Brundage DM et al: Pharmacokinetics of fentanyl in neonates. Anesth Analg 65:227-232, 1986
16. Gauntlett MB, Fisher DM, Hertzka RE et al: Pharmacokinetics of fentanyl in neonatal humans and lambs: Effects of age. Anesthesiology 69:683, 1988

17. Robinson S, Gregory GA: Fentanyl-air-oxygen anesthesia for patent ductus arteriosus in preterm infants. Anesth Analg 60:331-334, 1981

18. Greely WJ, de Bruijn NP: Changes in sufentanil pharmacokinetics within the neonatal period. Anesth Analg 67:86-90, 1988

19. Yaster M: The dose response of fentanyl in neonatal anesthesia. Anesthesiology 66:433-435, 1987

20. Anand KJ: Neonatal stress responses to anesthesia and surgery. Clin Perinatol 17:207-214, 1990

21. Anand KJ, Aynsley Green A: Measuring the severity of surgical stress in newborn infants. J Pediatr Surg 23:297-305, 1988

22. Anand KJ, Carr DB: The neuroanatomy, neurophysiology, and neurochemistry of pain, stress, and analgesia in newborns and children. Pediatr Clin North Am 36:795-822, 1989

23. Anand KJ, Hickey PR: Pain and its effects in the human neonate and fetus. N Engl J Med 317:1321-1329, 1987

24. Anand KJ, Sippell WG, Aynsley Green A: Randomised trial of fentanyl anaesthesia in preterm babies undergoing surgery: Effects on the stress response (erratum appears in Lancet 1:234, 1987). Lancet 1:62-66, 1987

25. Anand KJ, Hansen DD, Hickey PR: Hormonal-metabolic stress responses in neonates undergoing cardiac surgery. Anesthesiology 73:661-670, 1990

26. Jonmarker C, Westrin P, Larsson S et al: Thiopental requirements for induction of anesthesia in children. Anesthesiology 67:104-107, 1987

27. Lockhart CH, Nelson WL: The relationship of ketamine requirement to age in pediatric patients. Anesthesiology 40:507-508, 1974

28. Meakin G, McKiernan EP, Morris P et al: Dose-response curves for suxamethonium in neonates, infants and children. Br J Anaesth 62:655, 1989

29. Meretoja OA, Wirtavuori K: Influence of age on the dose-response relationship of atracurium in paediatric patients. Acta Anaesthesiol Scand 32:614, 1988

30. Meretoja OA, Wirtavuori K, Neuvonen PJ: Age-dependence of the balanced anesthesia. Anesth Analg 67:21, 1988

31. Goudsouzian NG, Ryan JF, Savarese JJ: The neuromuscular effects of pancuronium in infants and children. Anesthesiology 41:95, 1974

32. Blinn A, Woelfel SK, Cook DR et al: Pancuronium dose-response revisited. Presented at the American Academy of Pediatrics Anesthesiology Section, 1991

33. Bohn DJ: Ventilatory and blood gas parameters in predicting survival in congenital diaphragmatic hernia. Paediatr Surg Int 2:336, 1987

34. Bohn DJ, James I, Filler RM et al: The relationship between $PaCO_2$ and ventilation parameters in predicting survival in congenital diaphragmatic hernia. J Pediatr Surg 19:666, 1984

35. Bohn DJ, Tamura M, Perrin D et al: Ventilatory predictors of pulmonary hypoplasia in congenital diphragmatic hernia, confirmed by morphometry. J Pediatr 111:423, 1987

36. Bohn DJ: Ventilatory management and blood gas changes in congenital diaphragmatic hernia.   In Falkner F, Kretchmer N, Rossi E, eds.   Congenital diaphragmatic hernia.   (Modern problems in paediatrics, Vol 24.) Karger, Basel, 1989, p 76

37. Raynor AC, Capp MP, Sealy WC: Lobar emphysema of infancy. Ann Thorac Surg 4:374, 1967

FASTING AND PREMEDICATION IN INFANTS AND CHILDREN

J. Lerman

In this lecture, I shall discuss two very exciting aspects of pediatric anesthesia: 1) the development of a scientific basis for the fasting interval for infants and children scheduled for surgery, and 2) premedications, old and new. Both aspects are pertinent to clinical pediatric anesthetic practice today because our understanding of these issues has changed dramatically in the past few years. As I outline below, the changes will reduce the unpleasantness of the hospital visit and the amount of suffering infants and children in our care will have to endure, while we maintain a very high standard of care.

THE OPTIMAL FASTING INTERVAL

Fasting is considered a mandatory prerequisite to elective surgery in infants and children. If the purpose of fasting is to minimize the risk of regurgitation and the severity of pneumonitis, then it is important to determine the fasting interval that minimizes the incidence and/or severity of these complications. At the same time, however, excessive fasting may lead to hypoglycemia, hypotension, irritability, and excessive hunger. What follows is a review of the current literature on this subject that will help us to establish a consensus on an acceptable fasting interval for children.

ELECTIVE SURGERY

Investigators have demonstrated that more than 50% of healthy children under anesthesia are at risk of pneumonitis, should aspiration occur (1). This incidence was based on the following risk criteria: a gastric fluid pH <2.5 and a gastric fluid volume >0.4 ml/kg. Despite the prevalence of these risk factors, the incidence of aspiration in children remains very low: 1:10,000 (2) and 1:1,000 (3). These data support the

215

T.H. Stanley and P.G. Schafer (eds.), Pediatric and Obstetrical Anesthesia, 215-227.
© 1995 Kluwer Academic Publishers.

clinical impression that, while many children may be at risk for pneumonitis, aspiration is a very rare event in healthy children.

CLEAR FLUIDS

Several factors determine the rate of gastric fluid emptying. These include fluid volume and composition (osmolarity), pathological conditions (diabetes), and medications (narcotics). Gastric emptying of clear fluids follows an exponential decay with respect to the volume of fluid within the stomach. In adults, the elimination half-life of 7 ml/kg isotonic saline is 12 minutes (4). If the rate of gastric fluid emptying were at least as rapid in children, one would expect that a fluid load of isotonic saline would be eliminated within 5 half-lives, or 1 hour after ingestion. Data from preterm infants suggest that water is emptied extremely rapidly from the stomach, with a half-life of approximately 15 minutes (5). These data support the notion that clear fluids are eliminated rapidly from the stomach in infants and children.

The effects of the fasting interval on gastric fluid pH and volume have been the subject of several studies. The results have been consistent: clear fluids may be given orally up to 2 hours before surgery to children who are scheduled for elective surgery without increasing the risk of regurgitation, decreasing gastric fluid pH, or increasing gastric fluid volume (6,7). Furthermore, the volume of oral fluids that may be administered preoperatively may be as great as 10 ml/kg without affecting gastric fluid pH and volume (8). Administration of a sugar-containing solution may also allay the concerns of anesthetists, insofar as the risk of perioperative hypoglycemia is concerned. Finally, irritability and thirst are lessened when clear fluids are given 2-3 hours before induction of anesthesia compared with 6-8 hours before anesthesia(9). As we continue to critically review our fasting protocols, we may soon come full circle to the recommendation of Leigh and Belton who stated in 1948 that *clear fluids may be given (to healthy children) up to 1 hour before surgery* (10).

BREASTMILK/FORMULA

The safe time interval between breast feeding or formula and elective surgery in infants is poorly understood. However, it is known that gastric emptying is more rapid in preterm infants (33-37 weeks gestation at birth) who are less than 2 months of age than it is in full-term infants (1-6 months of age) (Figure 1) (11,12).

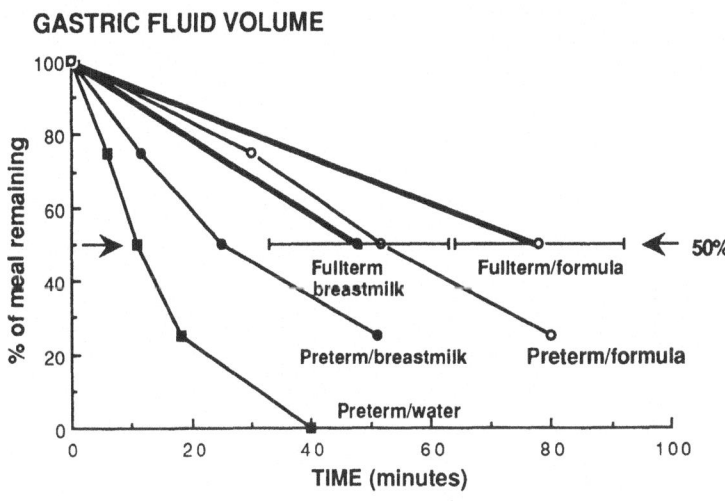

GASTRIC FLUID VOLUME

Figure 1. Percent of breast milk, formula, and water remaining after ingestion by full-term (solid lines) and preterm (dotted light lines) infants. Time to complete elimination of the meal is 4 half-lives (50% meal remaining). Data are means ± standard deviations (5,11,12).

The more rapid gastric emptying in preterm infants has been attributed to age-related differences in metabolic requirements and growth rate. Within each age group, the mean rate of gastric emptying after breast milk was almost 50% more rapid than after isocaloric commercial formula, although the variability (standard deviation) in the elimination half-lives was large (30% of the mean values) (Figure 1). The difference between the rates of gastric emptying of breast milk and formula has been attributed to differences in the lipid and protein content of the two semi-solid fluids. However, recent studies indicate that breast milk and whey hydrosylate feeds are emptied more rapidly than are casein-predominant and cow's milk feeds (Figure 2) (13,14).

The delayed gastric fluid emptying after casein-predominant meals may be attributed to three possible causes: 1) the casein content in the feeds, 2) casein-induced opioid inhibition of gastric motility, and 3) osmolarity of the feeds (13-15). In a clinical study of residual gastric feeds, 3% of infants (n = 1) who had been breast-fed 2.7 hours earlier, and 6% of those (n = 2) who had ingested commercial formula 2.7 and 4.3 hours earlier, had residual gastric fluid volumes >0.4 ml/kg at induction of anesthesia (16).

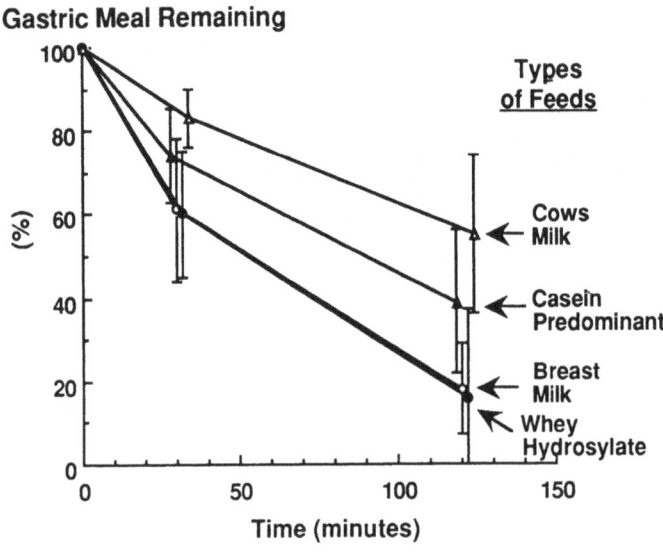

Figure 2. Percent of meal remaining in the stomach of infants 120 minutes after ingestion. Four different meals were evaluated. These meals varied in their casein content. Significantly less meal remained after ingestion of breast milk and whey hydrosylate compared with casein-predominant and cow's milk meals (13).

In addition to the rate of gastric emptying, the optimal fasting interval must also take into account the severity of pneumonitis that may result after aspiration of the breast milk or infant formula. Criteria for severe pneumonitis after aspiration include a pH <2.5 and a volume >0.4 ml/kg. A recent reappraisal of Roberts and Shirley's report (17), together with data from monkeys (18), suggests that these criteria should be revised to pH <2.5 and volume >0.8 ml/kg. Preliminary data from our department indicate that aspiration of non-acidified breast milk causes intrapulmonary shunting and histopathological changes in lung parenchyma that are similar to those of saline (19). Further studies are underway to quantitate the effects of acidified breast milk and formula on the lungs.

In summary, these data indicate that a fasting interval of 4 hours after breast feeding, 4 hours after feeding whey hydrosylate meals, or 6 hours after casein-predominant feeds is warranted. These recommendations will continue to evolve as further data becomes available.

EMERGENCY SURGERY

In contrast to the overwhelming evidence in favor of a brief fasting interval before elective surgery, there is a paucity of evidence supporting a brief fasting interval before emergency surgery. Although many clinicians delay emergency surgery (where possible) at least 6 hours after a meal, there is little evidence to support this strategy. Approximately 50% of injured children are at increased risk of aspiration pneumonitis after both 4-hour and 8-hour fasts (20,21). Olsson and Hallen concluded that the severity of the trauma is a more important determinant of gastric emptying than the duration of the fast (22). In one study of children requiring emergency surgery, regurgitation occurred only at extubation and not at induction of anesthesia. The authors concluded that there is no safe interval between ingestion of the last solid food and induction of anesthesia that reliably decreases the risk of pneumonitis if aspiration does occur in patients scheduled for emergency surgery. The effects of gastrokinetic and pH-modifying drugs in these cases remain unclear.

WHAT'S NEW IN PREMEDICATION FOR CHILDREN?

The ideal premedication for infants and children should satisfy several requirements, including accessibility, ease of administration, acceptable formulation, absence of side effects, and minimal monitoring. With the current emphasis on ambulatory surgery, premedication should also ensure: 1) a level of sedation/anxiolysis that facilitates a smooth separation from parents, and 2) rapid onset and short duration of action that does not extend the hospital stay (23). Although a wide range of drugs and routes of administration have been investigated, recent interest has focused on several newer drugs and routes of administration. These will be reviewed:

1. Nasal sufentanil
2. Nasal midazolam
3. Nasal ketamine
4. Oral transmucosal fentanyl citrate (OTFC)
5. Oral midazolam
6. Oral ketamine
7. Oral clonidine
8. Sublingual midazolam.

NASAL SUFENTANIL

The nasal route for administration of drugs has been almost totally neglected, save for local anesthetic administration. Its lack of popularity stems from its association with substance abuse and the fact that most children do not readily accept liquids dripped into the nose. Nonetheless, this route of drug administration produces very rapid absorption into the systemic circulation, avoids first-pass hepatic metabolism, and is relatively pain free.

Nasally administered sufentanil has been investigated as a preoperative sedative because its potency exceeds that of fentanyl, thereby permitting the instillation of a smaller volume of liquid in the nose. The optimal dose of sufentanil is 1.5 or 3.0 μg/kg (24). This dose sedates children sufficiently to facilitate a smooth separation from their parents within 10 minutes of administration and reduces the need for postoperative analgesics, without excessive complications or delays in discharge from the hospital.

Side effects, however, may limit the use of nasal sufentanil (24). Doses between 1.5 and 4.5 μg/kg produce: 1) drowsiness or deep sleep in 29% of children, 2) decreases in ventilatory compliance in 49% of children, and 3) hemoglobin oxygen desaturations to <95% in 5% of children. In addition, 5% (1 child) of those who received 1.5 μg/kg developed laryngospasm after extubation. Side effects, including chest rigidity, postoperative emesis, and postoperative respiratory depression, occurred frequently with 4.5 μg/kg.

The role of nasal sufentanil as a premedication in pediatric anesthesia will be limited by the vigilance required to ensure adequacy of ventilation and oxygenation and the greater acceptance of other premedications discussed below.

NASAL MIDAZOLAM

The parenteral formulation of midazolam is administered undiluted (5 mg/ml) into the nasal passages by dropper or needle-less syringe (25). The dose recommended for children 1.5-5 years of age is 0.2 mg/kg. Peak blood levels are achieved by 10 minutes; these levels are one-half those measured after IV administration (26).

Clinical effects of midazolam are apparent 10 minutes after administration. Midazolam produces a dissociative state; loss of consciousness is not a feature of this medication. Children are easily separated from their parents 10-15 minutes after premedication. The drawbacks of nasal midazolam include the lack of enthusiasm for the nasal route for drug administration and the bitter aftertaste. These two drawbacks will limit the enthusiasm for the routine use of nasal midazolam.

NASAL KETAMINE

Intranasal instillation of parenteral ketamine has been investigated in preschool children 2-5 years of age (27). A dose of 6 mg/kg, administered 20-40 minutes before surgery produced excellent or adequate sedation in virtually all children. Adverse responses to the instillation of ketamine were not reported. The recovery period was notable for the absence of emergence delirium, and for the similarity of emergence times after ketamine and a control premedication. Nonetheless, additional studies are required to fully characterize the effects of intranasal instillation of ketamine.

ORAL TRANSMUCOSAL FENTANYL CITRATE

Oral Transmucosal Fentanyl Citrate (OTFC) is one of the first attempts to deliver a premedication to children via the transmucosal oral route. OTFC is prepared by dissolving fentanyl citrate in a sucrose solution that is then molded into a lozenge with a handle. Unfortunately, this formulation was nicknamed the "fentanyl-lollipop" and engendered widespread opposition from activists, who argued that "opioid-tainted candy" is a poor example for children. Despite the "lollipop" nickname, OTFC actually resembles a suppository. Moreover, it is curious that fentanyl, a potent opioid and respiratory depressant, would be selected for its sedative properties, a side effect of the drug, as its main action in this preparation. Not surprisingly, this preparation of fentanyl has not been approved as a premedicant in Canada.

OTFC is available in a range of doses, between 10 and 25 μg/kg. The dose being recommended as a premedication is in the lower dose range of 10-15 μg/kg. Its onset of action is 10-20 minutes, with a duration of action of approximately 30 minutes (28-31). However, its effectiveness as a premedication is drastically reduced if it is chewed and swallowed rather than absorbed via the transoral route. Studies in adults indicate that its systemic bioavailability (0.52) is almost twice that after oral administration (0.32) (32). Absorption of fentanyl is more rapid after transmucosal absorption than after oral administration. Side effects and complications reported after OTFC include arterial oxygen desaturation (5%), decreases in respiratory rate, pruritus (80-90%), and postoperative nausea (11%) and emesis (26-65%) (28-31). These effects are dose dependent.

OTFC has also been effective in the postoperative period as an analgesic and for procedural pain relief. It decreases the analgesic requirements postoperatively and does not delay discharge from the hospital. Indeed, its major role in pediatrics may be for the management of painful procedures outside the operating room.

One of the difficulties with this premedication is that its administration is labor intensive. All opioids must be accounted for before, during, and after administration, and this includes OTFC. Any unused portion of the preparation must be returned and/or discarded appropriately. Parents or other children in the waiting area should not be allowed to consume any of the premedication. Furthermore, the patient must remain under constant observation to ensure that the OTFC is not chewed or given to others nearby and that side effects, such as arterial oxygen desaturation, do not occur.

This preparation of an opioid has raised much concern—not only because of the side effects produced, but also because of the plausible social implications from tainting "candy" with an opioid. Because of these and other concerns, the use of OTFC as a premedication remains limited in children.

ORAL MIDAZOLAM

Oral midazolam is rapidly becoming the most popular premedication for children. Midazolam induces a dissociative state after oral administration without loss of consciousness (33,34). We administer oral midazolam in a dose of 0.75 mg/kg for children 1-6 years old and 0.4 mg/kg for those 6-12 years old (34). It is prepared in our pharmacy by mixing midazolam (5 mg/ml concentration of the parenteral formulation) and a tutti-frutti syrup to produce a thick solution with a midazolam concentration of 3 mg/ml. Many vehicles have been used to mask the bitter aftertaste of midazolam (Coca-Cola, Kool-Aid, Jell-O), but none appears to have won universal acceptance. Because of this palatability problem, children must be encouraged to ingest the entire volume of the midazolam syrup in one fast swallow, lest they refuse to ingest the remainder. The bitter taste of midazolam remains its only significant drawback as a premedication for children.

Midazolam has a rapid onset of action (10-20 minutes) (35) and a short duration of action (34). It is reliable and without serious side effects (33-35). The bioavailability of midazolam after oral administration is 15% (for doses 0.45-1.0 mg/kg) to 27% (for a dose of 0.15 mg/kg) compared with 85-100% after parenteral administration (36). This may be explained by midazolam's extensive first-pass hepatic metabolism. Peak serum midazolam concentrations occur 50 minutes after oral administration. At this time, the blood levels of oral midazolam (0.45 mg/kg) are only slightly less than those of IV midazolam (0.15 mg/kg) (36). The elimination half-life after oral midazolam is 1.2 hours, less than that reported in adults. Its action is terminated by hydroxylation via hepatic microsomal oxidative pathways. The primary metabolite is 1-hydroxy midazolam, with smaller quantities of 4 and 1,4-hydroxy midazolam formed.

Serious side effects after oral midazolam are uncommon. Cardiorespiratory side effects were not observed in 90 children 1-6 years of age who received between 0.5 and 1.0 mg/kg (34,35). Airway complications did *not* occur. However, several minor complications have been observed, including loss of balance and head control in 20% of those given 0.75 mg/kg and in 25% of those given 1.0 mg/kg (34). Two children (3%) experienced dysphoric reactions before surgery. These side effects all resolved before discharge from the hospital.

Oral midazolam satisfies all requirements for the ideal premedication except for its palatability. It is ideal for circumstances when sedation without loss of consciousness is preferred immediately before surgery, and when intensive preoperative supervision is not immediately available.

ORAL KETAMINE

The oral route remains the preferred route for administration of premedicants, including ketamine, to children. To improve its palatability, ketamine, like midazolam, must be administered in a thick vehicle (ie., syrup). Preliminary studies indicate that oral ketamine in a dose of 6-10 mg/kg provides excellent sedation without complications in children 1-7 years of age (37,38).

In a dose of 6 mg/kg, ketamine sedates children within 10 minutes and exerts a maximum effect within 20 minutes (38).

Side effects after oral ketamine are dose related. After a 6 mg/kg dose, nystagmus occurred in 60% of children, random limb movements in 13%, and tongue faciculations in 20% (38). Increased secretions were noted in 33% of children. Surprisingly, emergence phenomena and nightmares have not been reported with this premedication.

When we compared the characteristics of oral ketamine 5 mg/kg with those of oral midazolam 0.5 mg/kg, we found that the sedative and anxiolytic effects of the two drugs were remarkably similar (39). However, recovery after midazolam was 20% more rapid than after ketamine. This was attributed to vomiting that occurred in several children who had received oral ketamine premedication. Interestingly, the only child who experienced nightmares after the surgery was in the midazolam group.

A cost/benefit analysis of the two premedications tends to favor midazolam over ketamine provided that the doses used differed by tenfold (39). Midazolam is less expensive than ketamine and provides a superior recovery profile.

In order to minimize the incidence of side effects from these premedications, some clinicians have recommended combination therapies of oral ketamine 3 mg/kg and midazolam 0.25-0.35 mg/kg. These combinations merit further attention before they are recommended for widespread use.

ORAL CLONIDINE

Clonidine, an α_2-adrenoreceptor agonist, has recently found favor as a premedication in children (40). Its role in this regard stems from the sedative side effect reported after its use in adults. In a study in children, investigators concluded that a dose of 4 μg/kg of clonidine is superior to both 2 μg/kg and diazepam 0.4 mg/kg for the quality of separation and acceptance of the face mask (40). Although the speed of onset was not studied, the authors noted that the onset of sedation was slow (approximately 1.5 hours). This may prove to be the "Achilles' heel" of this premedication. They found that a dose of 4 μg/kg attenuated the hypertensive and tachycardic responses to tracheal intubation without evidence of hypotension or bradycardia. Unless the onset of sedation proves to be faster than the 1.5 hours in this study, this premedication will hold little prospect of becoming the universal premedication for children.

SUBLINGUAL MIDAZOLAM

The sublingual route for administration of premedicants and coronary vasodilators in adults is well established. This does not, however, hold true for children. The reason for this difference in preference lies in the inability of young children to cooperate with instructions to hold medication under their tongue. Recently, Karl et al studied the role of sublingual midazolam (0.2 mg/kg) in infants and children 0.5-10 years of age (41). Liquid midazolam (5 mg/ml) was placed sublingually, and the subjects were asked not to swallow the liquid. Between 77% and 96% of the subjects were sedated within 10 minutes: however, the younger subjects tended to be non-compliant, spitting out or swallowing the midazolam prematurely. These latter subjects were inadequately sedated. The authors noted significantly less crying with sublingual midazolam than they did with nasal instillation of midazolam. Sublingual midazolam may be superior to intranasal midazolam, but I await further evidence of its success as a premedication.

REFERENCES

1. Coté CJ, Goudsouzian NG, Liu LM et al: Assessment of risk factors related to the acid aspiration syndrome in pediatric patients: Gastric pH and residual volume. Anesthesiology 56:70-72, 1982
2. Tiret L, Nivoche Y, Hatten F et al: Complications related to anesthesia in infants and children: A prospective study of 40,240 anaesthetics. Br J Anaesth 61:263-269, 1988
3. Borland L, Saitz E, Woefel S: Pulmonary aspiration: A 20 month experience. Amer Acad of Pediatrics (spring session) 37, 1990
4. Hunt JN: Some properties of an alimentary osmoreceptor mechanism. J Physiol (Lond) 132:267-288, 1956
5. Siegel M, Lebenthal E, Krantz B: Effect of caloric density on gastric emptying in premature infants. Pediatrics 104:118-122, 1984
6. Crawford M, Lerman J, Christensen S et al: Effects of duration of fasting on gastric fluid pH and volume in healthy children. Anesth Analg 71:400-403, 1990
7. Schreiner M, Triebwasser K, Keon T: Ingestion of liquids compared with preoperative fasting in pediatric outpatients. Anesthesiology 72:593-597, 1990
8. Splinter WM, Stewart J, Muir J: Large volumes of apple juice preoperatively do not affect gastric pH and volume in children. Can J Anaesth 37:36-39, 1990
9. Splinter WM, Stewart JA, Muir JG: The effect of preoperative apple juice on gastric contents, thirst and hunger in children. Can J Anaesth 36:55-58, 1989
10. Leigh MD, Belton MK: Pediatric anesthesia. New York, Macmillan, 1948, p 6
11. Cavell B: Gastric emptying in preterm infants. Acta Paediatr Scand 68:725-730, 1979
12. Cavell B: Gastric emptying in infants fed human milk or infant formula. Acta Paediatr Scand 70:639-641, 1981

13. Billeaud C, Guillet J, Sandler B: Gastric emptying in infants with or without gastro-oesophageal reflux according to the type of milk. Euro J Clin Nutr 44:577-583, 1990

14. Tolia V, Lin C-H, Kuhns LR: Gastric emptying using three different formulas in infants with gastroesophageal reflux. J Ped Gastr Nutr 15:297-301, 1992

15. Billeaud C, Senterre J, Rigo J: Osmolarity of the gastric and duodenal contents in low birth weight infants fed human milk or various formulae. Acta Paediatr Scand 71:799-803, 1982

16. Van der Walt JH, Foate JA, Murrell D et al: A study of preoperative fasting in infants aged less than three months. Anaesth Intens Care 18:527-531, 1990

17. Roberts RB, Shirley MA: Antacid therapy in obstetrics (letter). Anesthesiology 53:83, 1980

18. Raidoo DM, Rocke DA, Brock-Utne JG et al: Critical volume for pulmonary acid aspiration: Reappraisal in a primate model. Br J Anaesth 65:248-250, 1990

19. Shorten G, Cutz E, Lerman J: The effects of pulmonary aspiration of human breast milk and normal saline in the intubated rabbit. Can J Anaesth (Vol 5) 41:A57-B, 1994

20. Schurizek K, Rybro L, Boggild-Madsen N et al: Gastric volume and pH in children for emergency surgery. Acta Anaesth Scand 30: 404-408, 1986

21. Bricker S, McLuckie A, Nightingale D: Gastric aspirates after trauma in children. Anesthesia 44: 721-724, 1989

22. Olsson G, Hallen B, Habraeus-Jonzon K: Aspiration during anesthesia: A computer-aided study of 185,358 anaesthetics. Acta Anaesth Scand 30:84-92, 1986

23. Nicolson SC, Betts EK, Jobes DR et al: Comparison of oral and intramuscular preanesthetic medication for pediatric inpatient surgery. Anesthesiology 71:8-10, 1989

24. Henderson JM, Brodsky DA, Fisher DM et al: Preinduction of anesthesia in pediatric patients with nasally administered sufentanil. Anesthesiology 68:671-675, 1988

25. Wilton NC, Leigh J, Rosen DR et al: Preanesthetic sedation of preschool children using intranasal midazolam. Anesthesiology 69:972-975, 1988

26. Walbergh EJ, Wills RJ, Eckhert J: Plasma concentrations of midazolam in children following intranasal administration. Anesthesiology 74:233-235, 1991

27. Weksler N, Ovadia L, Muati G et al:. Nasal ketamine for paediatric premedication. CJA 40:119-121, 1993

28. Feld LH, Champeau MW, van Steennis CA et al: Preanesthetic medication in children: A comparison of oral transmucosal fentanyl citrate versus placebo. Anesthesiology 71:374-377, 1989

29. Nelson PS, Streisand JB, Mulder SM et al: Comparison of oral transmucosal fentanyl citrate and an oral solution of meperidine,

diazepam, and atropine for premedication in children. Anesthesiology 70:616-621, 1989

30. Stanley TH, Beiman BC, Rawal N et al: The effects of oral transmucosal fentanyl citrate premedication on preoperative behavioral responses and gastric volume and acidity in children. Anesth Analg 69:328-335, 1989

31. Streisand JB, Stanley TH, Hague B et al:..Oral transmucosal fentanyl citrate premedication in children. Anesth Analg 69:28-34, 1989

32. Streisand JB, Varvel JR, Stanski DR et al: Absorption and bioavailability of oral transmucosal fentanyl citrate. Anesthesiology 75:223-229, 1991

33. Feld L, Negus JB, White PF: Oral midazolam preanesthetic medication in pediatric outpatients. Anesthesiology 73:831-834, 1990

34. McMillan CO, Spahr-Schopfer IA, Sikich N et al: Premedication of children with oral midazolam. Can J Anaesth 39:545-550, 1992

35. Levine MF, Spahr-Schopfer IA, Hartley E et al: Oral midazolam premedication in children: The minimum time interval for separation from parents. Can J Anaesth 40:726-729, 1993

36. Payne K, Mattheyse FJ, Liebenberg D et al: The pharmacokinetics of midazolam in paediatric patients. Eur J Clin Pharmac 37:267-272, 1989

37. Stewart KG, Rowbottom SJ, Aitken AW et al: Oral ketamine premedication for paediatric cardiac surgery: A comparison with intramuscular morphine (both after oral trimeprazine). Anaesth Intens Care 18:11-14, 1990

38. Gutstein HB, Johnson KL, Heard MB et al: Oral ketamine preanesthetic medication in children. Anesthesiology 76:28-33, 1992

39. Alderson P, Lerman J: Oral premedication for paediatric ambulatory anesthesia: A comparison of midazolam and ketamine. Can J Anaesth 41:221-226, 1994

40. Mikawa K, Maekawa N, Nishina K et al: Efficacy of oral clonidine premedication in children. Anesthesiology 79:926-941, 1993

41. Karl HW, Rosenberger JL, Larach MG et al: Transmucosal administration of midazolam for premedication in pediatric patients. Anesthesiology 78:885-891, 1993

ANESTHESIA FOR THE EX-PREMATURE INFANT

J. M. Badgwell

Because of an increased survival rate in the neonatal intensive care unit (NICU), more and more "ex-preemies" are presenting to the operating room for surgical procedures. Remember that the premature infant is defined as being less than 37 weeks gestational age. Therefore, an "ex-preemie" by definition has now reached greater than 37 weeks conceptual age. This discussion will consider the anesthetic management of premature, as well as ex-premature, infants.

TYPICAL EX-PREMATURE CASE

You notice on the operative schedule that a 2-month old infant is listed for retinal cryotherapy *under MAC!* When you visit the child, you discover that his gestational age is 28 weeks and his postnatal age is 9 weeks, giving the child a conceptual age of 37 weeks. You further discover that the child had severe respiratory distress syndrome (RDS) and was "on a ventilator" for 2 weeks in the NICU.

As the anesthesiologist caring for this infant, you must first ask yourself, "Can I do this case as a MAC?" It has been my experience that most of these infants require general anesthesia to provide adequate surgical immobilization. Deep sedation would be hazardous because of the potential risk to the airway of obstruction and/or the development of apnea.

You must then determine the extent of pulmonary involvement. Does the infant have bronchopulmonary dysplasia? Bronchopulmonary dysplasia represents "chronic lung disease" of the premature and is essentially an x-ray diagnosis. It occurs in 10-20% of premature infants. Children with known bronchopulmonary dysplasia have been diagnosed and are usually being followed by a pediatrician. However, even without parent awareness or a radiographic diagnosis, some premature infants will have residual lung disease. These children can be diagnosed by asking the

229

T.H. Stanley and P.G. Schafer (eds.), Pediatric and Obstetrical Anesthesia, 229-243.
© 1995 *Kluwer Academic Publishers.*

parents if the infant had the "breathing done for him," and if the infant has had recurrent pulmonary infections.

Children with residual pulmonary involvement will have altered pulmonary function tests consisting of increased functional residual capacity, decreased pulmonary compliance, and increased airway resistance. These abnormalities will lead to altered arterial blood gases and may lead to spuriously low end-tidal PCO_2 measurements. Children with bronchopulmonary dysplasia often have a large difference in the arterial and end-tidal PCO_2 values due to loss of adventitial and vascular pulmonary tissue that results in an increased dead space ventilation.

PREOPERATIVE ASSESSMENT

The preoperative assessment should include a careful calculation of the patient's various ages. *Gestational age* is the time from conception to birth. *Postnatal age* is the time period from birth to the present time. *Conceptual age* is from conception to the present time. A term infant is defined as one with a gestational age of 37-42 weeks, whereas a preterm infant is less than 37 weeks gestational age. By my interpretation, an "ex-premature" infant is a preemie who has attained a postconceptual age of 40 weeks. Up until then, s/he is merely "premature." Term infants weighing less than 2500 g are defined as small for gestational age (SGA). These infants are prone to aspiration pneumonia and hypoglycemia. Preterm infants, on the other hand, have a high incidence of hyaline membrane disease and perioperative apnea. Newborn infants with the respiratory distress syndrome (RDS) exhibit tachypnea, inspiratory retraction, expiratory grunt, and oxygen hemoglobin desaturation.

INTRAOPERATIVE MANAGEMENT OF THE CHILD WITH BRONCHOPULMONARY DYSPLASIA

Intraoperative pulmonary care includes endotracheal intubation, controlled ventilation, and PEEP (2-4 mm H_2O). Chronic air trapping in preterm infants with bronchopulmonary dysplasia may preclude the intraoperative use of nitrous oxide. Excessive inflation pressures must also be avoided in infants with bronchopulmonary dysplasia. Intraoperative fluid therapy must be monitored carefully to avoid pulmonary edema, particularly in infants receiving diuretic therapy.

ENDOTRACHEAL INTUBATION

Rather than needing a reason to intubate premature and ex-premature infants, I usually need a good reason *not* to intubate them. It is generally safer to intubate these infants because they have: 1) a higher incidence of airway obstruction, 2) poorly developed respiratory control, 3) a biphasic response to hypoxia (initial increase in respiration, then apnea), and 4) a very compliant, circular rib cage with horizontal placement of the diaphragm. This latter factor causes the work of breathing to be increased in infants, especially if partial airway obstruction occurs. Furthermore, infants only have about 25% (10% in prematures) of the Type 1 anaerobic resistant fibers and, therefore, develop respiratory fatigue more easily than older infants and children. Finally, neonates and ex-prematures have an increased oxygen consumption, decreased functional residual capacity, and an increased closing volume compared to older infants and children. For these reasons, I intubate and control ventilation in all infants.

Should infants be intubated awake? Unless the infant is very sick or has a full stomach, I prefer to anesthetize him/her before intubation. If awake intubation is to be performed, it should be done using an oxyscope, a laryngoscope blade that allows delivery of supplemental oxygen. Topical lidocaine may be applied to the mucosa of the tongue and posterior pharynx by allowing the child to suckle lidocaine jelly. The disadvantage of awake intubation in infants is the potential development of bradycardia or hypertension. These factors may in turn lead to increased intracranial pressure and/or intraventricular hemorrhage. Most infants, unless they are critically ill, can tolerate anesthesia for intubation.

ENDOTRACHEAL EXTUBATION

These infants do better when their tracheas are extubated with the infant fully awake. If the infant is not fully awake at the end of the operation, s/he should be extubated in the postanesthesia care unit with the anesthesiologist in attendance. In small infants, extubation during early awakening and residual light anesthesia often is followed by breath holding or apnea, which may lead to sudden oxygen-hemoglobin desaturation and hypoxia bradycardia. Therefore, in neonates, it is much safer to delay extubation until they are fully awake. A fully awake infant moves his/her extremities purposefully and opens his eyes, the true sign of awakening. "Deep extubation," or tracheal extubation while the infant is deeply anesthetized, is inadvisable in infants but, rather, is reserved for older pediatric patients.

During extubation, infants may respond to laryngeal stimulation by breath holding or laryngospasm. If so, jaw thrust using the survival position (thumbs on the mask, fingertips behind the ramus of the mandible, applying anterior traction that usually dislocates the tempero-mandibular joint) and positive pressure ventilation using a "flutter" technique will eventually allow ventilation of the infant's lungs. If this maneuver does not work, reintubation facilitated by succinylcholine may be required.

CONSIDERATIONS FOR RETROLENTAL FIBROPLASIA

It is generally considered that preterm infants under 44 weeks of gestational age (the age when vascularization of the retina is completed) are at risk of retinopathy of prematurity (ROP). Recent studies, however, have identified a subpopulation at increased risk for ROP (1). The most important variable is apparently birth weight; those infants weighing less than 1000 g have a 45% chance of developing ROP (1). Nevertheless, gestational age is still a correlate because it determines the degree of retinal development.

It was once advised that PaO_2 must be maintained below 80 mm Hg. The role of oxygen, however, has become controversial. In 1951, oxygen therapy was described as a factor in the pathogenesis of ROP (2). In this study, a higher incidence of retinal problems was reported in a private nursery where oxygen was readily available. The premature babies of poorer families, cared for by the ward nursery, where oxygen was less readily available, had a lower incidence of ROP. In the 1960s, the risk for ROP was thought to be associated with an arterial oxygen tension greater than 100 mm Hg. Studies in the mid-1980s implicated the free radicals, oxygen$^-$ and OH$^-$, as well as hydrogen peroxide, in the genesis of ROP. Normally, enzymes such as superoxide dismutase and cytochrome oxidase protect susceptible cell membranes against these injurious products of oxygen-mediated reactions. The immature retina may be deficient in these enzyme systems and thus more vulnerable to the effects of hyperoxia (3). Studies now suggest a changing oxygen environment as a contributing factor in ROP. Other reports, however, describe premature infants who develop ROP despite not receiving supplemental oxygen (4). Furthermore, the disease has occurred in full-term infants of normal birth weight and in infants with cyanotic heart disease (5,6).

So, where to keep the SpO_2 of ex-premature infants? It would appear that the SpO_2 should be kept between 90-95% to prevent excessive oxygenation and retinal artery vasoconstriction. Below 90%, the oxygen-hemoglobin dissociation curve is very steep, and tissue oxygenation may be in jeopardy. To measure PaO_2 in the retina, arterial catheters or pulse oximetry must measure preductal oxygenation (right upper extremity or temporary artery).

SURGICAL TREATMENT OF ROP

The surgical treatment of ROP is directed at preventing its progression and repairing existing retinal defects (7,8). The immature avascular retina secretes an angiogenic factor in response to hypoxia. The angiogenic factor then stimulates a vasoproliferative reaction in the leading edge of the vascular retina. Surgical ablation of the avascular retina inhibits the release of angiogenic factor and thus minimizes neovascularization. Cryotherapy (or application of a cooled probe) is aimed at destroying the avascular retina. Cryotherapy is moderately successful in limiting the extent of retinal disease but is not uniformly effective in preventing eventual retinal detachment.

For a posterior retinal detachment, scleral buckling is indicated. In the buckling procedure, a silicone prosthesis is implanted in the sclera to secure the retina against the globe. If neovascularization has progressed into the vitreous, however, a scleral buckle alone is insufficient and vitrectomy is required. Vitrectomy is performed through either a "closed" approach or an "open-sky" approach. Surgical exposure is improved by removing the cornea and preserving it in tissue solution during the operation. The lens is removed, revealing the abnormal retrolental membranes, vascular vitreous, and detached retina. The membranes and vitreous are finely cut and aspirated, thus allowing the retina to be repositioned against the choroid. The cornea is then reattached, and saline is injected to re-establish the fluid nature of the anterior chamber.

DOSAGE CONSIDERATIONS FOR PRETERM INFANTS

VOLATILE AGENTS

Although the MAC for halothane in premature infants has not been studied, the anesthetic requirements of isoflurane have been investigated (9). The MAC of isoflurane in preterm neonates less than 32 weeks gestational age is 1.28 ± 0.17%, and in neonates of 32-37 weeks gestational age it is 1.41 ± 0.19%. In full-term neonates, the MAC for isoflurane is 1.60 ± 0.03%.

FENTANYL

There is little information available on the use of high-dose fentanyl anesthesia in preterm infants. There is, however, one pharmacokinetic study in infants who received fentanyl (30 µg/kg) at the start of surgery for repair of patent ductus arteriosus (10). In this study, the T1/2 Beta was 6-32 hours (17.7 ± 9.3), volume of distribution was between 2206 and 3896 ml/kg (2904 ± 517), and clearance was between 104.1 ml/kg/min (2.4 ± 1.3). These pharmacokinetic data are compared to older patients in Figure 1.

Although blood pressure remained stable throughout surgery, there was a gradual increase in heart rate at the time of skin closure (10). These findings correlate well with the clinical impression that towards the end of this operation, anesthesia becomes lighter after a single dose of fentanyl when no other anesthetic agents are given. Of particular interest was the lack of correlation between the prolonged elimination of fentanyl and the termination of its pharmacodynamic effect (10). At the end of surgery, most infants moved or breathed spontaneously despite high plasma concentrations of fentanyl (10). This phenomenon is explained by redistribution of fentanyl from the brain into fat and muscle. In summary, these studies suggest that a bolus of fentanyl (30 µg/kg) provides stable hemodynamics, but may not provide adequate analgesia during skin closure in these patients. It therefore seems reasonable to use fentanyl (30 µg/kg initially, followed by repeated doses as needed) as the sole agent in premature infants for repair of PDA. This regimen may delay onset of spontaneous respiration requiring mechanical ventilation continued into the immediate postoperative period.

The doses of fentanyl recommended above (30 µg/kg) may be appropriate for the preterm infant undergoing PDA ligation when postoperative ventilation is planned, but this dose may be excessive for the premature or ex-premature undergoing minor surgery (e.g., inguinal hernia repair) when early extubation or no endotracheal intubation is planned. In these cases, fentanyl may cause apnea or prolonged respiratory depression requiring continued intubation, especially if the preemies have been given other anesthetic agents.

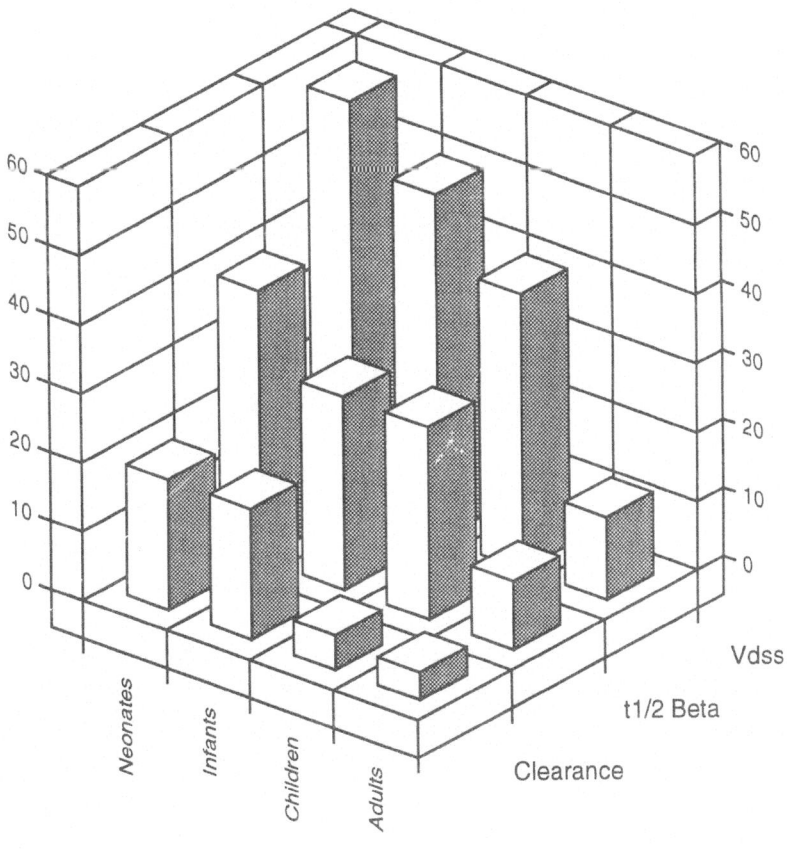

Figure 1.   The relationship of age and fentanyl pharmacokinetics. For the X-axis: Clearance = X value in ml/kg/min; T1/2 Beta = value x 10 min; and Vdss = value x 0.1 l/kg. Adapted from Collins (10) (Collins data = *) and Johnson (11).

ANESTHETIC TECHNIQUES FOR THE PREEMIE
OR THE EX-PREEMIE

GENERAL ANESTHESIA

If the airway is not a potential problem (e.g., if the infant does not have a "difficult" airway such as in Pierre-Robin Syndrome), I prefer to induce anesthesia in prematures with an intravenous technique using thiopental (5 mg/kg), atropine (0.02 mg/kg), and a muscle relaxant, followed by endotracheal intubation. If the infant has no IV access, I insert a #24 catheter into a dorsal hand, ventral wrist, or saphenous vein. Alternatively, a butterfly technique using a #27 butterfly needle may be used and a "real" IV started later. I prefer IV inductions in premature infants because it avoids potential complications that can occur during mask induction (breath holding, apnea, airway obstruction, laryngospasm, vomiting, and hypotension). At many leading institutions, however, anesthesia is induced using a face mask with spontaneous ventilation and maintained with a volatile agent without endotracheal intubation. This is an acceptable technique if one is able to recognize and treat the potential complications listed above.

REGIONAL ANESTHESIA WITH OR WITHOUT GENERAL ANESTHESIA

Caudal epidural blockade, with or without general anesthesia, may be used for intraoperative and postoperative analgesia after lower abdominal and genitourinary surgery in preterm infants. If general anesthesia is to be used, it is induced using either intravenous or inhalation technique. The trachea may or may not be intubated. Light anesthesia is maintained with nitrous oxide (60-70%) and halothane (0.2-0.5%). The infant is then turned on his side and given a caudal block with 0.5-1.25 ml/kg of 0.25% or 0.125% bupivacaine (maximum dose = 3 mg/kg) and epinephrine (5 μg/ml). If general anesthesia is not used, the block is induced using the same technique with the addition of gentle restraint for the infant. The infant is then given a sugar water nipple to suckle.

One must be very careful when using a combined general anesthetic with a volatile agent and a regional technique with bupivacaine. It has been shown that the volatile anesthetic agents enhance the toxic effects of bupivacaine when infused intravascularly in small subjects (12). Furthermore, it has been shown that hypoxia (13) and hypercarbia (Heavner et al, Reg Anesth, in press, 1994) that may occur secondary to airway obstruction also enhance the toxic effects of bupivacaine. Therefore, meticulous attention must be paid to airway patency when administering a combination anesthetic. For this reason, I prefer to intubate infants during the administration of combined general and regional anesthesia. The first sign of inadvertent intravascular injection of bupivacaine plus epinephrine is marked elevation of the T-wave on EKG (14).

The use of spinal anesthesia for hernia repair in premature infants less than 36 weeks gestational age recovering from RDS is reportedly a safe and satisfactory alternative to general anesthesia (15). Spinal anesthesia using hyperbaric tetracaine (0.4-0.6 mg/kg) inserted at the L_{4-5} level produces good analgesia with minimal cardiovascular instability.

TECHNICAL ASPECTS OF ANESTHESIA

THE ANESTHESIA MACHINE

Any anesthesia machine may be used in premature and ex-preemies if the machine has the capability to deliver oxygen and air using very low flows (see discussion below on fresh gas flows).

VENTILATORS

Of the many ventilators available for use in neonatal anesthesiology, four have proven to be very useful: the Sechrist Infant Ventilator Model IV-100B, the Ohmeda 7800, the Siemens-Elema 900C Servo, and the Drager Narcomed.

SECHRIST INFANT VENTILATOR

The Sechrist Infant Ventilator (SIV) is a "time-cycle, flow-controller," a fancy term for a "mechanical thumb." Closure of the expiratory valve ("the mechanical thumb") creates positive pressure in the breathing circuit and inflates the lungs. When pressure in the breathing circuit reaches the set pressure limit, an expiratory valve opens and gas within the breathing circuit is removed. Therefore, the SIV is a "pressure" ventilator. The SIV allows the user to set the peak inspiratory pressure (PIP), positive end-expiratory pressure (PEEP), respiratory rate (f) and I:E ratio. The SIV is applied to a Mapleson D breathing circuit simply by connecting the y-connector of the SIV breathing circuit to the end of either a Jackson-Rees circuit or a Bain circuit.

OHMEDA 7800 VENTILATOR

The Ohmeda 7800 ventilator is a volume controller with adult and pediatric bellows (300 ml maximum tidal volume). This ventilator may be connected to a circle system or a Bain circuit, both of which channel gas through a CO_2 absorber in the Ohmeda GMS system. We have used this ventilator with a pediatric breathing circuit with success in premature infants (as small as 500 grams), neonates, and ex-preemies.

Due to a large compression volume loss of gas in the system, initial set tidal volumes per kg are larger in neonates than older infants. [V_t: set: ~ 150 ml/kg for neonates ≤ 2 kg, ~ 75 ml/kg for infants ~ 5 kg, and ~ 25 ml/kg for infants ≤ 10 kg (Badgwell, unpublished data, 1994)]. This ventilator provides for accurate measurement of expired tidal volumes down to a minimum of 20 mls and allows for precise PEEP, PIP, and I:E ratio. It has an added safety feature—an adjustable PIP limiting dial that can be set as low as 20 cm H_2O.

In infants with very poor compliance (e.g., those with congenital diaphragmatic hernia), volume-controlled ventilation with a highly compliant breathing circuit, such as an adult circle system, may not adequately ventilate the infant's lungs. Should this situation occur, a pressure-limited ventilator may be used to provide adequate ventilation.

SIEMENS-ELEMA 900C SERVO VENTILATOR

This complex but useful ventilator allows for precise control of volume or pressure and PEEP and provides for a variety of ventilator modes (CPAP, pressure support, etc.). It is used by attaching the fresh gas flow (FGF) from the machine to the low pressure gas inlet on the Siemens. When FGF ≥ the set minute ventilation on the Siemens, sufficient working pressure (as indicated by a gauge on the ventilator) will be provided.

DRAGER NARKOMED

The ventilator on the Narkomed anesthesia machine may be used with either adult or pediatric bellows. When using the pediatric bellows, tidal volume is dependent on inspiratory flow (adjusted by turning the inspiratory flow dial) rather than by the preadjusted bellows height. A PIP limiting valve is present on the latest Narkomed, but there is no inherent or adjustable pressure limiting device on the earlier models. The absence of a pressure-limiting device may lead to barotrauma of small infants if excessive pressure on tidal volume is delivered inadvertently. The Drager measuring exhaled tidal volumes of 100 ml or greater.

MANUAL VENTILATION

There are times during surgery on neonates (e.g., tracheoesophageal fistula) when manual ventilation is required. For the most part, however, controlled ventilation with a ventilator is optimal. A recent report refutes the commonly held belief that the "educated hand" permits clinicians to detect subtle changes in pulmonary compliance in neonates during anesthesia (16). Steward has editorialized that, "in this day of reliable volume-cycled ventilators . . . mechanical ventilation provides very predictable and constant gas exchange over long periods of time"(17).

BREATHING CIRCUITS

For neonatal anesthesia, one may use either a Mapleson D (Jackson-Rees modification of the Ayre's t-piece or Bain circuit) breathing circuit or a circle system (pediatric or adult). Fresh gas flow requirements for Mapleson D circuits are 250 ml/kg/min as a starting point, in an attempt to provide an end-tidal PCO_2 of 38 mm Hg (18). When controlled ventilation is used in infants, the resistance and work of breathing added by inspiratory and expiratory valves in circle systems is not an issue. Compression volume loss is less in Mapleson D circuits than circle systems unless a CO_2 absorption canister is used with the Bain (e.g., the Ohmeda GMS system).

MONITORING

The essential monitors include rectal temperature, EKG, pulse oximetry, precordial or esophageal stethoscope, blood pressure, and capnography.

TEMPERATURE REGULATION AND MONITORING

One does not need to actively heat and humidify the breathing circuit (e.g., using a cumbersome cascade humidifier) to prevent heat and moisture loss in infants. The pediatric-sized heat and moisture exchangers (e.g., mini Humid-vents) are adequate to provide humidity and to preserve body temperature in infants (19).

BLOOD PRESSURE AND HEART RATE

The normal systolic blood pressure in newborn infants is about 80 mm Hg until around 2 hours of age, is about 70 mm Hg in the first day of life, returns to 80 mm Hg by 1 week, and then increases to about 100 mm Hg by 6 months of age. Heart rate is about 150 in the first day of life, 140 in the first week, and 160 in the first month. Bradycardia in the neonate is defined as a heart rate less than 130 beats per minute.

CAPNOGRAPHY

Accurate measurement of respiratory gases may be obtained in infants ventilated through a Mapleson D circuit using flow-through capnography (20), or by using aspiration capnography and sampling from anywhere in the endotracheal tube or from the narrowest portion of the endotracheal tube connector (20,21). Accurate measurements may be sampled from the elbow of the breathing circuit when using a pediatric circle system (including the Seimens-Elema Servo 900C ventilator) (22) or when using a Mapleson D circuit with a Sechrist Infant Ventilator (23).

POSTANESTHETIC RESPIRATORY COMPLICATIONS

POSTOPERATIVE APNEA

It is well-known that preemies and ex-preemies undergoing elective surgery are prone to develop perioperative respiratory complications (24). Preterm infants with a history of idiopathic apnea are more susceptible than full-term babies to develop life-threatening apnea in the postoperative period. Apnea is usually described as a cessation of breathing for 20 seconds or more resulting in cyanosis and bradycardia. This phenomenon occurs in 20-30% of preterm infants during the first month of life. Steward reported an 18% incidence of apnea in preterm infants during the first 12 hours after surgery (24). Liu and others reported an increased incidence of postanesthetic apnea in infants with a postconceptual age of less than 44 weeks (25). By contrast, Kurth observed postanesthetic apnea occurring in infants as old as 55 weeks conceptual age (26). These studies have led to the recommendation that infants younger than 44 weeks conceptual age who need surgery must be admitted to the hospital for 24-36 hours for postoperative monitoring and discharged only when they have been free of apnea for 12-24 hours.

OTHER CONSIDERATIONS TO PREVENT POSTOPERATIVE APNEA

Caffeine (10 mg/kg) infused at the time of induction may be used to reduce the risk of perioperative apnea (27). Preliminary results of a small number of infants indicate that spinal anesthesia without sedation is associated with less apnea than is general anesthesia or spinal anesthesia with ketamine sedation (28). Similarly, in former preterm infants given either a spinal or general anesthetic, postoperative arterial desaturation occurred with greater frequency and to greater degrees after general anesthesia (28,29). The incidence of apnea, however, was not significantly different (30). Finally, infants with anemia of prematurity, generally a benign condition, are at increased risk of developing postoperative apnea (30). Therefore, if anemia exists, it is preferable to delay elective surgery and give iron supplementation until the hematocrit is above 30%. If surgery cannot be delayed, one should be aware of the increased risk of postoperative apnea.

REFERENCES

1. Flynn JT: Acute proliferative retrolental fibroplasia: Multivariate risk analysis. Trans Am Ophthalmol Soc 81:549-591, 1983
2. Kinsey VE, Hemphill FM: Symposium: Retrolental fibroplasia (retinopathy of prematurity); etiology of retrolental fibroplasia; preliminary report of cooperative study of retrolental fibroplasia. Am J Ophthalmol 40:216-223, 1955
3. Patz A: The role of oxygen in retrolental fibroplasia. Trans Am Ophthalmol Soc 66:940-985, 1968
4. Adamkin DH, Shott RJ, Cook LN et al: Nonhyperoxic retrolental fibroplasia. Pediatrics 670:828-830, 1977
5. Brockhurst RJ, Chishti MI: Cicatricial retrolental fibroplasia: Its occurrence without oxygen administration and in full-term infants. Graefes Arch Clin Exp Ophthalmol 195:113-128, 1975
6. Kalina RE, Hodson WA, Morgan BC: Retrolental fibroplasia in a cyanotic infant. Pediatrics 50:765-768, 1972
7. Hirose T, Lou PL: Retinopathy of prematurity. Int Ophthalmol Clin 26:1-23, 1986
8. Flynn JT: Oxygen and retrolental fibroplasia: Update and challenge. Anesthesiology 60:397-399, 1984
9. LeDez KM, Lerman J: The minimum alveolar concentration (MAC) of isoflurane in preterm neonates. Anesthesiology 67:301-307, 1987
10. Collins C, Koren G, Crean P et al: The correlation between fentanyl pharmacokinetics and pharmacodynames in preterm infants during PDA ligation. Anesthesiology 61:A442, 1984

11. Johnson KL, Erickson JP, Holley FO et al: Fentanyl pharmacokinetics in the pediatric population. Anesthesiology 61:A441, 1984

12. Badgwell JM, Heavner JE, Kytta J: Bupivacaine toxicity in young pigs is age-dependent and is affected by volatile anesthetics. Anesthesiology 73:297, 1990

13. Heavner JE, Dryden DF, Sanghani V et al: Severe hypoxemia enhances central nervous system and cardiovascular toxicity of bupivacaine in lightly anesthetized pigs. Anesthesiology 77:142-7, 1992

14. Freid EB, Bailey AG, Valley RD: Electrocardiographic and hemodynamic changes associated with unintentional intravascular injection of bupivacaine with epinephrine in infants. Anesthesiology 79:394-398, 1993

15. Albajian JC, Mellish PWP, Browne AE et al: Spinal anesthesia for surgery in the high-risk infant. Anesth Analg 63:359, 1984

16. Spears RS, Yeh A, Fisher DM et al: The "educated hand": Can anesthesiologists assess changes in neonatal pulmonary compliance manually? Anesthesiology 75:55, 1991

17. Steward DJ: The "not-so-educated hand" of the pediatric anesthesiologist. Anesthesiology 75:555, 1991

18. Badgwell JM, Wolf AM, McEvedy BAB et al: Fresh gas flow formulae do not accurately predict end-tidal PCO_2 in paediatric patients. Can Anaesth 35:581-586, 1988

19. Bissonnette B, Sessler DI: Passive or active inspired gas humidification increases thermal steady-state temperatures in anesthetized infants. Anesth Analg 69:783, 1989

20. Badgwell JM, Heavner JE: End-tidal carbon dioxide pressure in neonates and infants measured by aspiration and flow-through capnography. J Clin Monit 7:285-288, 1991

21. Badgwell JM, McLeod ME, Lerman J et al: End-tidal PCO_2 measurements sampled at the distal and proximal ends of the endotracheal tube in infants and children. Anesth Analg 66:959-964, 1967

22. Badgwell JM, Heavner JE, May WS et al: End-tidal PCO_2 monitoring in infants and children ventilated with either a partial rebreathing or a non-rebreathing circuit. Anesthesiology 66:405-410, 1987

23. Hillier SC, Badgwell JM, McLeod ME et al: Accuracy of end-tidal PCO_2 measurements using a sidestream capnometer in infants and children ventilated with the Sechrist Infant Ventilator. Can J Anaesth 37:321, 1990

24. Steward DJ: Preterm infants are more prone to complications following minor surgery than are term infants. Anesthesiology 56:304-306, 1982

25. Liu LMP, Cote CJ, Goudsouzian NG et al: Life-threatening apnea in infants recovering from anesthesia. Anesthesiology 59:506-510, 1983

26. Kurth CD, Spitzer AR, Broennle AM et al: Postoperative apnea in preterm infants. Anesthesiology 66:483-488, 1987

27. Welborn LG, Hannallah RS, Fink R et al: High-dose caffeine suppresses postoperative apnea in former preterm infants. Anesthesiology 71:346-349, 1989

28. Welborn LG, Rice LJ, Broadman LM et al: Postoperative apnea in former preterm infants: Prospective comparison of spinal and general anesthesia. Anesthesiology 72:838-842, 1990

29. Krane EJ, Haberkern CM, Jacobsen CE: A comparison of spinal and general anesthesia in the former preterm infant. Anesthesiology 75:A912, 1991

30. Welborn LG, Hannallah RS, Higgins T et al: Does anemia increase the risk of postoperative apnea in former preterm infants? Anesthesiology 73:A1091, 1990

MANAGEMENT OF THE DIFFICULT PEDIATRIC AIRWAY

F. A. Berry

The ASA Task Force on the Difficult Airway developed an algorithm for the management of the difficult airway (Figure 1). A difficult airway is characterized by difficulty in both ventilation and intubation of the patient. The algorithm is divided into two major pathways. One of these strongly suggests the use of awake intubation. However, the pediatric patient is not a candidate, for the most part, for an awake intubation. Therefore, the path of the algorithm for general anesthesia includes the uncooperative patient and the pediatric patient, since almost all of them require general anesthesia for intubation.

The basic principles of the algorithm for the difficult airway apply to the pediatric patient, as well. The repeated warnings of "get help" and "consider awakening the patient" are true for all age groups. The rest of this discussion will focus on identification of the child with the difficult airway and the subsequent management thereof (1).

The approach to the difficult airway will be discussed under three main headings: 1) the anatomy of the airway, and of intubation; 2) the physiology and pharmacology of the protective airway reflexes; and 3) the clinical management. In talking with parents, any history of a difficult intubation, etc., is a red flag. The history of a difficult anesthetic experience can never be ignored, regardless of what the anesthesiologist considers his/her level of skill, since there are skilled anesthesiologists everywhere. There are various methods used for predicting the difficult airway but, in general, they depend upon three things: 1) the ability to extend the neck; 2) the ability to open the mouth; and 3) laryngoscopy.

Laryngoscopy involves displacement of the soft tissue of the oropharynx, which allows a line of vision to be developed from the teeth or mandibular alveolar ridge to the epiglottis and then the larynx. The soft tissue is displaced into potential space that is encompassed and, therefore, potentially restricted by an incomplete bony ring that is bound posteriorly by the hyoid bone, laterally by the rami of the mandible, and anteriorly by the mentum of the mandible. Any alteration in the shape or

245

T.H. Stanley and P.G. Schafer (eds.), Pediatric and Obstetrical Anesthesia, 245-252.
© 1995 Kluwer Academic Publishers.

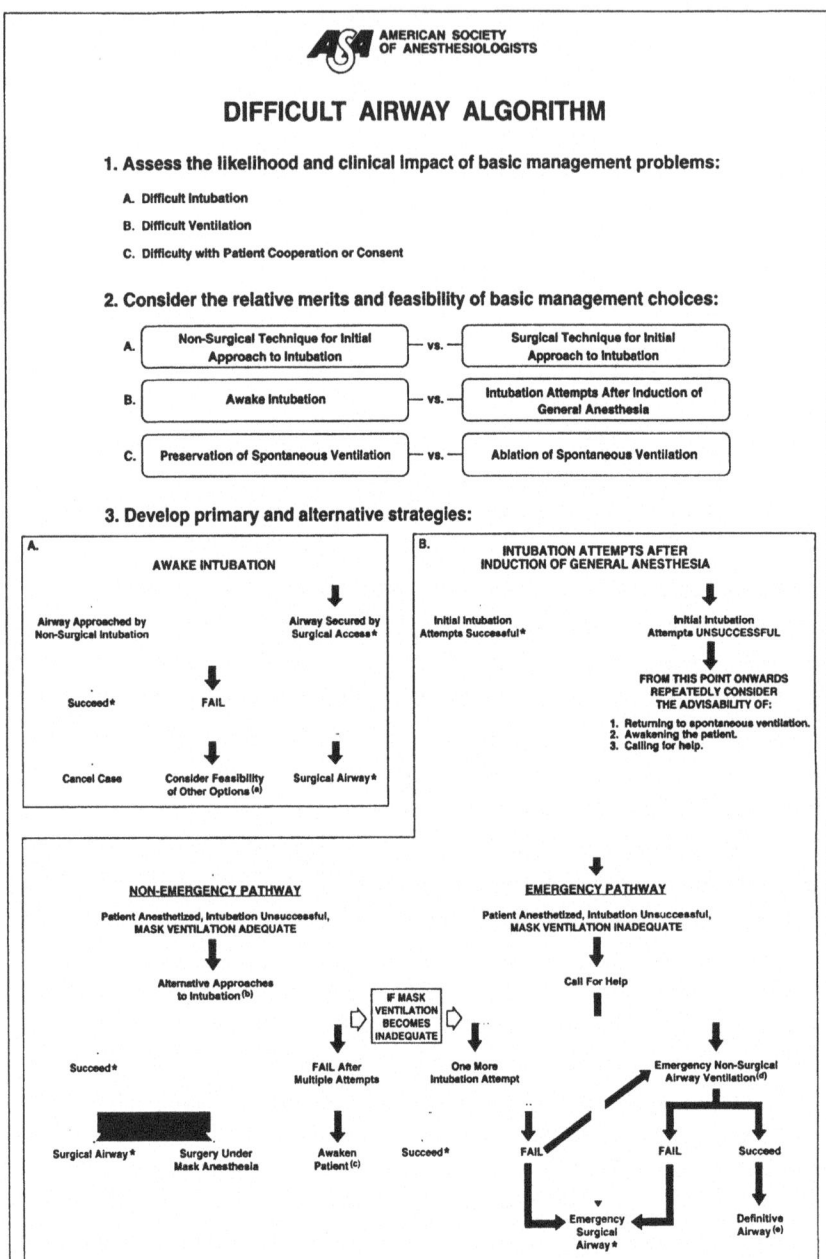

Figure 1. Difficult airway algorithm.

size of the bony structures results in a decrease in the space in which the soft tissue can be displaced with a laryngoscope. The potential displacement area may be normal, but there may be excessive soft tissue in the area that will have the same effect. This occurs in conditions such as cystic hygroma. This space can be evaluated by measuring the distance from the mentum of the mandible to the hyoid bone. The usual distance in an adult is 2-3 fingerbreadths, which is approximately 4-5 cms. In the infant, it is usually 2-3 cms.

PHYSIOLOGY AND PHARMACOLOGY OF THE PROTECTIVE AIRWAY REFLEXES

The protective airway reflexes, under normal circumstances, are reflexes that allow a remarkable coordination of vocalization, ventilation, and alimentation, while preventing any trespass by a foreign body, such as food, into the tracheobronchial tree. The partial activation of these reflexes during light levels of anesthesia often leads to laryngospasm, which is the major hazard of the difficult airway. Clinically, laryngospasm is usually characterized as either *partial* or *complete*. If there is partial laryngospasm, applying small degrees of positive-end expiratory pressure will often maintain the larynx in the open position, as well as increase the gradient of pressure, which will increase the ventilation of the patient. Excessive pressure can cause a barotrauma of the larynx, which may turn partial laryngospasm into complete laryngospasm. Patients in complete laryngospasm cannot be ventilated with any amount of positive pressure. The larynx will only open because of either severe hypoxia or pharmacological agents. Complete laryngospasm leads to hypoxia as the oxygen reserve of the functional residual capacity is consumed.

Control of the airway reflexes can be accomplished by the pharmacological depression of these reflexes. The three major techniques to control the reflexes are: 1) general anesthesia, 2) muscle relaxants to paralyze the muscles of the protective reflexes, and 3) topical anesthesia with local anesthetics.

CLINICAL MANAGEMENT OF THE DIFFICULT AIRWAY

Airway obstruction and hypoxia can occur with such alarming speed that a surgeon and equipment must be in the operating room before the induction of anesthesia if an emergency surgical airway is needed. There are three approaches to the surgical airway: 1) emergency tracheotomy, 2) emergency cricothyrotomy, and 3) emergency transtracheal ventilation. Emergency tracheotomy usually cannot be performed rapidly enough; therefore, the most rapid method for oxygenating the patient is by cricothyrotomy, or by transtracheal ventilation. Transtracheal ventilation is very difficult in infants because of the small airway.

PREMEDICATION

Patients with a suspected difficult airway, in general, should only be premedicated with an anticholinergic, which is useful to dry up the airway secretions. This can be administered orally 30 minutes before the procedure. At times, however, there may be difficulty in separating the child from his/her parents and achieving a peaceful induction. In those situations, moderate premedication under careful observation may be useful to accomplish a smoother separation and induction of anesthesia. The major drug that is used for this purpose is oral midazolam in a dose of 0.5 to 0.75 mg/kg. If the child has a history of difficulty in airway management, then the child should be in the operating room for the induction. Concerns about the psychological trauma that may occur with the separation of the parent and child at the time of anesthesia and surgery need to be recognized; but if there is a potential airway disaster, these needs may become secondary to the medical problem of a difficult airway.

INDUCTION AND MAINTENANCE OF ANESTHESIA

Induction techniques for the difficult airway should be the same as for any type of surgery and depend on the age of the child and the degree of cooperation. In general, an inhalation induction with spontaneous breathing results in what most consider to be the safest induction technique. However, the small child from 6-8 months up to 4-5 years may not cooperate, and other induction techniques may be indicated. This author prefers rectal methohexital (dose 30 mg/kg). At times, the child may be difficult, uncooperative, and combative. In this instance, a stunning dose of ketamine (3 mg/kg) is given in the triceps or deltoid muscle. Regardless of the technique to begin with, the hope for the maintenance of the anesthetic is to use primarily a volatile agent, anesthetizing the patient deep enough with assisted ventilation to allow laryngoscopy and, if possible, intubation. Cricoid pressure can be used to minimize gastric distention if ventilation becomes difficult. Positive pressure with 5-10 cm of water gently applied will increase the pressure gradient from the anesthesia circuit to the lungs, thereby speeding up induction. After the induction of anesthesia, an IV infusion should be started as quickly as possible. Anticholinergics can be administered and then, if the patient begins to cough, IV lidocaine in a dose of 1-1.5 mg/kg can be given and repeated in 5 minutes. Lidocaine will deepen anesthesia, depress the protective airway reflexes, and enable the anesthesiologist to proceed with a smoother anesthetic. The moment of truth arrives when the patient is deep enough to be laryngoscoped. If during attempts at laryngoscopy the patient breathholds, coughs, or exhibits any other antisocial behavior, s/he is not deep enough. The major reason for difficulty with a difficult airway is insufficient anesthetic depth.

INTUBATION TECHNIQUES

If any part of the airway can be visualized, various maneuvers can be used to facilitate intubation. If the glottis is easily visible, or at least the posterior glottis is easily visible, then the use of a stylet in the endotracheal tube will allow a successful placement of the endotracheal tube. Sometimes only the posterior arytenoids are visible. In this case, downward pressure on the larynx may well bring enough of the glottis into view to allow the passage of an endotracheal tube. At times, only the tip of the epiglottis is visible, and posterior pressure is not sufficient to allow visualization of the arytenoids or the glottis. In this case, a stylet with a fairly sharp curve is used in the endotracheal tube, which allows the endotracheal tube to be brought up under the tip of the visualized epiglottis. The anesthesiologist has to imagine in his/her mind's eye the location of the glottis and, listening to breath sounds through the tip of the endotracheal tube as well as condensation in the endotracheal tube, direct the tube anteriorly up and through the vocal cords. At times, if the breath sounds are clear, the endotracheal tube can be slipped off the stylet and slowly rotated so that the bevel of the endotracheal tube will not become hung up in the anterior commissure. After what is thought to be successful intubation, end-tidal CO_2 is determined to confirm endotracheal intubation.

ALTERNATIVE TECHNIQUES FOR INTUBATION

If laryngoscopy is unsuccessful, which is defined as the inability to visualize any part of the airway, several options are available (2-11). These techniques are: 1) blind oral or blind nasal intubation; 2) retrograde intubation; 3) fiberoptic intubation; 4) fiberoptic intubation through an LMA; 5) tracheostomy; or 6) aborting the surgery if the anesthesiologist does not feel confident to proceed, or if the patient is intermittently hypoxic and the anesthesiologist is having difficulty reestablishing rapid and complete saturation of the hemoglobin.

THE UNSUSPECTED DIFFICULT AIRWAY

As the anesthesiologist fine-tunes his/her practice of anesthesia and becomes more familiar with the various congenital and acquired airway problems, there will be fewer and fewer "unsuspected" difficult airways encountered. However, there are children who, in the initial examination, appear to be normal but actually have very difficult airways. The unsuspected difficult airway presents just as the name suggests. It may manifest itself early in the induction of anesthesia, with obstruction developing and becoming difficult to reverse. It may become evident at the time of laryngoscopy, with difficulty in visualizing the larynx or any other part of the airway. Various explanations for the difficulty enter the anesthesiologist's thoughts. One of the goals of an anesthesiologist must be a knowledge of his/her technical expertise, so that when a difficult airway occurs, a rapid evaluation of the situation should quickly pinpoint the difficulty. As soon as the anatomical problem is recognized, the anesthesiologist can sort out the situation and proceed with one of the techniques mentioned above or abort the surgery and come back at a later date.

TIMING OF EXTUBATION

The problems presented by the difficult airway do not end with the end of surgery. The last major hurdle is how and when to extubate the patient. Extubation should be accomplished when the patient is awake, and the protective reflexes are intact. For small children, I prefer to extubate them in the prone position. If there is any question, the endotracheal tube is left in place for hours, or perhaps overnight, and the situation reevaluated. The anesthetic technique used in a child with a difficult intubation is, in general, that of a volatile agent, minimizing the amount of narcotic that is administered. If the child is going to have severe pain at the time of recovery from anesthesia, small doses of narcotic are appropriate intraoperatively for the purpose of comfort in the immediate postoperative period. However, the use of large doses of narcotics in children with a difficult intubation often means that the child will not be awake enough at the end of surgery to be extubated. If narcotics are given and the child appears to be awake and alert at the end of surgery, a trial of extubation should be attempted. However, often stimulation of the endotracheal tube is enough stimulus that the child objects to the presence of the endotracheal tube; as soon as the endotracheal tube is withdrawn, the stimulus is also withdrawn, and the child may become obstructed. If narcotics have been given, it is appropriate to be ready with narcotic reversal agents, such as naloxone to immediately reverse the sedation and obstruction. If there is any doubt, the patient should remain intubated until the anesthesiologist feels comfortable extubating the patient. This may require that the anesthesiologist spend extra time in the recovery room.

POST-OBSTRUCTIVE PULMONARY EDEMA

Patients who become obstructed, and who make attempts to ventilate in spite of a closed glottis, are subject to developing what has been called "post-obstructive pulmonary edema," "post-hypoxic pulmonary edema," or "negative pressure pulmonary edema." The exact pathophysiology is not completely understood, but it takes a combination of hypoxia and obstruction. The most frequent time for post-obstructive pulmonary edema to occur is at the end of surgery, when premature extubation of the patient is followed by laryngospasm, hypoxia, and the ensuing pulmonary edema. This has often been called in the past, "silent aspiration." Obstruction and hypoxia may occur at the time of induction and intubation, and pulmonary edema may occur after this. The treatment for this condition is providing positive-end expiratory pressure on the airway. If the patient is still intubated and has gross pulmonary edema, the tube should remain in place, and the patient should be given sedation and oxygen and remain intubated for a period of time. When these patients develop pulmonary edema, it is very tempting to try to suction the edema fluid out. However, once the diagnosis is made, the treatment is application of end expiratory positive pressure. Interrupting this positive pressure to suction the patient out will only result in an increase in the amount of pulmonary edema. This is a difficult concept for most nurses to understand and accept, but it is mandatory to avoid suctioning in this condition. It becomes more problematic when the patient has been extubated and this occurs. The question of whether or not to reintubate depends on the degree of symptomatology and hypoxia. Some patients require reintubation and treatment with PEEP and sedation. There is no place for Lasix in the treatment of this condition.

POST-CASE ANALYSIS

Several things must be done after the difficult airway is encountered and, hopefully, successfully managed. An accurate, legible note must be included in the anesthetic record or progress note. The parents should be told of the problem, and a letter describing the problem and the method of its management should be given to them.

REFERENCES

1. Berry FA: Anesthesia for the child with a difficult airway. In: Berry FA, ed. Anesthetic management of difficult and routine pediatric patients. 2nd edition. New York, Churchill Livingstone, 1990
2. Audenaert SM, Montgomery CL, Stone B et al: Retrograde-assisted fiberoptic tracheal intubation in children with difficult airways. Anesth Analg 73:660-664, 1991
3. Baraka A, Muallem M: Bullard laryngoscopy for tracheal intubation in a neonate with Pierre-Robin syndrome. Paediatr Anaesth 4:111-113, 1994
4. Benumof JL: Intubation and extubation of the patient with Pierre-Robin Syndrome. Anesthesiology 77:401, 1992
5. Berthelsen P, Prytz S, Jacobsen E: Two-stage fiberoptic nasotracheal intubation in infants: A new approach to difficult pediatric intubation. Anesthesiology 63:457-458, 1985
6. Borland LM, Casselbrant M: The Bullard laryngoscope: A new indirect oral laryngoscope (pediatric version). Anesth Analg 70:105-108, 1990
7. Borland LM, Swan DM, Leff S: Difficult pediatric endotracheal intubation: A new approach to the retrograde technique. Anesthesiology 55:577, 1981
8. Gupta B, McDonald JS, Brooks JHJ et al: Oral fiberoptic intubation over a retrograde guidewire. Anesth Analg 68:517-519, 1989
9. Holzman RS, Nargozian CD, Florence FB: Lightwand intubation in children with abnormal upper airways. Anesthesiology 69:784-787, 1988
10. Stone DJ, Stirt JA, Kaplan MJ et al: A complication of lightwand-guided nasotracheal intubation. Anesthesiology 61:780, 1984
11. Sutera PT, Gordon GJ: Digitally assisted tracheal intubation in a neonate with Pierre Robin Syndrome. Anesthesiology 78:983-985, 1993

MUSCLE RELAXANTS IN INFANTS AND CHILDREN

D. R. Cook

Neuromuscular blocking agents (relaxants) are commonly used in infants and children to facilitate intubation, to provide surgical relaxation, and to control ventilation intraoperatively and perhaps postoperatively. Throughout infancy, the neuromuscular junction matures physically and biochemically, the contractile properties of skeletal muscle change, body fluid volumes decrease, the amount of muscle in proportion to body weight increases, the acetylcholine receptor changes configuration, and the neuromuscular junction is variably sensitive to neuromuscular-blocking drugs. The purposes of this lecture are to review the factors that influence the differences in the ED95 of relaxants in infants and children, and to review the factors that influence the choice of a specific relaxant for various procedures. In large part, the lecture will deal with ultra-short, short, and intermediate duration relaxants.

SUCCINYLCHOLINE

On a weight basis, more succinylcholine is needed in infants than in older children or adults to produce apnea, to depress respiration, or to depress neuromuscular transmission. Cook and Fischer (1) noted that in infants, succinylcholine (1 mg/kg) produced neuroblockade about equal to that produced by 0.5 mg/kg in children (6-8 years). At these equipotent doses, there is no statistically significant difference between the times to recover to 50% (T50) and 90% (T90) neuromuscular transmission in the two groups. Complete neuromuscular blockade develops in children given 1.0 mg/kg of succinylcholine. The ED95 of succinylcholine (the estimated dose of relaxant required to give 95% neuromuscular blockade) is higher in infants than in children or adults (1-3).

Goudsouzian and Liu (4) needed threefold higher infusion rates of succinylcholine (mg/kg/hr) to maintain 90% twitch depression in young infants than in older infants or children. Phase II block occurred after a slightly larger dose of succinylcholine in infants than in the other age

253

T.H. Stanley and P.G. Schafer (eds.), Pediatric and Obstetrical Anesthesia, 253-263.
© 1995 *Kluwer Academic Publishers.*

groups. Differences in cholinesterase activity, receptor sensitivity, or volume of distribution may explain these age-related differences in succinylcholine requirements.

The neonate has about one-half the pseudocholinesterase activity of the older infant, child, or adult. Thus, it is likely that augmented cholinesterase activity is responsible in part for the infant's resistance to succinylcholine. When succinylcholine was given in equal dose on a surface area basis (40 mg/m^2), Walts and Dillon (5) found no difference between infants and adults in the times to recover to 10%, 50%, or 90% neuromuscular transmission; this dose of succinylcholine produced complete neuromuscular blockade in all patients. Cook and Fischer (1) noted a linear relationship between the log dose on a mg/m^2 basis and the maximum intensity of neuromuscular blockade for infants, children, and adults. They also saw a linear relationship between the logarithm of the dose on a mg/m^2 basis and to either 50% or 90% recovery time for infants and children as a combined group. Because of its relatively small molecular size, succinylcholine is rapidly distributed throughout the extracellular fluid. The blood volume and extracellular fluid (ECF) volume of the infant are significantly greater than the child's or adult's, on a weight basis. Therefore, on a weight basis (mg/kg), twice as much succinylcholine is needed in the infant as in adults to produce 50% neuromuscular blockade. Since ECF and surface area bear a nearly constant relationship throughout life (6-8 l/m^2), it is not surprising that there is a good correlation between succinylcholine dose (in mg/m^2) and response throughout life. The data of Goudsouzian and Liu (4) suggest that relative resistance to succinylcholine persists in some infants, even when the dose is transformed to mg/m^2/min. These data suggest that the acetylcholine receptor matures with age.

MIVACURIUM

Mivacurium, a short-acting relaxant, is metabolized by plasma cholinesterase. In adults, when administered in doses less than 2 times the ED95, mivacurium appears to be devoid of cardiovascular effects; larger doses may be associated with a transient decrease in blood pressure from histamine release. Compared with adults, children require significantly more mivacurium (mg/kg) during comparable anesthetic backgrounds. When referenced to body surface area (mg/m^2), however, the dosage requirements are not significantly different. This suggests that age-related dosage requirements for mivacurium may be associated with age-related differences in volume of distribution. At equal potent doses, the onset time of mivacurium is faster in children than in adults; the clinical duration is likewise shorter in children. We observed cutaneous flushing in 3 children given high doses of mivacurium and a transient 32% decrease in mean arterial pressure in one of these patients. Flushing was not always associated with hypotension. Pseudocholinesterase activity influences the clearance and hence infusion roles in children. Mivacurium can be administered by infusion for several hours with no evidence of cumulation, and with rapid spontaneous or pharmacologically induced return of neuromuscular function after termination of the infusion. The mivacurium infusion rates are higher in infants and children than in adults (6).

ATRACURIUM

Atracurium, a muscle relaxant of intermediate duration, is metabolized by nonspecific esters and spontaneously decomposes by Hofmann degradation. Both processes are sensitive to pH and temperature. Under physiologic conditions, the breakdown of atracurium is mainly by ester hydrolysis; Hofmann elimination plays a minor role. Deficient or abnormal pseudocholinesterases have little or no effect on atracurium degradation (7,8).

We and other researchers have studied the effects of both age and potent inhalation agents on dose-response relationships of atracurium in infants, children, and adolescents (9-13). On a weight basis (mg/kg), the ED95 for atracurium was similar in infants (1-6 months of age) and adolescents, whereas children had a higher dose requirement. On a surface area basis ($\mu g/m^2$), the ED95 for atracurium was similar in children and adolescents; the ED95 ($\mu g/m^2$) for atracurium in infants was much lower.

At equipotent doses (1 x ED95), the duration of effect (time from injection to 95% recovery) was 23 minutes in infants and 29 minutes in children and adolescents, compared with 44 minutes in adults. The time from injection to T25 (25% neuromuscular transmission) was 10 minutes in infants, 15 minutes in children and adolescents, and 16 minutes in adults. At T25, supplemental doses are needed to maintain relaxation for surgery. At higher multiples of the ED95, the duration of effect (i.e., the time to T5) will be longer but the times from T5 to T25 will be the same. The shorter duration of effect in the infant may represent a difference in pharmacokinetics.

The pharmacokinetics of atracurium differ between infants, children, and adults (14). The volume of distribution is larger and the elimination half-life is shorter in infants than in children or adults. For both reasons, clearance in infants is more rapid. Although there is little difference in the kinetics of atracurium among children aged 2-10, there are age-related differences in the volume of distribution, elimination half-life, and clearance. The volume of distribution is higher in the younger patients and the elimination half-life shorter; clearance is little different.

In children, "light" isoflurane anesthesia (1% end-tidal) reduces the atracurium required by about 30% from that needed with thiopental-narcotic anesthesia. There was no statistically significant difference in the isoflurane or halothane dose response curve. For clinical purposes, both potent agents should be viewed as potentiating atracurium to the same degree (11).

We have recently used a continuous infusion of dilute atracurium (200 μg/ml) following a bolus to maintain neuromuscular blockade at 95 ± 5% (11). To maintain this degree of steady-state block, an infusion rate of 4-5 μg/kg/min was required during halothane or isoflurane anesthesia, and 8-10 μg/kg/min was required with thiopental-narcotic anesthesia following an initial bolus. No cumulation was seen with prolonged infusion; recovery of neuromuscular transmission was prompt. The recovery of neuromuscular transmission from the same degree of blockade was similar with all three anesthetics. From these infusion data one can estimate the removal of atracurium. At steady state, the infusion rate (Iss) equals the removal rate (Rss) of atracurium. Removal is directly related to the clearance and steady-state plasma concentration associated with 95% neuromuscular blockade (CPss95). Hence:

$$Iss = Rss = Clearance \times CPss95$$

From this relationship, one can estimate Cpss95 from clearance and the steady-state infusion rate. In children, during the potent anesthetics, CPss95 is about 1 μg/ml; during balanced anesthesia, it is about 2 μg/ml. Comparable studies are in progress in infants. Atracurium infusion requirements in children during nitrous oxide-narcotic anesthesia can be compared to those noted in several age groups of adults during similar anesthesia. D'Hollander and co-workers (15) noted that in patients 16-85 years old, the steady state atracurium infusion rate averaged 14.4 mg/m^2/hr; this corresponds to 240 μg/m^2/min. This value is similar to the 226 μg/m^2/min we noted.

VECURONIUM

Vecuronium, a steroidal relaxant related to pancuronium, is taken up largely by the liver, then excreted unchanged via the hepatobiliary system (40-50%) or alternatively excreted through the kidneys (4-14%). Limited biotransformation of vecuronium to the 3 hydroxy-, 17 hydroxy-, and 3, 17 dihydroxy- metabolites occurs. Only 3 hydroxy- vecuronium is known to have neuromuscular blocking effects (16). These routes of elimination may be affected by physiologic changes at the extremes of life (17,18).

The ED95 for vecuronium is somewhat higher in children than in infants and adults (17-19). At equipotent doses (2 x ED95) of vecuronium, the duration of effect was longest for infants (73 minutes) compared with that for children (35 minutes) and adults (53 minutes). Thus, vecuronium does not have intermediate duration in infants. Vecuronium is potentiated by potent inhalation anesthetics but not in a dose-dependent manner (20,21).

Fisher et al have recently determined the pharmacodynamics and pharmacokinetics of vecuronium in infants and children (22). The volume of distribution and mean residence time were greater in infants than in children. Clearance was similar in the 2 groups; the CPss50 was lower in infants than in children. The combination of a large volume of distribution in infants and fixed clearance results in a longer mean residence time. After a single dose of relaxant, recovery of neuromuscular transmission depends on both distribution and elimination. The combination of a longer mean residence time and a lower sensitivity for vecuronium explains the prolongation of neuromuscular blockade in infants.

It is now clear that critically ill patients treated with neuromuscular blocking drugs for long periods of time can develop profound muscle weakness, atrophy, and muscle necrosis. The myopathy appears to have several priming factors (e.g., glucocorticoids, myotrophic infections, and sepsis) and triggering factors (steroidal non-depolarizing relaxants and perhaps their metabolites).

ROCURONIUM

Rocuronium, an intermediate steroidal derivative of vecuronium, is less potent than vecuronium but has a shorter onset time of neuromuscular blockade and a similar duration of action. It has minimal cardiovascular effects. The ED95 of rocuronium in adults receiving balanced anesthesia is 300 μg/kg (23). At 2 times ED95, the onset time of complete neuromuscular blockade is about 1.5 minutes. At these doses, the clinical duration (i.e., time to T25) was 40 minutes which is comparable to that of vecuronium at equal multiples of the ED95. Cardiovascular changes were minimal. Woelfel et al (24) determined the ED50 and ED95 of rocuronium in children during halothane anesthesia to be 179 $\mu g \cdot kg^{-1}$ and 303 $\mu g \cdot kg^{-1}$ respectively. The initial recovery index (T10-T25) after an ED95 dose (given in incremental doses) was 3.2 minutes. Thus, the duration of neuromuscular blockade is somewhat shorter in children than in adults; the duration of blockade in infants is longer than in children (24).

PIPECURONIUM AND DOXACURIUM

Pipecuronium and doxacurium, new long-acting relaxants without cardiovascular effects, have recently been introduced into clinical practice. Both have a duration of action in adults and children similar to that of pancuronium; but unlike pancuronium they appear to be devoid of cardiovascular effects (25-28). Renal failure can prolong the effect of these relaxants (29,30). Children require higher doses of each relaxant than adults to achieve the same degree of neuromuscular blockade during equivalent anesthetic backgrounds. At equipotent doses of pipecuronium and doxacurium, the time to recovery of neuromuscular transmission to T25 is shorter in children than adults. Infants appear to be more sensitive to the neuromuscular blocking effects of pipecuronium. However, the clinical duration of action (T25) of pipecuronium following cumulative dosing is about 20 minutes in infants and 30 minutes in children. Spontaneous recovery indexes are not prolonged in the younger patients.

CARDIOVASCULAR EFFECTS OF RELAXANTS

Succinylcholine exerts variable and seemingly paradoxical effects on the cardiovascular system. Typically, IV succinylcholine produces initial bradycardia and hypotension, followed after 15-30 seconds by tachycardia and hypertension. In the infant and small child, profound and sustained sinus bradycardia (rates of 50-60 per minute) is commonly observed (31,32); rarely, asystole occurs. Nodal rhythm and ventricular ectopic beats are seen in about 80% of children given a single IV injection of succinylcholine; such dysrhythmias are rarely seen following intramuscular succinylcholine. Recently cardiac arrest from massive hyperkalemia has been reported following succinylcholine in infants and children with unsuspected muscular dystrophy. This has lead to re-examination of the role of succinylcholine in elective surgical procedures (33-36).

As in adults, the incidence of bradycardia and other dysrhythmias is higher in children following a second dose of succinylcholine. Atropine (0.1 mg) appears to offer adequate protection against these bradyarrhythmias in all age groups. In infants, vagolytic doses of atropine (0.03 mg/kg) are required for protection; in older children, adequate protection is provided by doses of 0.005 mg/kg.

We have seen several young infants who developed fulminant pulmonary edema following intramuscular (IM) succinylcholine (4 mg/kg) (37). The pulmonary edema occurred within minutes of the IM injection and responded to continuous positive pressure ventilation (CPAP). Since that report, we have collected additional cases of pulmonary edema and pulmonary hemorrhage following IV succinylcholine, as well. In each instance, the patient was lightly anesthetized. We speculate that this may represent a hemodynamic form of pulmonary edema from an acute elevation of systemic vascular resistance and an acute decrease in pulmonary vascular resistance. In addition, "leaky" capillaries appear to be involved. Whether these cardiovascular changes are mediated by succinylcholine itself or some other vasoactive substance (i.e., histamine) is not known.

The cardiovascular effects of the nondepolarizing relaxants are related to the magnitude of histamine release, ganglionic blockade, and vagolysis. In addition, the cardiovascular effects seem age related.

In infants and children, minimal cardiovascular effects are seen following atracurium, metocurine, and vecuronium at several multiples of the ED95. In adults, atracurium at 3 times the ED95 causes slightly less histamine release than 2 times the ED95 of metocurine and less than half as much histamine release as 1 times the ED95 of d-tubocurarine. Vecuronium (at any multiple of ED95) is not associated with histamine release. Infants and children appear less susceptible to histamine release following relaxants than adults. In a small series of infants, 5 times the ED95 of atracurium did not elicit flushing or alteration of heart rate or blood pressure. However, when atracurium is injected directly IV in infants and children, local signs of histamine release have been described. Rarely, flushing with or without mild hypotension is seen at high multiples of the ED95. At high doses, d-tubocurarine may cause hypotension and histamine release in children.

Keon and Downes (1979 unpublished data) compared changes in heart rate, changes in blood pressure, and differences in intubating conditions in infants (average age 5.6 months) "anesthetized" with nitrous oxide-oxygen following either d-tubocurarine (0.6 mg/kg) or pancuronium (0.1 mg/kg). None had received premedication. In both groups, there were modest increases in pulse rate; transient episodes of bradycardia occurred in some infants in both groups during intubation. No infant given pancuronium developed significant hypotension or hypertension (greater than 10% change from control levels). In contrast, 25% of the infants given d-tubocurarine experienced decreases in blood pressure greater than 10% from control (range 11-26%).

In children anesthetized with halothane and nitrous oxide, we noted that 1 times the ED95 of gallamine increases the heart rate by 42 beats per minute, and that 1 times the ED95 of pancuronium increases the heart rate by 19 beats per minute. Both drugs increase mean arterial pressure under these conditions by about 10 torr. At 2 times the ED95, further increases in heart rate were seen with pancuronium but not with gallamine. In contrast, we noted minimal effects of gallamine, pancuronium, or rocuronium on the heart rate in infants. Unless the heart rate had slowed from halothane, neither gallamine nor pancuronium exhibited any vagolytic effects. In an occasional infant, however, gallamine or pancuronium may cause a significant increase in heart rate. Since the infant responds to a variety of stimuli with bradycardia (e.g., potent inhalation agents, hypoxia, intubation), the potential vagolytic effects of pancuronium, gallamine, or rocuronium may be wanted side effects. For example, in adults, pancuronium is usually administered with high-dose fentanyl anesthesia to minimize the bradycardia seen with fentanyl; substitution of atracurium or vecuronium for pancuronium has resulted in profound bradycardia from the "fentanyls"—a totally predictable side effect. Whether profound bradycardia will be seen in infants anesthetized with deep halothane and given atracurium, vecuronium, doxacurium, or pipecuronium, remains to be seen. We have noted no significant change in heart rate and only a minimal (7 torr) decrease in blood pressure in infants anesthetized with halothane 1% end-tidal and nitrous oxide given 0.3 mg/kg of atracurium (9). No changes in heart rate or blood pressure have been noted after 70 µg/kg of vecuronium in pediatric patients also anesthetized with halothane and nitrous oxide (17).

REFERENCES

1. Cook DR, Fischer CG: Neuromuscular blocking effects of succinylcholine in infants and children. Anesthesiology 42:662-665, 1975

2. Cook DR, Fischer CG: Characteristics of succinylcholine neuromuscular blockade in infants. Anesth Analg 57:63-66, 1978

3. Meakin G, McKiernan EP, Morris P et al: Dose-response curves for suxamethonium in neonates, infants and children. Br J Anaesth 62:655-658, 1989

4. Goudsouzian NG, Liu LMP: The neuromuscular response of infants to a continuous infusion of succinylcholine. Anesthesiology 60:97-101, 1984

5. Walts LF, Dillon JB: The response of newborns to succinylcholine and d-tubocurarine. Anesthesiology 31:35-38, 1969

6. Brandom BW, Sarner JB, Woelfel SK et al: Mivacurium infusion requirements in pediatric surgical patients during nitrous oxide-halothane and during nitrous oxide-narcotic anesthesia. Anesth Analg 71:16-22, 1990

7. Stiller RL, Cook DR, Chakravorti S: In vitro degradation of atracurium in human plasma. Br J Anaesth 57:1085-1088, 1985

8. Stiller RL, Brandom BW, Cook DR: Determinations of atracurium by high-performance liquid chromatography. Anesth Analg 64:58-62, 1985

9. Brandom BW, Woelfel SK, Cook DR et al: Clinical pharmacology of atracurium in infants. Anesth Analg 63:309-312, 1984

10. Brandom BW, Rudd GD, Cook DR: Clinical pharmacology of atracurium in pediatric patients. Br J Anaesth 55:117s-121s, 1983

11. Brandom BW, Cook DR, Woelfel SK et al: Atracurium infusion in children during halothane, isoflurane, and narcotic anesthesia. Anesth Analg 64:471-476, 1985

12. Goudsouzian NG, Liu L, Cote CJ et al: Safety and efficacy of atracurium in adolescents and children anesthetized with halothane. Anesthesiology 39:459-462, 1983

13. Goudsouzian NG, Liu LMP, Gionfriddo M et al: Neuromuscular effects of atracurium in infants and children. Anesthesiology 62:75-79, 1985

14. Brandom BW, Cook DR, Stiller RL et al: Pharmacokinetics of atracurium in anesthetized infants and children. Br J Anaesth 58:1210-1213, 1986

15. D'Hollander AA, Luyckx C, Barvais L et al: Clinical evaluation of atracurium besylate requirement for a stable muscle relaxation during surgery: Lack of age-related effects. Anesthesiology 59:237-240, 1983

16. Durant NN: Norcuron, a new nondepolarizing neuromuscular blocking agent. Seminars in Anesthesia 1:47-56, 1982

17. Fisher DM, Miller RD: Neuromuscular effects of vecuronium (ORG NC45) in infants and children during N_2O, halothane anesthesia. Anesthesiology 58:519-523, 1983

18. D'Hollander AA, Massaux F, Nevelsteen M et al: Age-dependent dose-response relationship of ORG NC45 in anaesthetized patients. Br J Anaesth 54:653-657, 1982

19. Goudsouzian NG, Martyn J, Liu LMP et al: Safety and efficacy of vecuronium in adolescents and children. Anesth Analg 62:1083-1088, 1983

20. Rupp SM, Miller RD, Gencarelli PJ: Vecuronium-induced neuromuscular blockade during enflurane, halothane, and isoflurane in humans. Anesthesiology 60:102-105, 1984

21. Miller RD, Rupp SM, Fisher DM et al: Clinical pharmacology of vecuronium and atracurium. Anesthesiology 61:444-453, 1984

22. Fisher DM, Castagnoli K, Miller RD: Vecuronium kinetics and dynamics in anesthetized infants and children. Clin Pharm Ther 37:402-406, 1985

23. Foldes FF, Nagashima H, Nguyen HD et al: The neuromuscular effects of ORG9426 in patients receiving balanced anesthesia. Anesthesiology 75:191-196, 1991

24. Woelfel SK, Brandom BW, McGowan FX, Gronert BJ, Cook DR: Neuromuscular effects of 600 mg·kg^{-1} of rocuronium in infants during nitrous oxide-halothane anaesthesia. Paediatr Anesth 4:173-177, 1994

25. Churchill-Davidson HC, Wise RP: The response of the newborn infant to muscle relaxants. Can Anaesth Soc J 11:1-5, 1964

26. Donlon JV, Ali HH, Savarese JJ: A new approach to the study of four non-depolarizing relaxants in man. Anesth Analg 53:924-939, 1974

27. Goudsouzian NG, Liu LMP, Cote CJ: Comparison of equipotent doses of non-depolarizing muscle relaxants in children. Anesth Analg 60:862-866, 1981

28. Blinn A, Woelfel SK, Cook DR et al: Pancuronium dose-response revisitied. Paediatr Anesth 2:153-155, 1992

29. Goudsouzian NG, Liu LMP, Savarese JJ: Metocurarine in infants and children: neuromuscular and clinical effects. Anesthesiology 49:266-269, 1978

30. Goudsouzian NG, Ryan JF, Savarese JJ: The neuromuscular effects of pancuronium in infants and children. Anesthesiology 41:95-98, 1974

31. Digby-Leigh M, McLoyd D, Belton MK et al: Bradycardia following intravenous administration of succinylcholine in anesthetized children. Anesthesiology 18:698-702, 1957

32. Craythorne NWB, Turndorf H, Dripps RD: Changes in pulse rate and rhythm associated with the use of succinylcholine in anesthetized children. Anesthesiology 21:465-471, 1960

33. Rosenberg H, Gronert GA: Intractable cardiac arrest in children given succinylcholine (letter). Anesthesiology 77:1054, 1992

34. Berry FA: Succinylcholine and Duchenne muscular dystrophy (letter). Anesthesiology 79:401, 1993

35. Steizner J, Eberlin HJ, Schumucker I et al: Anaesthesia-induced cardiac arrest in two infants with unsuspected muscular dystrophy. Anaesthesist 42:44-46, 1993

36. Mehler J, Bachour H, Simona F et al: Cardiac arrest during induction of anesthesia with halothane and succinylcholine in an infant. Severe hyperkalemia and rhabdomyolysis due to a suspected myopathy and/or malignant hyperthermia. Anaesthesist 40:497-501, 1991

37. Cook DR, Westman H, Rosenfeld L et al: Pulmonary edema in infants: Possible association with intramuscular succinylcholine. Anesth Analg 60:220-223, 1981

NEW INHALATIONAL ANESTHETICS IN INFANTS AND CHILDREN

J. Lerman

The methyl ethyl ethers have proven to be a successful series of anesthetics because of several characteristics: molecular stability, non-flammability, lack of arrhythmogenicity, lack of neuronal excitation, cardiovascular stability, large lethal-to-anesthetic concentration ratio, and minimal end-organ effects (1,2). In this lecture, I shall review the pharmacology of the two new anesthetics, desflurane and sevoflurane, with a particular view to their future roles in pediatric anesthesia.

PHARMACOLOGY

Desflurane (difluoromethyl 1-fluoro—2,2,2—trifluoro-ethyl-ether) is a *methyl ethyl ether* compound that differs from isoflurane in only one substitution—a fluoride for a chloride ion at the alpha ethyl carbon (Table 1) (1). This substitution confers several differences in the physical properties of desflurane, which distinguishes it from the inhalational anesthetics currently available. First, it has a boiling point of 23.5°C, slightly above room temperature (Table 1). This precludes the use of the standard wick vaporizer. Second, it has a low blood solubility (comparable to that of nitrous oxide) and a mild odor (Table 1) (2). This low solubility should facilitate a rapid wash-in, but also, more importantly, a rapid wash-out (3). Finally, its chemical structure confers stability in terms of both in-vivo metabolism and degradation in the presence of soda lime (4).

In contrast to desflurane, sevoflurane (fluoromethyl 2,2,2-trifluoro-1-[trifluoromethyl] ethyl ether) is a *polyfluorinated methyl isopropyl ether* compound with physicochemical properties similar to the traditional ether anesthetics. However, there are three notable exceptions (Table 1) (5,6): 1) sevoflurane has low solubility in both blood (0.66) (5-7) and tissues; 2) sevoflurane has a pleasant, nonirritating odor (8-10); and 3) it is susceptible to both in-vivo metabolism (11,12) and in-vitro degradation

T.H. Stanley and P.G. Schafer (eds.), Pediatric and Obstetrical Anesthesia, 265-276.
© 1995 *Kluwer Academic Publishers.*

Table 1. Comparison of halothane, enflurane, isoflurane, sevoflurane, and desflurane.

PHARMACOLOGY:	Halothane	Enflurane	Isoflurane	Sevoflurane	Desflurane
Chemical Structure	F H F-C-C-Br F Cl	F F Cl H-C-O-C-C-H F F F	F Cl F H-C-O-C-C-F F H F	H CF3 F F-C-O-C-C-F H H F	F F F H-C-O-C-C-F F H F
Molecular weight	197.4	184.5	184.5	200.1	168
Boiling Point (°C)	50.2	56.5	48.5	58.6	23.5
Vapour Pressure (mmHg)	244	172	240	185	664
Odour	mild, pleasant	etheral	etheral	pleasant	etheral
SOLUBILITY:					
λb/g adults	2.4	1.2	1.4	0.66	0.42
λb/g neonates	2.14	1.78	1.19	0.66	---
λfat/b adults	51.1	---	45	48	27
MAC:					
MACadults	0.75	1.7	1.2	2.05	7.0
MACneonates	0.87	---	1.60	3.3	9.2

b/g refers to blood/gas
fat/b refers to fat/gas

(13). Thus, sevoflurane should provide a rapid, smooth inhalational induction and a rapid recovery from anesthesia in children, but it may also be degraded.

PHARMACOKINETICS

Desflurane has a blood/gas partition coefficient of 0.42 (one-sixth that of halothane and one-third that of isoflurane), which should speed the rise of alvcolar-to-inspired anesthetic partial pressures (Table 1) (3,14). Indeed, the wash-in of desflurane in adults is the most rapid of the potent inhalational anesthetics, but it lags behind nitrous oxide because of the concentration effect and the lower tissue solubility of nitrous oxide compared with desflurane.

The rate of rise of alveolar-to-inspired partial pressures of sevoflurane in adults is intermediate between desflurane and isoflurane (3). The slower wash-in of sevoflurane may be explained by its 50% greater solubility in blood and tissues compared to desflurane (Table 1).

Will the more rapid wash-in of halothane in children compared with adults also hold true for desflurane and sevoflurane? Yes, but the difference in the wash-in between children and adults will likely be less than that for halothane. The reason for the smaller difference with desflurane and sevoflurane may be attributed to differences in the effects of alveolar ventilation and cardiac output to the vessel-rich group on anesthetics of different solubilities. Alveolar ventilation and cardiac output affect the wash-in of less soluble anesthetics, like desflurane and sevoflurane, to a smaller extent than they do the more soluble anesthetics, such as halothane (14). Since, for the most part, these two factors account for the more rapid wash-in of inhalational anesthetics in children compared with adults, we can expect the difference in the wash-in of both desflurane and sevoflurane between children and adults to be less than with halothane.

Does a more rapid rate of rise of alveolar-to-inspired anesthetic partial pressures imply a more rapid induction of anesthesia with desflurane and sevoflurane than with halothane or the other ether anesthetics? No! Induction of anesthesia depends, not only on the rate of rise of alveolar-to-inspired anesthetic partial pressure, but also on the actual alveolar concentration of anesthetic (i.e., the over-pressure technique and irritation of the airway). Indeed, when the over-pressure technique is used with an anesthetic that lacks airway irritability (such as sevoflurane) and a properly designed vaporizer (preferably with a maximum inspired concentration of 8-10% sevoflurane), the rate of induction of anesthesia should be similar for *all* inhalational anesthetics (14).

The presence of right-to-left shunts will have a significant impact on the wash-in of the relatively insoluble anesthetics desflurane and sevoflurane. Right-to-left shunts slow the wash-in of anesthetics, less soluble anesthetics being affected to a greater extent than more soluble anesthetics (14). The effects of right-to-left shunts have not been of great clinical importance, since the only agent commonly used for inhalational inductions, halothane, is a relatively soluble anesthetic. However, this changes with the introduction of these less soluble anesthetics into pediatric anesthesia practice. In circumstances where right-to-left shunts exist (intrapulmonary or intracardiac shunts), the wash-in of desflurane and sevoflurane will lag behind that which would exist in the absence of the shunt.

PHARMACODYNAMICS

MAC

The MAC of desflurane in children is 5-6 times greater than that of isoflurane. MAC increases as age decreases, reaching a maximum value in infants 6-12 months of age, and then decreases with age to neonates (Figure) (15). The maximum MAC in infants 6-12 months of age is 9.9 ± 0.44%; in neonates it is 9.2 ± 0.02%. The MAC of desflurane decreases only 20% in the presence of 60% nitrous oxide (16).

Sevoflurane is 3-4 times more potent than desflurane. The MAC in children 1-12 years of age is constant at ≈2.5%, increasing slightly in infants 6-12 months, ≈2.7%, but leveling off at 3.2-3.3% in neonates and infants 1-6 months of age (10). Surprisingly, 60% nitrous oxide decreases the MAC of sevoflurane in children 1-3 years of age only 25% (10). This is less than the MAC reduction effects of nitrous oxide on isoflurane and halothane in children (17,18). This smaller effect of nitrous oxide on the MAC values of desflurane and sevoflurane in young children remains unexplained.

INDUCTION CHARACTERISTICS

The irritant effects of desflurane on the upper airway offset any potential advantages its lower blood solubility might confer during an inhalational induction. Induction of anesthesia with desflurane and

MAC DESFLURANE

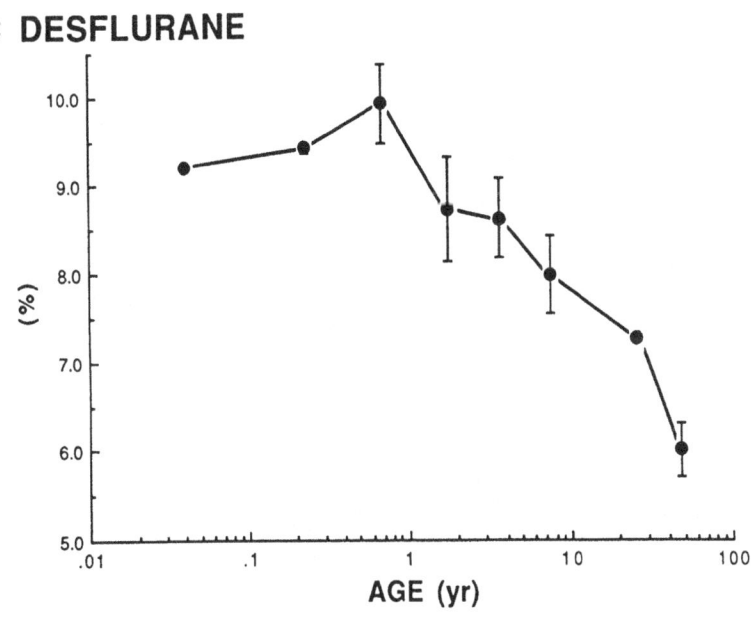

Figure.   MAC desflurane and age in neonates, infants, and children up to 12 years.
Data are means ± sd (15).

oxygen in infants and children is very stormy and disquieting. It is characterized by a 50% incidence of breath holding, a 36% incidence of coughing, and a 30% incidence of mild laryngospasm (19,20). This is reflected in similar times to loss of the eyelash reflex with desflurane (2.4 ± 1.2 min) and the more soluble anesthetic, halothane (2.1 ± 0.8 min) (19). Although the addition of adjuvant drugs might be expected to smooth the induction characteristics of an irritant anesthetic such as desflurane, clinical experience has failed to support this notion. Desflurane is not recommended for induction of anesthesia in infants and children.

In contrast to desflurane, induction of anesthesia with sevoflurane is smooth, pleasant, and rapid in infants and children of all ages (10). In a recent comparative study of adults, airway irritability occurred least frequently after sevoflurane when compared with halothane, enflurane, and isoflurane (21). These data are consistent with those published previously for halothane (22).

MAINTENANCE

Desflurane may be used as a maintenance anesthetic in children (15,19). If spontaneous ventilation is preferred, the child should be anesthetized first with halothane or an IV technique and only then switched to desflurane (23). Some investigators have suggested that, in this way, we can maximize the recovery characteristics and minimize the irritant effects of desflurane in children.

Sevoflurane may be used during the maintenance period but, in contrast to desflurane, it can also be used for induction of anesthesia. Spontaneous ventilation is easily accomplished with sevoflurane. However, it is a potent respiratory depressant, particularly at concentrations in excess of 1.5 MAC. Several instances of respiratory depression and apnea have been reported in children who were breathing sevoflurane spontaneously with an effective regional anesthetic in situ. The absence of stimulation may unmask the respiratory depressant effects of sevoflurane in children, and this must be monitored.

CIRCULATION

The circulatory responses to an inhalational induction with either desflurane or sevoflurane and to 1 MAC of both anesthetics under steady-state conditions are similar. For both anesthetics, systolic arterial pressure decreases ≈25% from awake values in all age groups before skin incision. Heart rate remains unchanged or decreases <10% from awake values at 1 MAC (10,19,20), although two preliminary reports suggested that heart rate may increase during light sevoflurane anesthesia in children (24,25). Arrhythmias are uncommon with both anesthetics (10,15,19,20).

EMERGENCE/RECOVERY

Just as desflurane's wash-in is rapid, so too is its wash-out (3). Recovery from inhalational anesthesia depends on the wash-out of the anesthetic from blood and tissues: the more rapid the wash-out, the more rapid the recovery. In rats, recovery from desflurane anesthesia was the most rapid of the inhalational anesthetics (26). In a noncontrolled study in infants and children, we noted that emergence from desflurane was extremely rapid (20). This was recently validated against halothane for ambulatory surgery in young children (23).

The wash-out of sevoflurane is intermediate between desflurane and isoflurane but more rapid than halothane (3). Recovery after sevoflurane anesthesia is more rapid than that after halothane after both brief (9) and extended (2.5 MAC-hr) periods of anesthesia (27).

Clinically, the rapid elimination of desflurane and sevoflurane is a two-edged sword. On the one hand, recovery is extremely rapid after both of these anesthetics. On the other hand, complete recovery leaves the child exposed to surgical sequelae, including unopposed pain. With both of these anesthetics, a strategy for managing postoperative pain must begin during the anesthetic. To optimize the speed of recovery, a regional anesthetic is preferable. Whatever the planned strategy for pain management, it must be initiated before recovery from anesthesia.

METABOLISM

Published data indicates that the metabolism of desflurane is small. In rats and swine, desflurane resists metabolism: it is degraded only one-fifth to one-tenth that of isoflurane (4). In humans, desflurane also resists metabolism, with serum inorganic fluoride concentrations ≤2 μM after 7.3 MAC-hr of desflurane (28).

In contrast to the stability of desflurane, sevoflurane is metabolized both in vivo and in vitro. The rate of metabolism of sevoflurane in vivo (3%) is similar to that of enflurane (8). Sevoflurane is metabolized in the liver by microsomal defluorination, via the cytochrome P450IIE1 isozyme system in humans, to hexafluoroisopropanol (HFIP) and inorganic fluoride (29). HFIP has been detected only in the urine in adults. The plasma profile of inorganic fluoride after sevoflurane is similar to that of enflurane: the plasma concentration of inorganic fluoride increases during sevoflurane anesthesia to reach a maximum value within the 60 minutes of discontinuing the anesthetic and then decreases to <10 μM by 4 hours (10,11). In children 1-12 years of age, the maximum plasma concentration of inorganic fluoride after ≈1 MAC-hr sevoflurane is 15-25 μM (10). The plasma profile of inorganic fluoride in children after 1-5 MAC-hr of sevoflurane suggests that the concentrations are well below the "nephrotoxic threshold" (30). In adult volunteers given 9.5 MAC-hr of sevoflurane, plasma inorganic fluoride concentrations peaked at 47 ± 3 μM but returned to ≤10 μM by 48 hours (31). Since previous data indicated that the plasma inorganic fluoride profile after methoxyflurane in children is attenuated, compared with a similar anesthetic exposure in adults (32), I expect the same will hold true for sevoflurane, even after long exposure. The plasma profile of inorganic fluoride, after sevoflurane anesthesia in children who have received enzyme-inducing drugs or who have renal insufficiency, has not been determined. Nonetheless, one of the redeeming features of this relatively insoluble anesthetic that distinguishes it from the more soluble anesthetic methoxyflurane is that its rapid wash-out decreases the probability of a sustained increase in the plasma concentration of inorganic fluoride.

To understand the relationship between nephrotoxicity and inhalational anesthetics, it seems reasonable to consider two new notions. First, consider the renal exposure to inorganic fluoride over time, rather than as an isolated plasma value, such as the maximum plasma concentration of inorganic fluoride ion. That is, we should be considering the area under the curve (AUC) of the plasma concentration of the fluoride-time profile for nephrotoxic risk after exposure to anesthetics. Second, we should also recognize differences in cytochrome P450 isozymes in rat and human renal parenchyma.

Our preliminary studies indicate that the AUC for inorganic fluoride after sevoflurane anesthesia in children is ≈10% of the area after a similar MAC exposure of methoxyflurane. Furthermore, the renal concentrating ability of adults who were given sevoflurane was similar to that of enflurane, despite a twofold greater plasma inorganic fluoride concentration after sevoflurane (31). Creatinine clearance and urinary n-acetyl-b-glucosaminidase concentration remained constant after both anesthetics. Recent evidence suggests that the nephrotoxic data from rats anesthetized with sevoflurane may be explained, in part, by the presence of microsomal isozymes within the renal parenchyma that are capable of degrading sevoflurane. These isozymes are not present in human renal tissues. At the present time, it would seem that plasma inorganic concentrations of fluoride are unlikely to determine the ultimate fate of sevoflurane in pediatric anesthesia.

Sevoflurane is unstable in soda lime absorbers (5,13,33). Although most inhalational anesthetics are only adsorbed in soda lime and baralyme, sevoflurane, like halothane, is also degraded. Two of the degradation products formed from sevoflurane are vinyl compounds (compound A and B). These compounds accumulate in very minute quantities in closed circuits and in even smaller quantities in low-flow and semi-closed circuits (34,35). Controversy still surrounds the risk of toxicity from compound A and, in particular, the threshhold concentration that produces renal cellular or functional toxicity in rats and humans (36,37,38). Thus far, the use of sevoflurane in circuits with soda lime has not been thoroughly investigated in children. Until further information is available, I would *not* recommend sevoflurane for use in closed circuit anesthesia in children. Sevoflurane may, however, be used with semiclosed circuits and is recommended without restriction for use with circuits that do not use carbon dioxide absorbers, such as the Mapleson D and F circuits.

VAPORIZERS

One important consideration for both of these anesthetics is the delivery system used to deliver a clinically acceptable concentration of anesthetic. The TEC 6 desflurane vaporizer has been designed to accommodate desflurane, an inhalational anesthetic with a boiling point just above room temperature. This vaporizer is a temperature-controlled, pressurized vaporizer that acts much like a fuel injection engine (39). The TEC 6 requires an external electrical source to maintain a steady concentration of desflurane in the effluent. In the event of a power failure, the effluent concentration decreases rapidly as the temperature within the vaporizer decreases. Consequently, I recommend both on-line agent analysis and a second vaporizer for backup, in the event of a failure of the vaporizer.

Sevoflurane can be delivered using a traditional wick-type vaporizer. However, the maximum deliverable concentration of sevoflurane on commercial vaporizers in Japan is only 5%. This precludes the effective use of the over-pressure technique and, consequently, induction of anesthesia may be delayed compared with halothane. In one center in Japan, two SevoTec vaporizers are used to deliver a 10% inspired concentration. Commercial vaporizers for sevoflurane in North America should be available to deliver 8% sevoflurane in the near future.

SUMMARY

Although desflurane will not play a significant role as an induction agent in children, it produces hemodynamic stability for maintenance of anesthesia. Its low blood and tissue solubility will facilitate rapid decreases in the depth of anesthesia and, at the conclusion of anesthesia, a rapid recovery. Desflurane resists degradation, both in vivo and in vitro, and therefore remains free of organ toxicity. Its unusual physicochemical properties require a pressurized electric vaporizer. In contrast, sevoflurane is the first anesthetic to challenge halothane as the induction agent of choice in infants and children. Its lack of irritant airway effects suggests that it can be used with either a mask or a tracheal tube for induction and maintenance of anesthesia. Elimination of sevoflurane and recovery from sevoflurane anesthesia are rapid, second only to desflurane. At the present time, prolonged anesthesia with sevoflurane is best avoided in children with renal insufficiency and in closed circuits until further data is available.

REFERENCES

1. Terrell RC: Physical and chemical properties of anesthetic agents. Br J Anaesth 56:3S-7S, 1984
2. Yasuda N, Targ AG, Eger EI II: Solubility of I-653, sevoflurane, isoflurane and halothane in human tissues. Anesth Analg 69:370-373, 1989
3. Yasuda N, Lockhart S, Eger EI II et al: Comparison of kinetics of sevoflurane and isoflurane in humans. Anesth Analg 72:316-324, 1991
4. Koblin DD, Eger I. II, Johnson BH et al: 1-653 resists degradation in rats. Anesth Analg 67:534-538, 1988
5. Wallin RF, Regan BM, Napoli MD et al: Sevoflurane: A new inhalational anesthetic agent. Anesth Analg 54:758-766, 1975
6. Halsey MJ: Investigations on isoflurane, sevoflurane and other experimental anesthetics. Br J Anaesth 53:435-475, 1981
7. Malviya S, Lerman J: The blood/gas solubilities of sevoflurane, isoflurane, and halothane and serum constituent concentrations in neonates and adults. Anesthesiology 72:793-796, 1990
8. Holaday PA, Smith FR: Clinical characteristics and biotransformation of sevoflurane in healthy human volunteers. Anesthesiology 54:100-106, 1981
9. Naito Y, Tamai S, Shingu K et al: Comparison between sevoflurane and halothane for pediatric ambulatory anesthesia. Br J Anaesth 67:387-389, 1991
10. Lerman J, Sikich N, Kleinman S et al: The pharmacology of sevoflurane in infants and children. Anesthesiology 80:814-824, 1994
11. Shiraishi Y, Ikeda K: Uptake and biotransformation of sevoflurane in humans: A comparative study of sevoflurane with halothane, enflurane, and isoflurane. J Clin Anesth 2:381-386, 1990
12. Frink Jr. EJ, Malan TP, Isner RJ et al: Renal concentrating function with prolonged sevoflurane or enflurane anesthesia in volunteers. Anesthesiology 80:1019-1025, 1994
13. Hanaki C, Fujii K, Morio M et al: Decomposition of sevoflurane by soda lime. Hiroshima J Med Sci 36:61-67, 1987

14. Lerman J: Pharmacology of inhalational anesthetics in infants and children. Pediatr Anesth 2:191-203, 1992
15. Taylor RH, Lerman J: Minimum alveolar concentration of desflurane and hemodynamic responses in neonates, infants and children. Anesthesiology 75:975-979, 1991
16. Fisher DM, Zwass MS: MAC of desflurane in 60% nitrous oxide in infants and children. Anesthesiology 76:354-356, 1992
17. Murray DJ, Mehta MP, Forbes RB et al: Additive contribution of nitrous oxide to halothane MAC in infants and children. Anesth Analg 71:120-124, 1990
18. Murray DJ, Mehta MP, Forbes RB: The additive contribution of nitrous oxide to isoflurane MAC in infants and children. Anesthesiology 75:186-190, 1991
19. Zwass MS, Fisher DM, Welborn LG et al: Induction and maintenance characteristics of anesthesia with desflurane and nitrous oxide in infants and children. Anesthesiology 76:373-378, 1992
20. Taylor R, Lerman J: Induction and recovery characteristics of desflurane in infants and children. Can J Anaesth 39:6-13, 1992
21. Doi M, Ikeda K: Airway irritation produced by volatile anesthetics during brief inhalation: Comparison of halothane, enflurane, isoflurane and sevoflurane. Can J Anaesth 40:122-126, 1993
22. Fisher DM, Robinson S, Brett CM et al: Comparison of enflurane, halothane, and isoflurane for diagnostic and therapeutic procedures in children with malignancies. Anesthesiology 63:647-650, 1981
23. Davis PJ, Cohen IT, McGowan FX et al: Recovery characteristics of desflurane versus halothane for maintenance of anesthesia in pediatric ambulatory patients. Anesthesiology 80:298-302, 1994
24. Piat V, Dubois MC, Murat I: Comparison of induction and recovery characteristics of sevoflurane and halothane in children (abstract). Br J Anaesth 72 (suppl 1) A178, 1994
25. Taivainen T, Meretoja OA, Tiainen P et al: Sevoflurane versus halothane in pediatric anesthesia (abstract). Br J Anaesth 72 (suppl 1) A177, 1994
26. Eger EI II, Johnson BH: Rates of awakening from anesthesia with I-653, halothane, isoflurane, and sevoflurane: A test of the effect of anesthetic concentration and duration in rats. Anesth Analg 66:977-982, 1987
27. Levine M, Sarner J, Lerman J et al: Emergence characteristics after sevoflurane anesthesia in children: A comparison with halothane. Anesth Analg 76:S221, 1993
28. Koblin DD: Characteristics and implications of desflurane metabolism and toxicity. Anesth Analg 75:S10-16, 1992
29. Kharasch ED, Thummel KE: Identification of cytochrome P450 2E1 as the predominant enzyme catalyzing human liver microsomal defluorination of sevoflurane, isoflurane, and methoxyflurane. Anesthesiology 79:795-807, 1993

30. Levine M, Sarner J, Lerman J et al: Plasma inorganic fluoride ion concentration in children after prolonged sevoflurane anesthesia. Can J Anaesth 40:A66, 1993

31. Frink EJ, Malan TP, Isner RJ et al: Renal concentrating function with prolonged sevoflurane or enflurane anesthesia in volunteers. Anesthesiology 80:1019-1025, 1994

32. Stoelting RK, Peterson C: Methoxyflurane anesthesia in pediatric patients: Evaluation of anesthetic metabolism and renal function. Anesthesiology 42:26-29, 1975

33. Wong DT, Lerman J, Volgyesi GA: Factors affecting the disappearance of sevoflurane in baralyme. Can J Anaesth 39:366-369, 1992

34. Frink EJ, Malan TP, Morgan SE et al: Quantification of the degradation products of sevoflurane in two CO_2 absorbants during low-flow anesthesia in surgical patients. Anesthesiology 77:1064-1069, 1992

35. Bito H, Ikeda K: Closed circuit anesthesia with sevoflurane in humans: Effects on renal and hepatic function and concentrations of breakdown products with soda lime in the circuit. Anesthesiology 80:71-76, 1994

36. Mazze RI. The safety of sevoflurane in humans (editorial). Anesthesiology 77:1062-1063, 1992

37. Gonsowski CT, Laster MJ, Eger EI II et al: Toxicity of compound A in rats: Effect of a 3-hour administration. Anesethesiology 80:556-565, 1994

38. Gonsowski CT, Laster MJ, Eger II EI et al: Toxicity of compound A in rats: Effect of increasing duration of administration. Anesthesiology 80:566-575, 1994

39. Weiskopf RB, Sampson D, Moore MA: The desflurane (TEC 6) vaporizer: Design, design considerations, and performance evaluation. Br J Anaesth 72:474-479, 1994

STRESS RESPONSES IN PEDIATRIC ANESTHESIA

P. R. Hickey

Survey of the neuroanatomical, neurophysiological, and neurochemical development of the nociceptive pathways in the central nervous system of the human fetus and newborn has shown that the structural and functional machinery necessary for the perception of pain and the production of stress responses is present at birth (1). Substantial cardiovascular, humoral, metabolic, and behavioral responses to painful and stressful stimulation have been documented in newborns and infants (1-4). These data contradict traditional beliefs that infants do not possess the physiological machinery to feel pain, that they are somehow "protected" from pain and operative stress by unexplained endogenous mechanisms, or that neonates do not perceive nociceptive stimuli as painful. On a humane basis alone, these data argue that all small children, infants, and neonates need control of stress responses and adequate anesthesia and analgesia in the perioperative period. Thus modulation of stress responses is an important goal of pediatric anesthesia and may be of particular importance in the youngest of patients, infants and neonates.

EFFECTS OF PAIN AND STRESS IN INFANTS

The cardiopulmonary, hormonal, metabolic, and behavioral responses of infants and small children to painful stimuli during and after operations have been shown to be deleterious in at least some cases. Increases in heart rate and blood pressure, and increases in intracranial pressure, along with high osmotic loads caused by high blood glucose levels, which result from stress in the operating room and intensive care unit, have been suggested as a cause of intracranial hemorrhage in newborn infants. Deleterious decreases in arterial oxygen saturation and increases in serum cortisol levels result from the stress of circumcision in the unanesthetized infant (5,6).

Hormonal and metabolic responses after thoracotomy in premature infants have been documented to continue for several days post-

277

T.H. Stanley and P.G. Schafer (eds.), Pediatric and Obstetrical Anesthesia, 277-282.
© 1995 *Kluwer Academic Publishers.*

operatively (2-4). Responses in beta-endorphins, catecholamines, growth hormone, cortisol, glucagon, and insulin all have been documented. These hormonal responses result in changes in oxygen consumption and alterations in blood glucose, lactate, pyruvate, tissue glycogen levels, and protein metabolism. Particularly during and after major operative procedures, the magnitude of stress responses in neonates and older infants may reach levels considered pathologic, resulting in protein breakdown and negative nitrogen balance, impaired immune responses, hypercoagulable states, and poor tissue perfusion.

Recent evidence from clinical studies suggests that anesthetic techniques directed at reducing stress responses intraoperatively and postoperatively, such as high-dose narcotic techniques and epidural techniques for procedures in the lower half of the body, can modify stress responses and result in improved hospital morbidity in both adults and children (2-6). These deleterious stress responses, when unmodified by adequate anesthesia, may be associated with postoperative complications, or even death, in the human neonate (4-6). From the viewpoint of the anesthesiologist who is trying to preserve normal homeostasis during the perioperative period, anesthesia and stress control for the fetus, neonate, and infant is mandatory, particularly during and after major operative procedures, when substantial physiological derangements are expected to occur.

POSTOPERATIVE STRESS

In the postoperative period, stress responses can continue; and anesthetic/analgesic techniques designed to minimize postoperative stress responses can be important in preventing complications. In infants undergoing major cardiac surgery, critical hemodynamic crises may be triggered by inadequate pain control. High-risk infants who have had complex intracardiac repairs and high pulmonary vascular resistance frequently have pulmonary hypertensive crises in the early postoperative period that result in severe systemic hypotension and sometimes sudden death. These are seen most frequently in agitated children, and they often respond to sedative and analgesic agents that block the stress of tracheal suctioning (11,12). Thus control of pain and stress in the postoperative period can potentially prevent deleterious hemodynamic crises, in addition to playing a role in attenuating metabolic and hormonal stress responses.

INFANT STRESS RESPONSES AND
POSTOPERATIVE OUTCOME

The concept of anesthetic technique having an impact on postoperative morbidity and mortality in an uncomplicated anesthetic and surgical procedure through modulation of stress responses is relatively novel and by no means universally accepted. However, it is becoming clear that extremes of stress and pain, in addition to modulating classic humoral and metabolic responses through activation of the sympathetic nervous system, also affect the immune system, cytokine production by various cell populations, protein synthesis and wound healing, coagulation, and tissue energy stores. These effects all have been demonstrated in isolated systems and in some clinical studies. All or some of these mechanisms might well mediate effects on mortality and morbidity.

Studies of neonates undergoing cardiac surgery at our institution show that in cases of extreme stress in neonates, morbidity and even hospital mortality may be affected by how well pain and stress are controlled in the perioperative period (4). In these studies, patients randomized to receive deep levels of opiate anesthesia and postoperative analgesia had a statistically lower incidence of both morbidity and mortality than those receiving light levels of inhalation with halothane, which is known to be ineffective in attenuating stress responses. Prior to the era of high-dose narcotic anesthesia, there was some question about whether sick neonates and infants could tolerate levels of anesthesia adequate to suppress stress responses (9). However, a number of recent studies have documented the safe use of high-dose narcotic anesthesia in neonates, infants, and small children (3,4,10,11).

STRESS RESPONSES AND OUTCOME IN FETAL SURGERY

With the coming era of fetal surgery, considerations of pain and stress responses in the human fetus have important potential clinical applications. Despite a lack of universal acceptance that modulation of stress responses can impact postoperative mortality, even in critically ill neonates undergoing high-risk surgical procedures, recent experimental studies published in fetal surgery literature unequivocally link anesthetic technique and postoperative mortality. These studies support the notion that unmodulated stress responses, even in the fetus, can result in postoperative mortality (13-15). Using total spinal anesthesia and indomethacin to inhibit fetal stress responses and block placental vasoconstriction, surgical procedures and cardiac bypass can be performed at 80% of full gestational age in fetal lambs, with subsequent continuation of the pregnancy to full-term and normal delivery. Other anesthetic techniques used in these studies that did not inhibit fetal stress led to progressive placental vasoconstriction after cardiac bypass, resulting in decreased cardiac output and placental gas exchange. The outcome of this process included progressive increases in arterial PCO_2, decreases in arterial pH, and finally, fetal death. Inhibition of stress responses by appropriate anesthetic management in this experimental fetal surgery was critical to postoperative fetal survival.

THE ROLE OF STRESS RESPONSES IN MINOR SURGERY

In cases of relatively minor surgery in the infant and neonate, the importance of modulating stress responses is less certain, and few data are available. Certainly, studies of circumcision in neonates have shown that substantial stress responses to such "minor" procedures occur, but their significance, other than documented short-term behavioral changes, remains unknown (1,7,8). Because the mechanisms by which stress responses affect postoperative morbidity and recovery are poorly understood, it is difficult to detect the subtle effects of inadequate protection from stress on the intra- and postoperative clinical course. Whether or not perioperative control of pain and stress are equally valuable and important factors in morbidity resulting from minor surgical procedures in infants and neonates is a question that will require considerable investigation in very large numbers of patients. Nevertheless, both clinical and experimental data clearly show that substantial and clinically significant stress responses result from surgical procedures in the infant, and even in the fetus, and that such stress responses can alter the postoperative outcome after uncomplicated anesthesia and surgery.

SUMMARY

Stress responses to surgical procedures are important considerations in pediatric anesthesia because even the youngest of neonates, prematurely born infants, have been shown to mount substantial classical stress responses to surgical procedures. Appropriate anesthetic techniques in infants and neonates have been shown to modulate these stress responses to both minor and major surgical procedures. In the case of major surgical procedures in neonates, the postoperative outcome has been shown to be linked to stress responses and can be modified by anesthetic techniques attenuating stress responses. In experimental fetal surgery procedures, anesthetic techniques inhibiting fetal stress responses are critical in averting postoperative mortality. The role of stress responses and their modulation by anesthetic techniques in postoperative morbidity resulting from minor surgical procedures remains unknown.

REFERENCES

1. Anand KJS, Hickey PR: Pain and its effects in the human fetus and neonate. New Engl J Med 317:1321-1329, 1987
2. Anand KJS, Sippell WG, Aynsley-Green A: Randomized trial of fentanyl anaesthesia in preterm babies undergoing surgery: Effects on the stress response. Lancet 1:243-248, 1987
3. Anand KJS, Hansen DD, Hickey PR: Hormonal-metabolic stress responses in neonates undergoing cardiac surgery. Anesthesiology 73:661-670, 1990
4. Anand KJS, Hickey PR: Halothane-morphine vs. high-dose sufentanil anesthesia and postoperative analgesia: Stress responses and clinical outcome in neonatal cardiac surgery. New Engl J Med 326:1-9, 1992
5. Tuman KJ et al: Effects of epidural anesthesia and analgesia on coagulation and outcome after major vascular surgery. Anesth Analg 73:696-704, 1991
6. Yeager MP et al: Epidural anesthesia and analgesia in high-risk surgical patients. Anesthesiology 66:729-736, 1987
7. Maxwell LG et al: Penile nerve block for circumcision. Obst-Gynecol 70:415-419, 1987
8. Stang HJ et al: Local anesthesia for circumcision: Stress and cortisol responses. JAMA 259:1507-1511, 1988
9. Berry FA, Gregory GA: Do premature infants require anesthesia for surgery? Anesthesiology 67:291-293, 1987
10. Yaster M, Koehler RC, Traystman RJ: Effects of fentanyl on peripheral and cerebral hemodynamics in neonatal lambs. Anesthesiology 66:524-530, 1987
11. Hansen DD, Hickey PR: Anesthesia for hypoplastic left heart syndrome: Use of high dose fentanyl in 30 neonates. Anesth Analg 65:127-132, 1986
12. Del Nido PJ, Williams WG, Villamater J et al: Changes in pericardial surface pressure during pulmonary hypertensive crises after cardiac surgery. Circulation 76:93-96 (supplement III), 1987
13. Fenton KN, Heinemann MK, Hickey PR et al: The stress response during fetal surgery is blocked by total spinal anesthesia. Surg Forum 43:631-634

14. Fenton KN, Heinemann MK, Hickey PR et al: Inhibition of the fetal stress response improves cardiac output and gas exchange after fetal cardiac bypass. J Thorac Cardiovasc Surg 107:1416-1422
15. Fenton KN, Zinn HE, Heinemann MK et al: Long-term survivors of fetal cardiac bypass in lambs. J Thorac Cardiovasc Surg 107:1423-1427

PERIOPERATIVE FLUID AND BLOOD VOLUME
MANAGEMENT IN INFANTS AND CHILDREN

D. R. Cook

Intraoperative fluid therapy may involve the initiation of fluid management or, alternatively, may be a continuation of ongoing fluid therapy. It can be as simple as replacing the deficits from the preoperative NPO status and providing maintenance fluids or as complex as correcting preoperative abnormal deficits, intraoperative translocated fluids, and variable blood loss, in addition to providing maintenance fluids.

Because of their high metabolic rate and water turnover, significant hypoglycemia and dehydration may occur in infants who are allowed to fast for prolonged periods of time (1-3). The fluid deficit incurred during fasting should be replaced during anesthesia. Assuming that a healthy child is in water and electrolyte balance at the time oral feedings are discontinued, the fluid deficit at the start of anesthesia can be estimated by multiplying the child's hourly maintenance fluid requirement by the number of hours that have elapsed since the last feeding. This deficit may be replaced by giving half of the calculated volume during the first hour of anesthesia and the other half over the next 2 hours (4), in addition to intraoperative maintenance fluids. Five percent dextrose in quarter-normal saline (5% dextrose/0.25 NS) is frequently used for maintenance fluid.

The literature reveals conflicting data about the intraoperative use of glucose. Infants under 4 years of age who are kept fasting for over 6 hours may become hypoglycemic and irritable (5). Other studies (6) failed to demonstrate hypoglycemia in infants below 2 years of age, including those who fasted for 6-8 hours; however, a tendency toward metabolic acidosis was demonstrated. Since the metabolic rate and oxygen consumption of infants and small children is significantly greater than older children and adults, it has been recommended to provide 5% dextrose for all infants at risk of hypoglycemia (serum glucose <40 mg/dl) from preoperative starvation. It must be remembered, however, that preterm infants receiving glucose infusions should be monitored carefully

283

T.H. Stanley and P.G. Schafer (eds.), Pediatric and Obstetrical Anesthesia, 283-289.
© 1995 *Kluwer Academic Publishers.*

for *hyperglycemia*, since their kidneys are unable to hyperfiltrate in the presence of hyperglycemia (7). The metabolic need for glucose in the infant age group is 5 gm/kg/day.

Hyperglycemia (glucose >200 mg/dl) has also been noted in older infants and children given 5% dextrose in lactated Ringer's as an intraoperative maintenance fluid. Elevated blood glucose concentrations may lead to an osmotic diuresis and may exacerbate neurologic injury associated with a cardiac arrest or other cerebral insults: (i.e., cerebral ischemia and asphyxia). The clinical significance of postoperative hyperglycemia in otherwise healthy children would seem to be minimal. However, in major surgical cases such hyperglycemia and osmotic diuresis may complicate or confuse ongoing fluid therapy, or may be hazardous (i.e., intracranial surgery). Therefore, blood glucose control is a reasonable goal for many cases and a critical goal in a few.

Blood glucose control can be achieved in several ways. Most children receiving glucose-free intravenous fluids during surgical procedures demonstrate an increase in their blood glucose concentration. Physiologic factors accounting for the hyperglycemic response to anesthesia and surgery include increased sympathoadrenal activity leading to a decrease in glucose tolerance, decreased glucose utilization, and increased gluconeogenesis. However, about 12% of patients who receive glucose-free solutions fail to increase their blood glucose concentrations. Since hypoglycemia may be undetected during anesthesia, it would seem prudent to measure intraoperative glucose concentrations if glucose-free solutions are used and to treat hypoglycemia if diagnosed. It seems paradoxical, however, to be depending on the stress of surgery to increase glucose at a time when "stress-free" anesthetics are being advocated.

In general, we advocate the use of glucose-containing solutions. One way to avoid hyperglycemia with a 5% dextrose solution is to decrease the infusion rate, but this may contribute to hypotension in fluid depleted children. A less concentrated glucose solution (e.g., 2.5% dextrose in lactated Ringer's) given at recommended infusion rates provides adequate glucose for healthy children (300 mg/kg/hr) and adequate volume replacement, while avoiding hyperglycemia and hypoglycemia. Since 2.5% dextrose in lactated Ringer's is not commercially available, it can easily be made by the individual practitioner with 50% dextrose solution.

INTRAOPERATIVE THIRD-SPACE LOSSES

Surgical trauma, blunt trauma, burns, infections, and a host of surgical conditions are associated with the isotonic transfer of fluids from the extracellular fluid compartment (and to a lesser extent from the intracellular compartment) to a nonfunctional interstitial compartment (8). This acute sequestration of fluid to a nonfunctional compartment has been called third-space loss; if these volumes are not replaced, they will decrease. The magnitude of third-space loss varies with the surgical procedure and is usually highest in infants undergoing intra-abdominal intestinal surgery. In addition, failure to cover the exposed gut and the use of heat lamps may increase evaporative loss. In infants, estimated third-space loss during intra-abdominal surgery varies from 6-10 ml/kg/hour; in intrathoracic surgery it is less (4-7 ml/kg/hour); in superficial surgery or neurosurgery it is negligible (1-2 ml/kg/hour) (9). Generally, lactated Ringer's solution, normal saline, or plasmalyte is used to restore third-space losses (10-12). The composition of these solutions approximates the content of the interstitial fluid compartment. The high chloride content of normal saline may be too much for premature infants and, consequently, other solutions may have to be used. Third-space requirements are estimated by the clinical response to fluid administration, with appropriate replacement being a sustained, appropriate blood pressure, adequate tissue perfusion, and adequate urine volume (0.5 ml/kg/hr).

BLOOD AND BLOOD COMPONENT THERAPY

Pediatric patients undergoing major procedures (e.g., tumor resection, reconstructive surgery, cardiac surgery, organ transplantation, trauma surgery, or surgery for burns) will invariably require some form of blood volume replacement. Indications for blood or blood component therapy are not always clearcut, hence the anesthesiologist must formulate a preoperative plan of management utilizing scientific rationale for a decision on blood therapy. Factors on which this decision is based include the patient's blood volume estimates, preoperative hematocrit, general medical condition, and ability to provide adequate oxygen transport to the tissues, as well as the nature of the surgical procedure, and the risks vs. benefits of transfusion.

All blood loss in neonates, infants, and children should somehow be replaced. An accurate measurement of blood loss and an accurate assessment of acceptable blood loss in the child are vital to any replacement regimen. Calculation of sponge weight, the use of calibrated miniaturized suction bottles, and a visual estimation (combined with a "guess factor") make it possible to define the magnitude of the blood loss. "Davenport's law"—that intraoperative blood loss of less than 10% requires no replacement, while that exceeding 20% must be replaced—is unsatisfactory in that it does not consider the starting blood volume, hemoglobin, or hematocrit of the patient. We find the concept of allowable red-cell loss or allowable blood loss preferable as a guide to blood replacement (13-14). Normovolemic hemodilution to a predetermined hematocrit can be achieved with crystalloid or colloid solutions. Blood volume is age-related. The neonatal blood volume has been reported to vary widely from 65 to 129 ml/kg, depending on the magnitude of the placental transfusion (15).

ESTIMATING ALLOWABLE BLOOD LOSS

Several methods have been proposed for estimating allowable blood loss from the blood volume, weight, and hematocrit (13,14). The formulas range from the simple to the complex, but all involve an estimate of blood volume. The safest hemoglobin or hematocrit that is allowed during surgery is debatable and clearly depends on the type of surgery, the patient's postoperative activity and his/her underlying medical condition. As a general rule, we accept hematocrits of 28-30 as the lowest acceptable hematocrit. In the newborn, 40% is the lowest acceptable hematocrit.

The estimated blood volume can be used with the following equation to calculate allowable blood loss (ABL):

$$ABL = Wt \times EBV \times [H_0 - H_1] / [H]$$

In this equation, H_0 is the original hematocrit, H_1 is the lowest acceptable hematocrit, and H is the average hematocrit $(H_0 + H_1) / 2$; all hematocrits are decimal values (i.e., 0.6, 0.5, etc.).

There is controversy as to whether the blood volume should be supported with crystalloid or colloid while the hematocrit is being allowed to decrease. If colloid (i.e., albumin, fresh frozen plasma) is used, then ongoing blood loss is replaced milliliter for milliliter. If isotonic crystalloid is administered, Furhman et al recommend replacing ongoing blood loss with an equal volume of lactated Ringer's solution until the serum protein concentration approaches 5 g/dl (13); after this point, blood volume is maintained with 5% albumin until the allowable blood loss has been exceeded. Others replace blood loss with 2-4 times the volume of lactated Ringer's solution. However, with these large volumes of crystalloid replacement, hypoproteinemia may result.

We replace blood loss with volumes of crystalloid 2 times the measured or calculated loss. In major surgery involving 1-2 body cavities, intravascular albumin may be transiently depleted or translocated. Consequently, we follow serum protein levels and begin replacing with 5% albumin when serum protein levels approach 5.0 g/dl.

BLOOD COMPONENT THERAPY

Blood component therapy depends on the clinical setting and the availability of various blood products. Bleeding from thrombocytopenia is rare with a platelet count of more than 50,000; serious bleeding is usual below 20,000. Normal adult values for clotting factors are attained between 1 and 12 months of age, depending on the specific factor. Fresh whole blood (less than 4 hours old) has a limited availability. If predicted blood loss is greater than or equal to 40% of blood volume, it is helpful to supply platelets and clotting factors. Component therapy is usually the rule, however (16-17). Packed red blood cells have a hematocrit of between 70% and 80%. An average of 1 ml/kg packed cells increases the hematocrit by 1.5%. Units of packed cells can be subdivided into pediatric packs of 80-100 ml. The fluid of these cells is relatively hyperkalemic (K^+, 15-20 mEq/l), acidotic (pH <7.0), and low in ionized Ca^{++}. When the maximum allowable blood loss is approached, consider transfusion with packed fresh red cells (PRBC) to adjust the hematocrit to about 30%.

When the amount of blood lost approaches one blood volume, labile clotting factors are greatly reduced; normal clotting requires 5-20% of Factor V and 30% of Factor VIII. All of the coagulation factors except platelets are present in normal quantities in fresh frozen plasma. We prefer to give 2:1 volumes of lactated Ringer's solution and packed cells (hematocrit 35-40%) to patients with massive blood loss (i.e., ≥1 blood volume). This ratio of cells and crystalloid can be varied to produce any desired hematocrit.

In patients with clinical signs of bleeding or documented abnormal clotting studies, crystalloid is replaced with fresh frozen plasma. The FFP is then administered with equal volumes of packed cells. The therapeutic value of FFP is related to volume expansion and provision of procoagulants. FFP contains 70% or more of the procoagulant factors of

288

fresh plasma (18) and is best utilized to replace depleted clotting factors in patients with Von Willibrand's disease, hemophilia A, and liver disease. It is also used in association with massive blood transfusion and perhaps DIC. The latter two conditions do not always represent clearcut indications for FFP transfusion. The National Institute of Health recommendations for FFP administration include reversal of oral anticoagulant, replacement of factor deficiencies as determined by the laboratory, treatment of immunodeficiencies, treatment of thrombotic thrombocytopenia purpura, treatment in antithrombin III deficiency, and massive blood transfusion (when factor V and VIII are less than 25% of normal) (19). The use of FFP carries with it risks of transfusion-transmitted diseases, as is the case with any blood product.

The need for platelets intraoperatively may be predicted from the preoperative platelet count. Platelets can be mobilized from the spleen and bone marrow as bleeding occurs. An infant with a high preoperative count (>250,000) may not need a platelet transfusion until 2-3 blood volumes are lost, whereas an infant with a low count (<150,000) may need platelets after only 1 blood volume is lost (16,17,20). One platelet pack per 10 kg is usually adequate.

REFERENCES

1. Pildes RS: Carbohydrate metabolism in the mother, fetus, and neonate. In Behrman RE, ed. Neonatal perinatal medicine. St. Louis, CV Mosby, 1977.
2. Cornblath M, Schwartz R: Disorders of carbohydrate metabolism in infancy. Philadelphia, WB Saunders, 1976, pp 345-443
3. Pildes RS: Management of acute metabolic problems in the neonate. In Aladjem S, Brown AK, eds. Perinatal intensive care. St. Louis, CV Mosby, 1977, pp 294-324
4. Liu LMP: Pediatric blood and fluid therapy. In Hersey SG, ed. Refresher courses in anesthesiology, Vol 12. Philadelphia, JB Lippincott, 1984, pp 109-120
5. Thomas DKM: Hypoglycemia in children before operations: Its incidence and prevention. Br J Anaesth 46:66, 1974
6. Nilsson K, Lavsson EL et al: Blood-glucose concentrations during anaesthesia in children. Br J Anaesth 56:375, 1984
7. Brodehl J, Franken A, Glissen K: Maximal tubular reabsorption of glucose in infants and children. Acta Paediatr Scand 61:413, 1972
8. Shires T, Williams J, Brown F: Acute changes in extracellular fluids associated with major surgical procedures. Ann Surg 154:803-810, 1961
9. Bennett EJ: Fluid balance in the newborn. Anesthesiology 43:210-224, 1975

10. Rowe MI, Arango A: The neonatal response to massive fluid infusion. J Pediatr Surg 6:365-371, 1971

11. Rowe MI, Arango A: The choice of intravenous fluid in shock resuscitation. Pediatr Clin North Am 22:269-274, 1975

12. Rowe MI, Arango A: Colloid versus crystalloid resuscitation in experimental bowel obstruction. J Pediatr Surg 11:635-643, 1976

13. Furhman EB, Roman DG, Lemmer LAS et al: Specific therapy in water, electrolyte, and blood-volume replacement during pediatric surgery. Anesthesiology 42:187-193, 1975

14. Bourke DL, Smith TC: Estimating allowable hemodilution. Anesthesiology 41:609-612, 1974

15. Oh W, Blankenship W, Lind J: Further study of neonatal blood volume in relation to placental transfusion. Ann Pediatr 207:147, 1966

16. Buchholz DH: Blood transfusion: Merits of component therapy I. J Pediatr 84:1-15, 1974

17. Buchholz DH: Blood transfusion: Merits of component therapy II. J Pediatr 84:165-172, 1974

18. Schmidt PJ: Component therapy. In Stehling LC, ed. Techniques of blood transfusion. Int Anesthesiol Clin 20:23-43, 1982

19. National Institute of Health: Fresh frozen plasma: Indication and risks consensus development conference statement. Vol 5, No 5, 1984

20. Coté CJ, Liu LMP, Szyfelbein SK et al: Changes in serial platelet counts following massive blood transfusion in pediatric patients. Anesthesiology 62:197-201, 1985

REGIONAL ANESTHESIA IN THE PEDIATRIC PATIENT

L. J. Rice

In the last 5 years, regional anesthesia has progressed from a novelty to a routine part of modern pediatric anesthesia practice (1-4). This renaissance of pediatric regional anesthesia paralleled the general recognition that children feel pain and require analgesia at least as much as adults do (5). Regional anesthesia can provide complete analgesia with minimal physiologic derangement. Regional anesthesia, when added to a light general anesthetic, provides profound analgesia with a decreased need for narcotics, a rapid and pain-free recovery, and earlier ambulation and discharge. In addition, continuous catheter techniques may be utilized to provide prolonged analgesia for hospitalized patients.

There are, however, some possible disadvantages to the use of regional blockade in the pediatric patient. When used in conjunction with a light general anesthetic, many techniques require a skilled "extra pair of hands" to support the airway and monitor the patient during placement of the block. In addition, do combining local anesthetics and general anesthetics increase the risk of anesthesia? Is it possible to detect local anesthesia toxicity early in a heavily sedated or anesthetized patient? Finally, why bother to add a regional anesthetic to a perfectly good general anesthetic?

These disadvantages seem to be mostly theoretical rather than real. Using regional anesthesia as an adjunct to general anesthesia seems to be similar to using intravenous opioids or neuromuscular blocking agents to supplement a volatile agent—it can be a valuable part of a balanced anesthetic plan.

PHARMACOLOGY AND PHARMACOKINETICS

Little work has been done regarding toxic blood levels of local anesthetics in children; at this time, adult levels are the references that are used. When considering how much local anesthetic to administer, one must consider not only how much of, but also where, the local anesthetic

T.H. Stanley and P.G. Schafer (eds.), Pediatric and Obstetrical Anesthesia, 291-302.
© 1995 *Kluwer Academic Publishers.*

is to be administered. Toxicity of local anesthetics will depend on rapidity of absorption, as well as the total dose of the drug administered. The relatively rapid increase to peak blood concentrations following intercostal, tracheal, and interpleural injections of local anesthetics requires caution in both children and adults.

Protein binding, drug metabolism, and intravascular injection have similar effects in patients of all ages, with a few exceptions. Neonates and infants less than 3 months of age have immature metabolic pathways and significantly decreased liver blood flow.

These factors affect both clearance and elimination of local anesthetics. Furthermore, the proteins that usually bind these drugs (albumin and alpha-1 acid glycoprotein) are also reduced in neonates (6). Esters, such as tetracaine, are metabolized by pseudocholinesterase. Even though infants less than 6 months of age have half the adult level of pseudocholinesterase, elimination of ester drugs is not delayed. For these reasons, systemic toxicity can occur more easily when injecting amide drugs, such as bupivacaine.

Absorption, distribution, and elimination of local anesthetics have been evaluated in children following virtually every regional anesthetic technique. There is rapid absorption and redistribution of local anesthetic followed by a slow elimination phase after caudal and lumbar epidural blockade (2 blocks commonly employed in pediatric patients). Elimination half-lives of lidocaine and bupivacaine are approximately 2 and 4.5 hours, respectively (7,8). Most regional blocks can be performed safely with 2.5-3 mg/kg of bupivacaine (1 ml/kg of bupivacaine 0.25%) or with 1 ml/kg of lidocaine 1% (9,10). However, when using a continuous catheter technique, one must employ smaller doses of local anesthetic for infusion (0.4 mg/kg/hr of bupivacaine or 1.5 mg/kg/hr of lidocaine) (11).

TOPICAL ANESTHESIA

EMLA cream (Eutectic Mixture of Local Anesthetics) is the first local anesthetic that will penetrate intact skin. Available in Europe for more than 10 years, it has recently become approved for use in the United States. This combination of lidocaine and prilocaine provides anesthesia to a depth of 5 mm when applied to intact skin, covered with an occlusive dressing, and left for an hour (12-14). EMLA is an effective anesthetic for venepuncture, and it can be used as the superficial topical anesthetic for lumbar puncture as well (15). Lidocaine must be injected to anesthetize more deeply prior to lumbar puncture or bone marrow sampling. EMLA has also been employed for neonatal circumcision, immunizations, and laser ablation for port-wine stains. The greatest impact of EMLA has been in the treatment of pediatric patients who must undergo repeated invasive procedures, such as oncology or dialysis patients. These patients, and others who face repeated invasive procedures, frequently can separate the emotional component of pain from the needle stick. As with other topical anesthetics, the child often will not believe that pain will be reduced or eliminated the first time EMLA is employed; emotional support and encouragement is still important. Frequently, however, the child will not allow subsequent invasive procedures without the use of EMLA.

Other topical anesthetic techniques will be discussed under the penile and ilioinguinal technique sections.

PENILE BLOCK

Local anesthetics are well absorbed by exposed mucous membranes. EMLA, lidocaine preparations, and bupivacaine have been used to provide adjunct intraoperative anesthesia, as well as postoperative analgesia, following circumcision (16-18).

Tree-Trackarn and others found significant differences between methods of postoperative analgesia in boys ages 1-13 undergoing circumcision (16). The children who received topical lidocaine spray, ointment, or jelly uniformly had analgesia similar to those boys who received dorsal penile nerve blocks—analgesia better than that provided by morphine 0.2 mg/kg IM. A second study compared postoperative analgesia in boys and men (17). This double-blind study compared the use of topical lidocaine jelly 2% with a placebo (the jelly base without lidocaine). The investigators found significant reductions in both pain (with movement) and tenderness (at rest) between the patients who had received the local anesthetic and those who had received the placebo. Moreover, reapplication of the cream was made at 6-hour intervals following discharge from the hospital, and the groups continued to show significant differences for 48 hours following surgery. The investigators noted no incidence of infection but cautioned that the dried jelly did alter the wound appearance.

Andersen showed that irrigation of the glans penis (exposed mucous membrane) with lidocaine 2% following amputation of the foreskin allowed halothane to be eliminated and the remainder of the surgical procedure to be performed simply using inhaled nitrous oxide and oxygen (18). Lidocaine also provided better postoperative analgesia than did saline in this double-blind study.

Blockade of the dorsal nerve of the penis provides effective analgesia for hypospadias repair and circumcision, both of which are commonly performed in infants and children.

ANATOMY

The distal two-thirds of the penis is innervated by the dorsal nerves, which are bilateral and adjacent to the midline. The dorsal nerves are distal twigs of the pudendal nerves, which arise from the sacral plexus (S2,3,4). At the base of the penis, they divide into multiple filaments that encircle the shaft before reaching the glans. These nerves are covered by Buck's fascia and lie alongside the dorsal artery and veins of the penis, also midline structures. The base and proximal part of the penis are innervated by the genitofemoral and ilioinguinal nerves.

TECHNIQUE

Broadman described the subcutaneous ring block, consisting of subcutaneous infiltration around the root of the penis with 0.25% bupivacaine (19). This block is the simplest approach to blocking the penile nerves.

A more complicated approach to the penile block involves injection of local anesthetic near the dorsal nerves of the penis. Dorsal penile nerve block involves 1 or 2 injections of 1-2 ml of local anesthetic deep to Buck's fascia. Maxwell and co-workers employed a block in the newborn involving 0.4 ml of local anesthetic injected at the 10:30 and 1:30 positions at the base of the penis (20). Brown and colleagues, investigating the anatomic basis of this block by using injected radiologic contrast medium and dissection techniques, noted that the double-injection technique provided a more satisfactory diffusion of local anesthetic than a single injection (21). However, there have been case reports of gangrene of the tip of the glans penis using this technique (22).

ILIOINGUINAL-ILIOHYPOGASTRIC NERVE BLOCK

Topical analgesia has been successfully employed here as well. Although there is no exposed mucous membrane here, the ilioinguinal and iliohypogastric nerves are exposed during the dissection and are easy to block with a simple instillation of bupivacaine 0.25% (23). The local anesthetic may simply be used as an irrigation, but it must be left in place for 1 minute to allow the tissues and the exposed nerve to absorb it.

There are several ways to perform this simple block, which is effective for postoperative analgesia following inguinal hernia repair, as well as hydrocelectomy and orchidopexy.

ANATOMY

Three nerves—the iliohypogastric, the ilioinguinal, and, to some degree, the genital branch of the genitofemoral—supply the inguinal area. The ilioinguinal nerve runs between the transverse and internal oblique muscles and is an L1 branch of the lumbar plexus. It becomes more superficial proximal to the superficial inguinal ring, supplying sensation to the skin of the scrotum. The iliohypogastric nerve, which is also a branch of L1, runs superficial to the inguinal muscles close the anterior superior iliac spine. It supplies the skin immediately above the inguinal ligament.

TECHNIQUE

The ilioinguinal and iliohypogastric nerves can easily be blocked by infiltration of the abdominal wall in the area medial to the anterior superior iliac spine. A 25-gauge needle is used to puncture the skin one-half inch medial and one-half inch inferior to the anterior superior iliac spine, just above the inguinal ligament. Three "pops" will be felt as the skin and external and internal oblique fasciae are pierced. Then three fan-shaped injections are made as the needle is withdrawn, leaving a subcutaneous weal. If the block is performed at the completion of surgery, the area to be infiltrated may be approached through the lateral edge of the groin incision.

Langer and colleagues performed a double-blind study where ilioinguinal and iliohypogastric nerve blocks were performed by the surgeon, comparing bupivacaine to normal saline infiltration following induction of general anesthesia but prior to the start of the surgery (24). They found a significant decrease in the number of children requiring supplemental analgesia following inguinal hernia repair, both in frequency and dosage of codeine necessary in the ambulatory surgery area in the bupivacaine group. This significant difference persisted in the amount of acetaminophen required at home up to 48 hours after surgery.

Perhaps the benefits of regional anesthesia outlast the pharmacology of the local anesthetic!

Occasionally this block is accompanied by a transient motor block of the femoral nerve. Authors who use a more dilute solution to perform the block have noted no such complication. In some studies, the blocks were performed by the surgeon prior to closing the incision. Patients receiving both caudal and regional nerve blocks showed significantly better pain relief than the unblocked patients.

CAUDAL ANESTHESIA/ANALGESIA

Caudal analgesia is the most useful and popular pediatric regional block used today. Circumcision, hypospadias repair, anal surgery, and clubfoot repair are common indications for caudal blocks. There are very few problems with "single-shot" caudals, although it is possible to reach the dura via the caudal epidural space. It was thought at one time that caudals might cause urinary retention, but Fisher and others, as well as Dalens and colleagues, demonstrated that most children void within 6-8 hours of a "single-shot" caudal, and there is no difference in voiding time (or analgesia) between caudal and ilioinguinal-iliohypogastric nerve blocks (25,26).

Continuous caudal blockade has been employed, not just to provide prolonged analgesia, but to provide continuous sympathetic blockade in children with vascular insufficiency secondary to intense vasoconstriction (e.g., meningococcal purpura fulminans) (27). Complications are rare but do occur. Unlike adults, hypotension is almost unheard of in children under 8 years of age, even with high thoracic blockade (28). Local anesthetic accumulation is a real risk with patients receiving continuous infusions of local anesthetic, and doses must be watched carefully (29). Addition of opioid may lead to respiratory depression, particularly in younger children (30).

ANATOMY

The sacral hiatus is extremely easy to identify in infants and young children under 8 years of age. The coccyx lies immediately caudal to the sacral hiatus. The hiatus is covered by the sacrococcygeal membrane. In infants and prepubertal children, these landmarks are easily palpable or even visible through the skin because of the absence of the large sacral pad of fat that usually develops at puberty.

The dural and subarachnoid sacs may extend to the third or fourth sacral vertebrae in infants. Moreover, since the sacral hiatus is relatively more cephalad, the distance between the sacral hiatus and the end of the dural sac is relatively short. The epidural fat in the infant and small child has a gelatinous, spongy appearance, which offers less of an obstacle to the cephalad spread of injected local anesthetics or catheter advancement than that of the adult.

SINGLE-SHOT TECHNIQUE

The lateral position is most often employed. After careful skin preparation, the sacral hiatus is identified using firm pressure by the left index finger. Asepsis is maintained, whether by gloving or palpating the skin through a sterile alcohol swab. The caudal space is entered using a short (1-inch), 23-gauge needle that has been attached to a syringe containing the appropriate volume of local anesthetic solution. The needle must be placed exactly in the midline and inserted at a 60-degree angle to the coronal plane, perpendicular to all other planes. As the needle is advanced, the bevel should be facing anteriorly to minimize the chance of piercing the anterior sacral wall (the most common reason for aspirating blood). A distinct "pop" is felt as the sacrococcygeal membrane is pierced. The angle of the needle is then lowered to 20 degrees and advanced an additional 2-3 mm to make sure that all the bevel surface is in the caudal space. Further advancement of the needle is not necessary and will increase the chances of dural puncture. After repeatedly demonstrating the absence of blood or CSF following attempted aspiration, the appropriate amount of local anesthetic solution is injected, and the child is placed in the supine position.

AGENTS/DOSAGE

Volume, total dose, and concentration of the drug determine the quality, duration, and extent of a caudal block. There is currently no general agreement, however, on whether age or weight is the better criterion for achieving the desired level of analgesia in children. Bupivacaine 0.125% and bupivacaine 0.25% both provide identical intraoperative and postoperative analgesia following hernia repair; it is not known if the more concentrated solution is required for other surgical procedures. When diluting local anesthetics, remember to use *preservative-free normal saline.*

The easiest formula for dose calculation is that of Armitage (31). Using the desired local anesthetic solution, Armitage maintains that a volume of 0.5 ml/kg will result in an adequate sacral block; 1 ml/kg is used to block the lower thoracic nerves; and 1.25 ml/kg is necessary to reach the mid-thoracic region. The total mg/kg dosage must always be checked to ensure that it is within the acceptable safe dose of the drug selected.

CONTINUOUS CAUDAL

Several techniques are possible for infusion of local anesthetics or local anesthetic/opioid combinations. Standard adult equipment can be used in children of all ages, but the length of the needle makes using this technique awkward in small children. Several companies (Preferred Medical Products, Portex) make special equipment for use in children— both 20-gauge needles with 24-gauge catheters and short 18-gauge needles with 20-gauge catheters. Problems with the smaller catheters include kinking at the skin and inability of an infusion pump to pump against the very high resistance.

Placement of a caudal catheter is very similar to placement of an epidural catheter in adults. How much catheter to insert depends on the size of the child and the site of the surgical procedure. Both Bösenberg and Gunther have demonstrated that because of the loose gelatinous fat in the young child's epidural space, a 20-gauge catheter can frequently be passed from the caudal space as far as the thorax (32,33).

SPINAL ANESTHESIA

The neonatal spinal cord can end anywhere from T12 to L3. It is therefore preferable to perform the lumbar puncture in children below the L3 interspace. At that level, the subarachnoid space is located approximately 1-1.5 cm from the skin.

TECHNIQUE

A standard, disposable spinal anesthesia tray, a 1-ml syringe, a 22-gauge 3.5 cm or 25-gauge 2.25 cm pediatric Quincke needle, and a clear, fenestrated operative drape are required. The child is placed in the lateral or sitting position with the back maximally flexed. The infant's neck must remain extended, since flexion of the neck of a premature infant may decrease the transcutaneous PO_2 by as much as 28 mm Hg. Sedation with ketamine 1-2 mg/kg IM prior to placement of the block may be desirable in vigorous infants over 52 weeks conceptual age; younger patients rarely require sedation.

CLINICAL USE

In 1984, Abajian and others reported on 81 surgeries in 78 patients under 1 year of age in whom spinal anesthesia was used for surgery below the diaphragm; 36 of these infants were categorized as "high risk" (34). They concluded that spinal anesthesia can be safely and reliably performed, even in high-risk infants. More recently, others have reported similar success with spinal and caudal anesthesia in children, as well as in infants. Both spinal and caudal anesthetic techniques may be particularly useful in children in whom one wishes to avoid airway manipulation.

PERIPHERAL NERVE BLOCKS

Peripheral nerve blocks can provide anesthesia and analgesia in areas where central blocks are inappropriate, such as the upper extremity. They are useful for management of chronic pain and can also be employed where prolonged sympathectomy is desirable. A successful peripheral block depends on injecting an appropriate amount of local anesthetic solution close to the nerve to be blocked (Table). While the approach to these blocks is similar in children to that in adults, special considerations must be kept in mind.

A peripheral nerve stimulator (PNS) is a critical tool for these blocks. Since most blocks in children are placed after the child is asleep or heavily sedated, paresthesia cannot be elicited. The PNS is an invaluable means of identifying the nerve bundle in these cases. The standard, unsheathed needle connected to a nerve stimulator has the greatest density of radiated electrical current at its tip; little current flows from its shaft. Ordinary needles are therefore suitable for regional anesthesia. On a PNS such as Professional Instruments Model NS-3A, which has a 1-10 analog scale, a setting of 1-3 is useful. The suggested volumes are shown in the Table. It is important to calculate the total mg/kg of local anesthetic agent desired, to ensure that the total dose employed is in the safe range.

Table. Volume of local anesthetic for peripheral nerve blocks in children.

Block	Volume (ml/kg)
Axillary brachial plexus	0.33
Interscalene brachial plexus	0.25
Sciatic nerve	0.15-0.2
Inguinal paravascular ("3-in-1" block)	0.5

CONCLUSION

Regional anesthesia now occupies almost as valuable a place in pediatric anesthesia as in grownup anesthesia! The skills learned in adult patients can be easily translated into regional blocks in pediatric patients. Some regional techniques (caudal) are actually easier in pediatric patients than they are in adults.

REFERENCES

1. Rice LJ, Britton JT: Neural blockade for pediatric pain management. In Sinatra RS, Hord AH, Ginsberg B, eds. Acute pain, mechanisms and management. St. Louis, CV Mosby Company, 1992, pp 483-507
2. Sethna NF, Berde CB: Pediatric regional anesthesia. In Gregory G, ed. Pediatric anesthesia, 2nd edition. New York, Churchill Livingstone 1994, pp 281-319
3. Rice LJ, Britton JT: Pediatric postoperative analgesia. Sem in Anesth 12:27-36, 1993
4. Yaster M: Pediatric regional anesthesia. American Society of Anesthesiologists Annual Refresher Courses 216, 1993
5. Acute pain management in infants, children and adolescents: Operative and medical procedures, Rockville, MD. Agency for Health Care Policy and Research, US Department of Health and Human Services. DHHS Publication no. 92-0020
6. Burrows FA, Lerman J, LeDez KM et al: Alpha-1 acid glycoprotein and the binding of lidocaine in children with congenital heart disease. Can J Anaesth 37:883-888, 1990
7. Ecoffey C, Desparmet J, Berdeaux A et al: Pharmacokinetics of lignocaine in children following caudal anesthesia. Br J Anaesth 56:1399-1402, 1984
8. Ecoffey C, Desparmet J, Maury M et al: Bupivacaine in children: Pharmacokinetics following caudal anesthesia. Anesthesiology 63:447-448, 1985

9. Eyres RL, Oppenheimer R, Brown TCK: Plasma bupivacaine concentrations in children during caudal epidural analgesia. Anaesth Intens Care 11:20-22, 1983

10. Bricker SRW, Telford RJ, Booker PD: Pharmacokinetics of bupivacaine following intraoperative intercostal nerve block in neonates and infants aged less than 6 months. Anesthesiology 61:942-947, 1989

11. Berde CB: Convulsions associated with pediatric regional anesthesia. Anesth Analg 75:164-166, 1992

12. Maddi R, Horrow JC, Mark JB et al: Evaluation of a new cutaneous topical anesthesia preparation. Reg Anes 15:109-111, 1990

13. Hopkins CS, Buckley CJ, Bush GH: Pain-free injection in infants: Use of a lidocaine-prilocaine cream to prevent pain at intravenous injection of general anesthesia in 1-5 year old children. Anaesthesia 43:188-201, 1988

14. Soliman IE, Broadman LM, Hannallah RS: Comparison of the analgesic effects of EMLA (Eutectic Mixture of Local Anesthetics) to intradermal lidocaine prior to venous cannulation in unpremedicated children. Anesthesiology 68:804-806, 1988

15. Halperin DL, Koren G, Attias D et al: Topical skin anesthesia for venous, subcutaneous drug reservoir, and lumbar punctures in children. Pediatrics 84:281-284, 1989

16. Tree-Trackarn T, Piryavaraporn S: Postoperative pain relief for circumcision in children: Comparison among morphine, nerve block, and topical analgesia. Anesthesiology 62:519-522, 1985

17. Tree-Trackarn T, Piryavaraporn S, Lertakyamanee J: Topical anesthesia for relief of post-circumcision pain. Anesthesiology 67:395-398, 1987

18. Andersen KH: A new method of analgesia for relief of circumcision pain. Anaesthesia 44:118-120, 1989

19. Broadman LM, Hannallah RS, Belman AB et al: Post-circumcision analgesia—a prospective evaluation of subcutaneous ring block of the penis. Anesthesiology 67:399-402, 1987

20. Maxwell LG, Yaster M, Wetzel RC: Penile nerve block for newborn circumcision. OB Gyn 70:415-419, 1987

21. Brown TCK, Weidner NJ, Bouwmeester J: Dorsal nerve of penis block—anatomical and radiological studies. Anaesth Intens Care 17:34-38, 1989

22. Sara CA, Lowry CJ: A complication of circumcision and dorsal nerve block of the penis. Anesth Intens Care 13:79-85, 1984

23. Casey WF, Rice LJ, Hannallah RS: A comparison between bupivacaine instillation versus ilioinguinal-iliohypogastric nerve block for postoperative analgesia following inguinal herniorrhaphy in children. Anesthesiology 72:636-639, 1990

24. Langer JC, Shandling B, Rosenberg M: Intraoperative bupivacaine during outpatient hernia repair in children: A randomized double-blind trial. J Pediatr Surg 22:267-270, 1987

25. Fisher QA, McComiskey CM, Hill JL et al: Postoperative voiding interval and duration of analgesia following peripheral or caudal nerve blocks in children. Anesth Analg 76:173-177, 1993

26. Dalens B, Hasnaoui A: Caudal anesthesia in pediatric surgery: Success rate and adverse effects in 750 consecutive patients. Anesth Analg 68:83-89, 1989

27. Anderson CT, Berde CB, Sethna NF et al: Meningococcal purpura fulminans: Treatment of vascular insufficiency in a 2-yr-old child with lumbar epidural sympathetic blockade. Anesthesiology 71:463-464, 1989

28. Dohi S, Naito H, Takahashi T: Age-related changes in blood pressure and duration of motor block in spinal anesthesia. Anesthesiology 50:319-322, 1979

29. McCloskey, JJ, Haun SE, Deshpande JK: Bupivacaine toxicity secondary to continuous caudal epidural infusion in children. Anesth Analg 75:287-290, 1992

30. Valley RD, Bailey AG: Caudal morphine for postoperative analgesia in infants and children: A report of 138 cases. Anesth Analg 72:120-124, 1991

31. Armitage EN: Local anaesthetic techniques for prevention of postoperative pain. Br J Anaesth 58:790-799, 1986

32. Bösenberg AT, Bland BAR, Shülte-Steinberg O et al: Thoracic epidural anesthesia via the caudal route in infants. Anesthesiology 69:265-269, 1988.

33. Gunther JB, Eng C: Thoracic epidural anesthesia via the caudal approach in children. Anesthesiology 76:935-938, 1992

34. Abajian JC, Mellish RWP, Brown AF et al: Spinal anesthesia for surgery in the high-risk infant. Anesth Analg 63:359-364, 1984

POSTOPERATIVE NAUSEA AND VOMITING IN CHILDREN

J. Lerman

Postoperative nausea and vomiting (PONV) is one of the most common and distressing complications after anesthesia and surgery in children. With the increasing emphasis on ambulatory surgery and early discharge from the hospital of inpatients, PONV has been identified as a very common impediment to early ambulation. Accordingly, great effort and expense have been invested in understanding the mechanism of PONV and developing effective management strategies to prevent it in children. In this lecture, I shall briefly review the pathophysiology of PONV, the perioperative factors associated with PONV, and a series of management strategies that are aimed at preventing PONV in children.

PATHOPHYSIOLOGY

The physiology of the vomiting reflex was first described by Borison and Wang in 1942 (1). This reflex enables the body to rid itself of toxins from the gastrointestinal tract and to respond to chemotherapy, radiotherapy to the trunk, specific disease states, and anesthesia and surgery. The vomiting reflex is comprised of a series of afferent and efferent communication systems that inform the brain of the need to vomit and then execute the response. Afferent receptors within the gastrointestinal tract include the chemoreceptors in the mucosa of the upper GI tract (which contains enterochromaffin cells) and the mechanoreceptors of the muscular layer of the GI tract. These sensors activate afferent vagal pathways that terminate in the chemotrigger zone (CTZ) in the area postrema (AP) in the brain stem. Parallel vagal pathways originate in the hepatic arterial vasculature. These receptors may be activated by the presence of circulating toxins within the liver. Alternatively, these circulating toxins may bathe the CTZ and directly trigger the vomiting reflex. The motor efferent pathways involved in the emetic reflex include actions by the GI tract, as well as the cardiac,

303

T.H. Stanley and P.G. Schafer (eds.), Pediatric and Obstetrical Anesthesia, 303-314.
© *1995 Kluwer Academic Publishers.*

respiratory, and sympathetic nervous systems. These pathways, which will be described briefly, converge to produce the propulsive regurgitation that characterizes an emetic episode.

Our understanding of the pathophysiology of the vomiting reflex has led to many new and exciting developments in prevention of the reflex. For example, the stimulus to vomit after chemotherapy is directly attributable to the specific chemotherapeutic agent. Animal models were developed to explore the mechanisms and pathways associated with chemotherapy-induced vomiting. In contrast, our understanding of PONV has been sadly lacking. In part, this may be explained by the absence of an animal model for PONV. The pathophysiology of PONV in humans remains poorly understood, although several afferent pathways have been identified (Figure 1) (2)

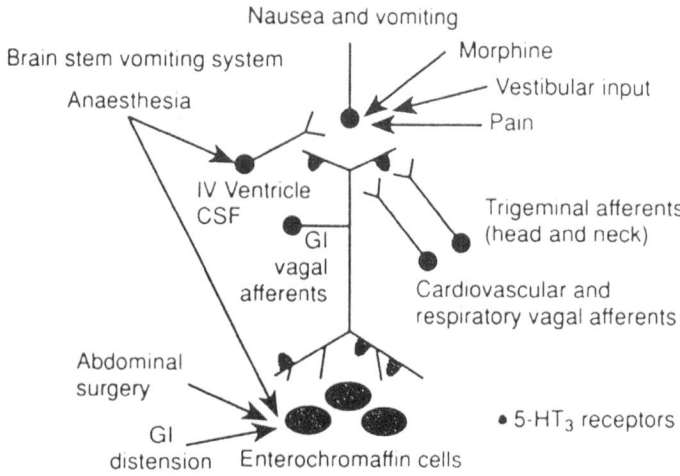

Figure 1.   Afferent pathways involved in anesthesia and surgery that may initiate the vomiting reflex. Stipled (5-HT3) dots indicate possible sites of action of 5-HT3 receptor antagonists. From Naylor RJ and Rudd JA (37).

PATIENT AND SURGICAL FACTORS

AGE

When all types of surgery are considered, the incidence of PONV increases with age throughout infancy and childhood, reaching a maximum value in children 6-16 years old and decreasing thereafter (3). This relationship between age and PONV may be explained in part by the nature of the surgery and in part by the changing threshold for emesis in the pediatric age groups.

GENDER

In adults, the incidence of postoperative vomiting is 2-4 times greater and more severe in females than it is in males (3,4). This has been associated with changes in hormones in females during the menstrual cycle (5). In contrast, in the prepubertal child, gender does not affect the incidence or severity of PONV (3,6).

HISTORY OF PONV/MOTION SICKNESS

PONV occurs up to 3 times more frequently in subjects with a history of PONV after previous surgery. Subjects with a history of motion sickness also appear to be susceptible to PONV (3).

OBESITY

Although obesity has been associated with PONV, the data are conflicting. To date, there are no controlled studies of the incidence of PONV in obese subjects.

DELAYED GASTRIC EMPTYING

This situation occurs in infants with pyloric stenosis, women who are pregnant, patients who have diabetes or increased intracranial pressure, and those with bowel obstruction. Delayed gastric emptying increases the likelihood of PONV.

Types of Surgery

In children, the incidence of PONV is greatest in strabismus surgery (40-80%), followed closely by tonsillectomy and adenoidectomy (40-60%), and then superficial abdominal and intra-abdominal surgery. The smallest incidence of PONV occurs in superficial peripheral surgery (10-15%) (3).

Emesis after strabismus surgery occurs 2-24 hours after surgery and is often triggered by ingestion of fluids. The stimulus for PONV after strabismus surgery is believed to arise from stimulus of the oculo-emetic reflex during traction on the extraocular muscles. Other mechanisms, including the effects of acute correction of the visual axes and vestibular-induced emesis, have been proposed. We studied the effect of patching the surgical eye after surgery and found that the incidence of PONV was no less in children whose eyes were patched than it was in children whose eyes were not patched (unpublished data).

The stimulus for PONV after tonsillectomy and adenoidectomy has been attributed to the chemical irritant effects of blood in the upper gastrointestinal tract, effects of traction on the tonsillar fossa or hypopharynx, and/or opioid administration.

POSTOPERATIVE FACTORS

Opioid and nitrous oxide anesthesia is associated with a greater incidence of PONV than inhalational anesthesia (7). Neuraxial (intrathecal and epidural) narcotics have also been associated with PONV.

Ingestion of clear fluids has, until recently, been a mandatory prerequisite for discharge from the ambulatory unit in most children's hospitals. Recent evidence suggests that early administration of fluids leads to a greater incidence of emesis in the hospital and overall than when fluids are administered only if demanded by the patient (8). Many anesthetic departments are now easing up on the need for children (excluding infants <1 year of age) to ingest clear fluids before discharge from the hospital. Recommended guidelines for fluid administration to children undergoing ambulatory surgery are now being formulated. They specify intraoperative IV fluids, such as lactated Ringer's solution (up to 20 ml/kg), for minor surgery and postoperative oral fluids for children at home (when requested by the child).

PHARMACOLOGICAL RISK FACTORS

PREMEDICATION

Intramuscular droperidol (100 µg/kg) has been associated with a low incidence of PONV in adults undergoing strabismus surgery (9).

INDUCTION AGENTS

Nausea and vomiting have been associated with the traditional drugs, etomidate, methohexital, and thiopental (10), although the newer agent, propofol, is thought to be less emetogenic (11). Indeed, it has been suggested that propofol has anti-emetic properties that are independent of its intralipid medium. Published studies in children have documented a salutary effect of propofol on the incidence of PONV after strabismus surgery when it was used for both induction and maintenance, although the effect was short-lived in one report (12-15). Unfortunately, data from some of these studies have been difficult to interpret because intraoperative narcotics were used.

INHALATIONAL AGENTS, INCLUDING NITROUS OXIDE

Potent inhalational anesthetics are associated with PONV. Nitrous oxide has also been associated with PONV, particularly after gynecological, gastrointestinal, and middle ear surgery (3,16). The mechanism of PONV after nitrous oxide remains speculative but includes gastrointestinal distention, middle ear pressure, and/or a central nervous system direct effect. However, many of these studies were flawed by a multitude of factors. Conclusive evidence implicating nitrous oxide in PONV remains unavailable.

MUSCLE RELAXANTS

Muscle relaxants per se have not been associated with PONV. However, reversal agents in atropine and anticholinesterases have been implicated in PONV.

AUTHOR'S VIEW

To minimize the likelihood of PONV when required, I use propofol with nitrous oxide and muscle relaxants. I prefer a regional blockade for pain management in deference to narcotics, although NSAIDS and acetaminophen may be used where appropriate for postoperative pain.

PROPHYLACTIC THERAPY

DROPERIDOL

This butyrophenone mediates its anti-emetic properties via dopamine receptor antagonism. Its long half-life has provided several hours of anti-emetic action after emetogenic surgeries such as strabismus and tonsillectomy. The dose of droperidol recommended for prophylaxis in strabismus surgery (75 µg/kg) (17) far exceeds that recommended for prophylaxis in adult surgeries (5-20 µg/kg). Although smaller doses of droperidol have been studied (3), there is no uniform agreement on the effectiveness of these smaller doses. Nevertheless, side effects including sedation, extrapyramidal movements (i.e., oculogyric crises), and delayed discharge from hospital have limited the use of droperidol.

METOCLOPRAMIDE

This benzamide acts via dopamine and serotonin receptor antagonism, the latter mechanism being important only with larger doses of metoclopramide, such as those used in chemotherapy (1-2 mg/kg). Few studies have been published with metoclopramide in children. The effective dose for prophylaxis for PONV after strabismus surgery in children is 0.15-0.25 mg/kg IV (18,19). This dose has not been associated with reports of extrapyramidal reactions, sedation, or delayed discharge from hospital.

LORAZEPAM

In a dose of 10 µg/kg IV, lorazepam decreased the incidence of PONV after strabismus surgery in children 3-13 years by 50% compared with placebo (20). The mechanism of anti-emetic action of lorazepam remains to be defined.

PROPOFOL

Several studies have documented the effectiveness of propofol anesthesia as a prophylactic measure to decrease the incidence of PONV in children. When used solely as an induction agent, propofol has not been uniformly effective in decreasing the incidence of PONV. However, when it also constitutes the maintenance phase of anesthesia (in the absence of narcotics), the 24-hour incidence of PONV (at least in strabismus surgery) is small (24%) (15). When it is used as a therapeutic measure in adults, IV propofol (0.15 mg/kg) decreases the frequency of repeated emetic episodes (21). When we studied the same dose of propofol in children undergoing tonsillectomy and adenoidectomy, we found that it did not affect the incidence of repeated episodes of emesis within 4 hours of the intervention (unpublished data). Propofol decreases the incidence of PONV in children, although its effectiveness in a therapeutic capacity remains to be clarified.

DIMENHYDRINATE

This old anti-emetic/sedative (Gravol®) has been used for many years without documented clinical efficacy in children. It is available in parenteral (IV and IM), oral, and rectal preparations. Recently, we studied its use for PONV after tonsillectomy and adenoidectomy. The incidence of PONV was 65% in the placebo group and 30% in the dimenhydrinate group (22). This anti-emetic suffers from the same drawback as the other traditional anti-emetics, with sedation being common, but is very inexpensive.

SEROTONIN RECEPTOR ANTAGONISTS

Recognition of the plausible role of serotonin in the pathogenesis of PONV followed observations that high-dose metoclopramide effectively prevented cisplatin-induced emesis. It was postulated that with these large doses, metoclopramide prevented emesis by blocking both serotonin and dopamine receptors. Subsequently, radioligand binding studies identified the presence of high concentrations of serotonin (5-HT_3) receptors on presynaptic vagal afferents in the enterochromaffin cells of the upper gastro-intestinal tract. Large amounts of serotonin have been located in two sites in humans: in enterochromaffin cells of the GI tract, and in platelets.

In the past decade, four subtypes of serotonin receptors have been identified: $5\text{-}HT_1$, $5\text{-}HT_2$, $5\text{-}HT_3$ and $5\text{-}HT_4$. Each of these serotonin receptor subtypes confers physiologic responses, although only the $5\text{-}HT_3$ receptors are involved in nausea and vomiting. Several specific $5\text{-}HT_3$ receptor antagonists, characterized by up to a 1000-fold greater affinity for $5\text{-}HT_3$ receptors than for other 5-HT receptors and other non-5-HT receptors (dopamine and other receptors), have been developed, with ondansetron being the first available for clinical use (Figure 2).

Ondansetron has been proven to be effective for the prevention of emesis after chemotherapy (particularly cisplatin) and radiotherapy in adults and children, and for PONV in adults (23-26). Possible sites of action of ondansetron in chemotherapy-induced emesis include a central site in the CTZ and a peripheral site in either the enterochromaffin cells or the vagus/splanchnic nerves. Radiotherapy-induced emesis occurs more frequently after truncal rather than peripheral extremity treatment. Radiotherapy-induced effects are likely mediated via the enterochromaffin cells and vagal nerves of the gastrointestinal tract. Possible sites of action of $5\text{-}HT_3$ receptor antagonists in the prevention of PONV include both central (chemoreceptor trigger zone) and peripheral (enterochromaffin cells and vagal nerve fibers) receptors.

The pharmacokinetics of ondansetron have been thoroughly investigated. Factors that alter the kinetics of ondansetron include gender (adult females clear ondansetron more slowly than male counterparts), age, and hepatic impairment. These will be discussed in detail. Ondansetron is 70-75% protein bound in plasma, likely to albumin and, to a lesser extent, α_1 acid glycoprotein.

The oral preparation of ondansetron is rapidly absorbed but undergoes first-pass hepatic metabolism, resulting in a 50-70% bioavailability. The bioavailability increases with age in adults.

The parenteral preparation has been investigated in both children and adults. Between 3 and 80 years of age, total plasma clearance of ondansetron decreases, whereas the elimination half-life increases from 2.5-5.5 hours (27,28). The volume of distribution at steady state remains constant for all ages between childhood and the elderly at 1.8 l/kg.

The major route of clearance of ondansetron is metabolism via hepatic microsomal enzymes, with hydroxylation being the most important pathway. The metabolites are conjugated and eliminated via the kidneys, with <5% of the original drug eliminated unchanged. Accordingly, the elimination half-life of ondansetron is markedly prolonged in the presence of severely impaired hepatic function. Hepatic

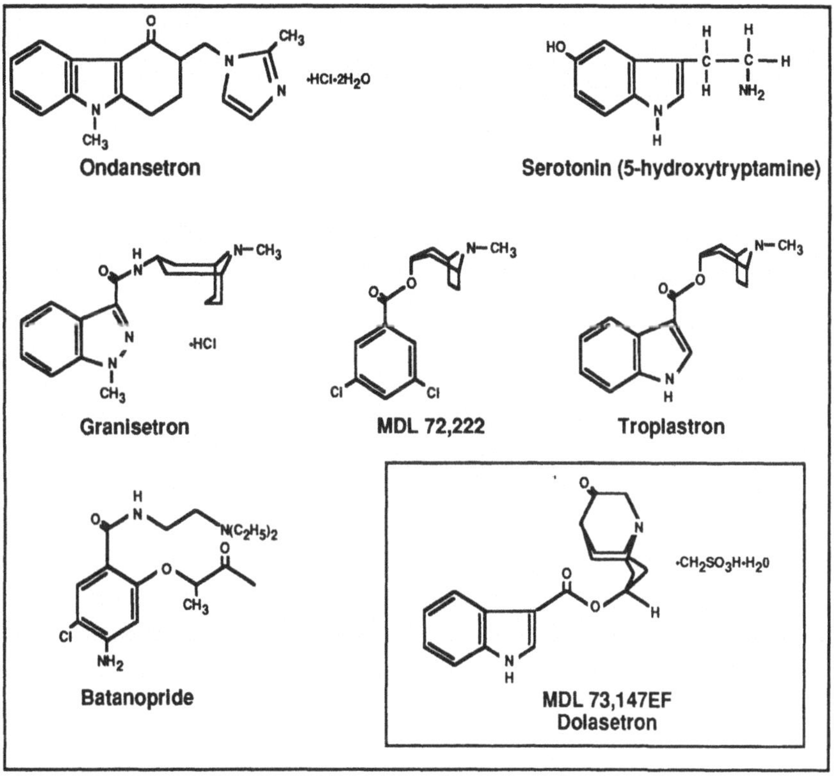

Figure 2.   Chemical structure of serotonin and several 5-HT3 receptor antagonists.
Ondansetron and granisetron are both available for clinical use,
dolasetron is currently under investigation, and tropisetron is no longer
under development. Figure courtesy of Nordic Merrell Dow, Canada,
Inc.

microsomal enzyme induction increases the rate of metabolism of
ondansetron and, therefore, decreases its half-life in vivo.

Side effects associated with ondansetron (and the whole class of 5-
HT_3 receptor antagonists) include headaches, constipation, and (very
rarely) allergic reactions. Prolongation of the QT interval on the ECG has
been reported after dolasetron administration.

Based on the pharmacokinetic study of ondansetron in children, we
postulated that a dose of 0.10 mg/kg should provide comparable blood
levels of ondansetron to those in adults. In a preliminary communication, a dose-response study of IV ondansetron in children undergoing
strabismus and tonsillectomy reported that 0.05 mg/kg was as effective as
0.10 and 0.15 mg/kg (29). To date, the doses of ondansetron used in clinical
studies range from 0.10 to 0.15 mg/kg IV. This will be a crucial issue when

we determine the cost-effectiveness of ondansetron and other 5-HT$_3$ antagonists.

The clinical efficacy of ondansetron in PONV in children is currently under investigation (30-35). To date, only one study has been published (36). Litman et al found that ondansetron 0.15 mg/kg IV decreased the incidence of PONV within the first 24 hours after tonsillectomy and adenoidectomy, from 73% in the placebo group to 27% in the ondansetron group (personal communication). In an unpublished, multi-centered, placebo-controlled study of 240 children undergoing strabismus surgery in Canada, ondansetron (0.10 mg/kg IV) decreased the 24-hour incidence of PONV from 65% in the placebo group to 30% in the ondansetron group. These studies demonstrate the superiority of ondansetron compared to placebo for strabismus surgery in children.

Development of 5-HT$_3$ receptor antagonists continues at a rapid rate. Figure 2 includes the chemical structures of some of the newer 5-HT$_3$ receptor antagonists, with dolasetron being the newest to launch clinical studies. This 5-HT$_3$ receptor antagonist is unique, in that its primary metabolite is approximately 100 times more potent an anti-emetic than its parent compound and has a half-life of 6-10 hours. Indeed, the 5-HT$_3$ receptor antagonist that will corner the clinical market will most certainly be the one that is most effective (and longest acting, i.e., up to 24 hours) for the least cost.

AUTHOR'S VIEW

Studies are required to compare the efficacy of the 5-HT$_3$ receptor antagonists to other anti-emetics. Only then will the cost/benefit ratio be calculable. Until such time, IV metoclopramide (0.15 mg/kg) remains the agent I prefer for prophylaxis against PONV in ambulatory surgery. For strabismus surgery, I still use IV droperidol 0.075 mg/kg.

REFERENCES

1. Borison HL, Wang SC: Physiology and pharmacology of vomiting. Pharmacol Rev 5:193-230, 1953
2. Andrews PLR: Physiology of nausea and vomiting. Br J Anaesth 69:2S-19S, 1992
3. Lerman J: Surgical and patient factors involved in postoperative nausea and vomiting. Br J Anaesth 69:24S-32S (suppl.), 1992
4. Belville JW, Bross IDJ, Howland WS: Postoperative nausea and vomiting IV: Factors related to postoperative nausea and vomiting. Anesthesiology 21:186-193, 1960

5. Beattie WS, Lindblad T, Buckley DN et al: The incidence of postoperative nausea and vomiting in women undergoing laparoscopy is influenced by the day of the menstrual cycle. Can J Anaesth 38:298-302, 1991

6. Rowley MP, Brown TCK: Postoperative vomiting in children. Anesth Intensive Care. 10:309-313, 1982

7. Zuurmond WWA, van Leeuwen L: Recovery from sufentanil anesthesia for outpatient arthroscopy: A comparison with isoflurane. Acta Anaesthesiol Scand 31:154-156, 1987

8. Schreiner MS, Nicolson SC, Martin T et al: Should children drink before discharge from day surgery? Anesthesiology 76:528-533, 1992

9. Meyers EF, Tomeldan SA. Glycopyrrolate compared with atropine in prevention of the oculocardiac reflex during eye-muscle surgery. Anesthesiology 51:350-352, 1979

10. Clarke RSJ. Nausea and vomiting. Br J Anaesth 56:19-27, 1984

11. Rabey RG and Smith G. Anaesthetic factors contributing to postoperative nausea and vomiting. Br J Anaesth 69:40S-45S (suppl. 1), 1992

12. Watcha MF, Simeon RM, White PF et al: Effect of propofol on the incidence of postoperative vomiting after strabismus surgery in pediatric outpatients. Anesthesiology 75:204-209, 1991

13. Reimer EJ, Montgomery CJ, Bevan JC et al: Propofol anesthesia reduces early postoperative emesis after paediatric strabismus surgery. Can J Anaesth 40:927-933, 1993

14. Larsson S, Asgeirsson B, Magnusson J: Propofol-fentanyl anesthesia compared to thiopental-halothane with special reference to recovery and vomiting after pediatric strabismus surgery. Acta Anaesthesiol Scand 36:182-186, 1992

15. Weir PM, Munro HM, Reynolds RI et al: Propofol infusions and the incidence of emesis in pediatric outpatient strabismus surgery. Anesth Analg 76:760-764, 1993

16. Felts JA, Poler M, Spitznagel EL: Nitrous oxide, nausea, and vomiting after outpatient gynecologic surgery. J Clin Anesth 2:168-171, 1990

17. Lerman J, Eustis S, Smith DR: Effect of droperidol pretreatment on postanesthetic vomiting in children undergoing strabismus surgery. Anesthesiology 65:322-325, 1986

18. Broadman LM, Ceruzzi W, Patane PS et al: Metoclopramide reduces the incidence of vomiting following strabismus surgery in children. Anesthesiology 72:245-248, 1990

19. Lin DM, Furst SR, Rodarte A: A double-blinded comparison of metoclopramide and droperidol for prevention of emesis following strabismus surgery. Anesthesiology 76:357-361, 1992

20. Khalil SN, Berry JM, Howard G et al: The antiemetic effect of lorazepam after outpatient strabismus surgery in children. Anesthesiology 77:915-919, 1992

21. Borgeat A, Wilder-Smith OHG, Saiah M et al: Subhypnotic doses of propofol possess direct antiemetic properties. Anesth Analg 74:539-541, 1992

22. Vener D, Carr A, Sikich N et al: Does dimenhydrinate control vomiting in children after outpatient strabismus surgery? Anesthesiology (abstracts) 1994 (in press)

23. Marty M, Pouillart P, Scholl S et al: Comparison of the 5-hydroxytryptamine$_3$ (serotonin) antagonist ondansetron (GR 38032F) with high-dose metoclopramide in the control of cisplain-induced emesis. N Engl J Med 322:816-821, 1990

24. Alon E, Himmelseher S: Ondansetron in the treatment of postoperative vomiting: A randomized, double-blind comparison with droperidol and metoclopramide. Anesth Analg 75:561-565, 1992

25. Gan TJ, Collis R, Hetreed M: Double-blind comparison of ondansetron, droperidol and saline in the prevention of postoperative nausea and vomiting. Br J Anaesth 72:544-547, 1994

26. Milne RJ, Heel RC: Ondansetron. Therapeutic use as an antiemetic. Drugs 41:574-595, 1991

27. Pritchard JF, Bryson JC, Kernodle AE et al: Age and gender effects on ondansetron pharmacokinetics: Evaluation of healthy aged volunteers. Clin Pharmacol Ther 51:51-55, 1992

28. Lerman J, Spahr-schopfer I, Sikich N et al: Pharmacokinetics of intravenous ondansetron (a 5-HT$_3$ antagonist) in healthy children. Can J Anaesth 40:A24, 1993

29. Lawhorn CD, Brown Jr RE, Huggins DP et al: Ondansetron dose response curve in pediatric patients. Anesth Analg 78:S240, 1994

30. Carr AS, Splinter WM, Bevan J et al: Ondansetron reduces postoperative vomiting in pediatric strabismus surgery. Anesthesiology (abstracts) 1994 (in press)

31. Conroy JM, Mahaffey JE, Wilson ME et al: Prevention of emesis following strabismus surgery. Anesthesiology 79:A10, 1993

32. Ummenhofer W, Frei FJ, Kern C et al: Ondansetron reduces postoperative nausea and vomiting in children. Anesthesiology 79:A1192, 1993

33. Lawhorn CD, Brown Jr RE, Schmitz ML et al: A comparative evaluation of ondansetron, droperidol, and placebo in prevention of postoperative vomiting following tonsillectomy and adenoidectomy in the pediatric patient. Anesthesiology 79:A1195, 1993

34. Lawhorn CD, Brown Jr RE, Schmitz ML et al: Prevention of postoperative vomiting in pediatric outpatient strabismus surgery. Anesthesiology 79:A1196, 1993

35. Furst SR, Rodarte A, Demars P: Ondansetron reduces postoperative vomiting in children undergoing tonsillectomy. Anesthesiology 79:A1197, 1993

36. Litman RS, Wu CL, Catanzaro FA: Ondansetron decreases emesis after tonsillectomy in children. Anesth Analg 78:478-481, 1994

37. Naylor RJ, Rudd JA: Pharmacology of ondansetron. Euro J Anaesthesiology 9:3-10 (suppl. 6), 1992

AN UPDATE ON MALIGNANT HYPERTHERMIA AND DUCHENNE'S MUSCULAR DYSTROPHY

F. A. Berry

There has been a tremendous change in the concepts of malignant hyperthermia (MH) over the past 25 years. The incidence of malignant hyperthermia back then was thought to be 1 in 15,000 (1). Today it is recognized that the frequency of MH is probably much closer to 1 in 200,000 (2). What happened to change the incidence? Well, several things. Twenty years ago, it was first appreciated that MH was accelerated metabolism under anesthesia, a cytogenetic disease. It was also recognized that the trigger agents were the volatile anesthetics and succinylcholine. Later, two other major things happened. One of these was the discovery that dantrolene was able to interrupt the cellular leak of calcium from the sarcoplasmic recticulum. This was thought to be the basic defect in MH. Early on, malignant hyperthermia was (appropriately) overdiagnosed because it was recognized that if one waited until the clinical findings of malignant hyperthermia were present, it was usually associated with a death rate that approached 50-60%. Therefore, the basic medical dictum of "the earlier the diagnosis, the easier the treatment" was certainly supported. However, with the recognition of accelerated metabolism under anesthesia and the use of end-tidal CO_2 and blood gas measurements, the diagnosis of the disease is much more accurate (3). Perhaps one of the major changes in the diagnosis of malignant hyperthermia is the recognition that masseter spasm as a clinical entity does not exist (4,5). The importance of this is that, in the clinician's attempts to find an early indicator of malignant hyperthermia, masseter spasm was thought to be important (6). As a matter of fact, by muscle testing for malignant hyperthermia susceptibility, 59% of patients who had a history of masseter spasm were found to be malignant hyperthermia susceptible. Now it is finally being appreciated that masseter spasm is actually masseter contracture and it occurs in all patients who are given succinylcholine (4,5,7). Most anesthesiologists agree that with isolated "masseter spasm," the anesthetic can be continued with trigger agents (8).

T.H. Stanley and P.G. Schafer (eds.), Pediatric and Obstetrical Anesthesia, 315-321.
© 1995 Kluwer Academic Publishers.

It has been suggested by some authors that a $PaCO_2$ >50 mm/Hg with controlled ventilation, a pH ⊥ 7.25, and a base deficit of >8 mEq/l represents clinical malignant hyperthermia (6). However, in the study of Littleford et al, these findings were frequent without the development of malignant hyperthermia (7). Children often run a base deficit of -6 to -10 during anesthesia and surgery.

The time of the most intense contracture of the masseter muscle comes at the end of fasciculation, when the nerve stimulator would indicate that the neuromuscular junction is paralyzed (5). Many anesthesiologists have been taught that this is the time to intubate. However, masseter contracture has nothing to do with the neuromuscular junction but is concerned with the intramyocellular contracture. The same type of contracture is found in eye muscles.

Another of the confounding factors that added to the confusion of the diagnosis of malignant hyperthermia is that patients with Duchenne's muscular dystrophy (DMD), when given succinylcholine, occasionally develop hyperkalemia. In some cases this is fatal. In addition, it was found that patients with unrecognized myopathies who were given succinylcholine occasionally developed hyperkalemia, often with a fatal outcome (9). It was not infrequent for these episodes to be called malignant hyperthermia. Now we know the clinical problem is that of hyperkalemia secondary to up-regulation of the acetylcholine receptors because of the muscle destruction of Duchenne's muscular dystrophy (10).

Be that as it may, the signs of malignant hyperthermia are directly related to accelerated metabolism under anesthesia secondary to volatile anesthetics and succinylcholine (11). In patients who are breathing spontaneously, an increase in ventilation will initially balance any increase in production of carbon dioxide. If a patient is suspected of having malignant hyperthermia, s/he should be paralyzed and a constant minute ventilation achieved. If the CO_2 goes up in the face of a constant minute ventilation, this would indicate malignant hyperthermia. At that point, the treatment is to immediately stop all volatile anesthetics and use a very high rate of fresh gas flow (in the neighborhood of 15-20 l/min) to wash the volatile anesthetics out of the patient and the machine. Treat with dantrolene 2-3 mg/kg while at the same time administering a large fluid load of 15 ml/kg of balanced salt solution. If there was an increase in muscle tone, referred to as muscle rigidity, then with successful therapy the muscle rigidity should cease. If the heart rate remains high and rigidity remains, continue to titrate dantrolene in up to 10 mg/kg. If urine output cannot be increased with a fluid load, then diuretics should be used. Hyperkalemia is a late finding in malignant hyperthermia. There will be enormous increases in CPK, as these patients undergo rhabdomyolysis. These patients need to be followed in an intensive care unit for 24 hours because of the problems of recrudescence.

DUCHENNE'S MUSCULAR DYSTROPHY (DMD)

The recent decision by the FDA, to rewrite the package insert to state that succinylcholine is contraindicated in infants, children, and adolescents in routine intubation, has caused considerable consternation in the pediatric anesthesia world (12-16). The rare but often fatal outcome of cardiac arrest with succinylcholine, in either recognized Duchenne's muscular dystrophy (DMD) patients or patients who were previously unrecognized, has been acknowledged for some time (17,18). There have been 20 or 30 case reports over the past 5-10 years that document this problem. For reasons that are not clear, the FDA decided to take this extraordinary step, in view of the fact that it may only occur in 1 in 500,000 anesthetics. Succinylcholine is still approved for either the rapid securing of an airway or if there are problems with the airway. In addition, the issue of intramuscular succinylcholine was totally ignored in the package insert. At any rate, the clinician still needs to know how to recognize hyperkalemia when it occurs and how to treat it. The clinician should also be aware that the use of nondepolarizing muscle relaxants before succinylcholine will greatly reduce the hyperkalemia that may occur in the presence of pathological neuromuscular systems (19).

The following short discussion of DMD will provide some background for understanding the disease. DMD occurs in 1 in 3600 live-born males. It only rarely occurs in females, and then only in females with genetic diseases such as Turner's syndrome. Approximately 25% of all patients with DMD are the result of a genetic mutation, which means that there will be no family history of anybody with DMD. DMD usually becomes clinically apparent at the age of 2-3 years in some subtle ways and, later, in some not-so-subtle ways. Some children with DMD are not diagnosed until age 6-8, but this is infrequent. By the age of 2-3, the child may not be quite as well coordinated as his peers and may have a slight delay in reaching milestones. The CPK is always elevated, even at birth. If the child should have an anesthetic in the neonatal or infant period and has cardiovascular problems with succinylcholine, then DMD should be suspected. Most children will develop coordination problems and classic

DMD by the time they are 3-5 years of age. Becker's muscular dystrophy patients may also have hyperkalemia with succinylcholine. The basic problem in DMD is a deficiency of dystrophin, which is an encoded protein. Cardiomyopathy is a constant feature of this disease, and its severity is not related to the severity of the neuromuscular disease. Intellectual impairment will occur in the vast majority of these patients, since the dystrophin is also absent from the brain. Also, dystrophin is missing within the conduction system of the heart, and this may explain why some of these children have arrhythmias and are difficult to resuscitate.

One of the ways that DMD may become evident is in association with anesthetics, and this is what prompted the FDA to ban succinylcholine. One of the reasons is that this hyperkalemia was thought to occur in "seemingly normal" children (13). However, it is of interest that in some of the cases that the FDA depended upon, the children were symptomatic at the time that the drugs were given (20). Part of our education system needs to be directed at informing clinicians of what to look for in the young child, aside from the family history. This includes any degree of delayed development, clumsiness, or not being able to keep up with peers.

HYPERKALEMIA WITH SUCCINYLCHOLINE IN NEUROMUSCULAR DISEASE

It is now recognized that the problem with patients with either recognized or unrecognized neuromuscular disease, trauma, etc., is that there is an up-regulation of the acetylcholine receptors with an increase in the number of acetylcholine receptors that are extra-junctional. The result is that, when succinycholine is given, hyperkalemia in varying degrees may occur. The problem is that the anesthesiologist at the time the hyperkalemia often occurs, which is within 2 or 3 minutes, is busy with intubation, taping in the endotracheal tube, checking the breath sounds, etc., and has not been watching the EKG, which may well have shown a peaked "T" wave. The first time the clinician becomes aware of a problem is when, all of a sudden, the EKG indicates that the rate has doubled. It has doubled because the "T" wave is now read by the EKG as a beat. This pseudotachycardia is then often treated with lidocaine, which is not the drug of choice. If the clinician has a precordial stethoscope, the true rate will be obvious from that. Also, the pulse oximeter will indicate the true heart rate. At that point, hyperkalemia should be treated with varying drugs. Calcium 10-15 Bg/kg (in a dilute solution) will help to reverse the effects of potassium. In addition, sodium bicarbonate 1-2 mEq should be given. If the circulation becomes unstable and the patient develops bradycardia and/or hypotension, then epinephrine 5-10 Bg/kg should be administered. This will enhance the movement of potassium into the cell as well as help to stabilize the circulation. The use of glucose and insulin should be reserved until the child has a stable circulation. Because of the problems of hyperkalemia, it is obvious that in a known patient with Duchenne's muscular dystrophy, succinylcholine should not be administered. If an unsuspected child develops hyperkalemia following succinylcholine, some form of neuromuscular disease should be suspected.

MYOCARDIAL DISEASE AND DMD

Myocardial disease is a constant finding in patients with Duchenne's muscular dystropy. One of the problems is evaluating the degree of myocardial disease in these patients. By the time they develop their myocardial disease, they usually also have a degree of neuromuscular disease, which means that they are usually wheelchair bound, and it is impossible to do a stress test. There has been a recent verbal report of the use of a "nonstress-stress test." This is done by evaluating cardiac output following the intravenous administration of a β-agonist such as isuprel. In this series of patients for elective surgery, if the cardiac output went up, then it was felt there was sufficient cardiac reserve to justify elective surgery. However, in about 20% of the patients, either the cardiac output did not go up or in some cases went down, and it was felt that these patients were not suitable candidates for elective surgery. This type of testing may well aid the anesthesiologist in determining the degree of myocardial disease in the patient.

MODIFICATION OF HYPERKALEMIA WITH SUCCINYLCHOLINE

What can be done to moderate the hyperkalemia in patients with unsuspected myopathies who appear normal? Gronert and Theye some 20 years ago found, in an isolated limb prep, that using small doses of nondepolarizing muscle relaxants before the administration of succinylcholine would greatly reduce the degree of hyperkalemia that occurred (19). It would then seem appropriate to consider this approach in children. In addition to decreasing myalgias and CPKs, it would seem appropriate to use a small dose of nondepolarizing muscle relaxant, such as Curare (0.05 mg/kg), 2-3 minutes before succinylcholine. The occurrence of hyperkalemia with succinylcholine is so rare that it will be difficult for any clinician to determine whether this has been effective treatment, but at least from an experimental viewpoint, this approach seems to be well justified.

SUMMARY

Malignant hyperthermia and Duchenne's muscular dystrophy continue to be a challenge for the anesthesiologist. This is because of their relatively infrequent occurrence and the potential disasters that may occur. It is hoped that our anesthetic management will be based on solid scientific evidence and that continued research and development of drugs will help to minimize some of the dangers.

REFERENCES

1. Kalow W, Britt BA, Chan FY: Epidemiology and inheritance of malignant hyperthermia. Int Anesthesiol Clin 17:119-139, 1979
2. Ording H: Incidence of malignant hyperthermia in Denmark. Anesth Analg 64:700-704, 1985
3. Van Der Spek AFL: Triggering agents continued after masseter spasm: There is proof in this pudding! Anesth Analg 73:358-370, 1991
4. Van Der Spek AFL, Fang WB, Ashton-Miller JA et al: Increased masticatory muscle stiffness during limb muscle flaccidity associated with succinylcholine administration. Anesthesiology 69:11, 1988
5. Leary NP, Ellis FR: Masseteric spasm as a normal response to suxamethonium. Br J Anaesth 64:448-492, 1990
6. O'Flynn RP, Shutack JG, Rosenberg H et al: Masseter muscle rigidity and malignant hyperthermia susceptibility in pediatric patients. Anesthesiology 80:1228-1233, 1994
7. Littleford JA, Patel LR, Bose D: Masseter muscle spasm in children: Implications of continuing the triggering anesthetic. Anesth Analg 72:151-160, 1991
8. Berry FA: Masseter spasm in perspective (editorial). Paedr Anaest 1:61-63, 1991
9. Rosenberg H, Gronert GA: Intractable cardiac arrest in children given succinylcholine. Anesthesiology 74:1054, 1992
10. Martyn JAJ, White DA, Gronert GA et al: Up-and-down regulation of skeletal muscle acetylcholine receptors. Anesthesiology 76:822-843, 1992
11. Strazis KP, Fox AW: Malignant hyperthermia: A review of published cases. Anesth Analg 77:297-304, 1993
12. Package Insert: Anectine (Succinylcholine Chloride) Injection, USP. Burroughs Wellcome Company, June 1993

13. Badgwell JM, Hall SC, Lockhart C: Revised label regarding use of succinylcholine in children and adolescents: II (letter). Anesthesiology 80:243, 1994

14. Morrell RC, Berman JM, Royster RL et al: Revised label regarding use of succinylcholine in children and adolescents: I (letter). Anesthesiology 80:242, 1994

15. Kent RS: Revised label regarding use of succinylcholine in children and adolescents: I and II (reply). Anesthesiology 80:244-245, 1994

16. Lerman J, Berdock SE, Bissonnette B et al: Succinylcholine warning. Can J Anaesth 41:165, 1994

17. Sethna NF, Rockoff MA: Cardiac arrest following inhalation induction of anaesthesia in a child with Duchenne's muscular dystrophy. Can Anaesth Soc J 33:799-802, 1986

18. Smith CL, Bush GH: Anaesthesia and progressive muscular dystrophy. Br J Anaesth 57:1113-1118, 1985

19. Gronert GA, Theye RA: Pathophysiology of hyperkalemia induced by succinylcholine. Anesthesiology 43:89-99, 1975

20. Miller ED, Sanders DB, Rowlingson JC et al: Anesthesia-induced rhabdomyolysis in a patient with Duchenne's muscular dystrophy. Anesthesiology 48:146-148, 1978

PEDIATRIC OUTPATIENT ANESTHESIA

R. S. Hannallah

Children are excellent candidates for outpatient (ambulatory) surgery. The typical pediatric surgical patient has no serious systemic disorder. Furthermore, most surgical procedures in children are simple and require less complicated techniques than those used in adults. From the child's perspective, the two greatest advantages of ambulatory surgery are the minimization of parental separation and the reduction of exposure to hospital-acquired infections.

PATIENT SELECTION CRITERIA

A successful outpatient surgical program requires that well-defined patient selection criteria be established and strictly adhered to by all surgeons who have admitting privileges in the facility. The three primary factors that must be considered when selecting a child for ambulatory surgery are the condition of the patient, the attitude of the parents, and the type of surgical procedure to be performed. These factors must be balanced with the capability of the surgical facility and the ability of its staff to deal with any expected or unexpected complications.

THE PATIENT

The child should be in good health; if not, any systemic disease s/he has must be under good control. Some anesthesiologists still restrict ambulatory surgery to patients classified as ASA physical status 1 and 2, while others accept ASA physical status 3 or even 4 patients, provided that their medical condition is well controlled.

Many *children with chronic diseases* are appropriate candidates for ambulatory surgery, as long as their diseases are under control. Physically handicapped, psychologically disturbed, or mentally retarded children are especially comforted by the continued presence of a parent or guardian that is usually fostered in ambulatory surgical facilities.

323

T.H. Stanley and P.G. Schafer (eds.), Pediatric and Obstetrical Anesthesia, 323-333.
© 1995 *Kluwer Academic Publishers.*

The *premature infant*, however, is not a suitable candidate for ambulatory surgery because of potential immaturity of the respiratory center, temperature control, and gag reflexes. Recent studies have reported a high incidence of perioperative complications, such as apnea, in these infants.

The age at which the premature infant attains physiologic maturity and no longer presents an increased risk for postoperative apnea must be considered individually. Criteria on which these decisions are based include growth and development; persistent problems during feeding; time to recovery from upper respiratory infections; history of apnea; and presence or absence of metabolic, endocrine, neurologic, or cardiac disorders.

It is generally considered that infants younger than 46 weeks postconceptual age (PCA) with a preoperative history of apnea are at greatest risk, although some authors have reported apnea in infants as old as 60 weeks PCA. As the child matures, the tendency toward apnea greatly diminishes; however, the age when all infants may be safely anesthetized on an ambulatory basis is unknown. Until more extensive, prospective studies are carried out, it seems prudent to admit to the hospital all ex-premature infants less than 50 weeks postconceptual age so that they may be monitored postoperatively for apnea, bradycardia, and oxygen desaturation. The choice of this particular age is rather arbitrary. It is best to individualize this decision and, when in doubt, to err on the conservative side. If the infant has bronchopulmonary dysplasia (BPD) or other neonatal problems, this period may need to be extended. Should any questions arise, inpatient care and postoperative monitoring are recommended.

THE PARENT

Parents of pediatric ambulatory patients should be capable of understanding, and willing to follow, specific instructions related to ambulatory surgery. In most cases, it is up to the physician to educate them and make them feel secure and comfortable.

THE PROCEDURE

The planned surgical procedure should be associated with only minimal bleeding and minor physiologic derangements. Superficial procedures are selected most often. The length of the procedure is not in itself a significant drawback. Most experts believe that almost any operation that does not require a major intervention into the cranial vault, abdomen, or thorax can be performed on an ambulatory basis. Patients with infected lesions are not good candidates because of the need for separate facilities in the recovery area.

The 5 most frequently performed ambulatory surgical procedures at Children's National Medical Center (CNMC) during the past 2 years were herniorrhaphy, myringotomy, adenoidectomy with or without myringotomy, circumcision, and eye-muscle surgery. Recent experience indicates that ambulatory adenotonsillectomy is also safe and cost-effective, and that there is little benefit in keeping these patients in the hospital more than a few hours after surgery. Young children (<3 years) who are undergoing tonsillectomy for the relief of severe airway obstruction, with or without sleep apnea, continue to suffer from the same symptoms in the immediate postoperative period and should, therefore, be admitted to the hospital for close observation and monitoring postoperatively.

PREOPERATIVE REQUIREMENTS AND SCREENING

The preoperative requirements for safe conduct of anesthesia in pediatric ambulatory patients are the same as those for inpatients, including a complete history and physical examination, appropriate laboratory tests, consultations when indicated, and an appropriate fasting period. In order to minimize delays and cancellations, it is desirable to complete as many of these requirements as possible before the day of surgery.

Many ambulatory surgical units actively participate in the preoperative screening of their patients. The degree of involvement varies from a simple telephone call to the parents 1 or 2 days prior to surgery, to the establishment of a formal screening clinic to clear all patients before admission into the operating suite. At CNMC, the parents of each child are contacted by telephone shortly after the operation is scheduled. A second call is made 48 hours or less before surgery. During the initial call, information is sought concerning past or present risk factors, such as a history of prematurity or cardiac or respiratory problems. This information helps to determine if additional preoperative evaluation or consultation is required prior to the day of surgery. In some cases, it may lead to a reevaluation of the appropriateness of scheduling the procedure on an ambulatory basis. During the second phone call, an assessment of the child's present health is made. NPO orders are reinforced, and practical matters related to parking, what to bring to the hospital, and expected duration of stay are explained.

On the day of surgery, all patients are screened for acute illness and NPO status. Vital signs are recorded. Any consultation reports are evaluated, and the need for special preoperative psychological or pharmacologic treatment is considered, before the child arrives in the operating room area.

With careful preoperative screening, the final preanesthesia evaluation of the pediatric ambulatory patient should result in no surprises; however, this is not always the case. Acute illnesses (e.g., an upper respiratory infection) may be present, or a previously undiagnosed heart murmur may be heard. These two conditions deserve a brief consideration.

THE CHILD WITH A RUNNY NOSE

A child who presents with a runny nose may have a completely benign, noninfectious condition (e.g., seasonal or vasomotor rhinitis), in which case elective surgery may safely be performed. On the other hand, the runny nose may be a prodrome to, or actually be, an infectious process, in which case elective surgery should be postponed. Since an estimated 20-30% of all children have a runny nose a significant part of the year, every child with a runny nose must be evaluated on an individual basis.

The preanesthetic assessment of these patients consists of a complete history, a physical examination, and an interpretation of certain laboratory data. Early in the clinical course of disease, the history will be the most important factor in the differential diagnosis. Specifically, allergic problems should be actively sought. Parents can usually tell whether their child's runny nose is "the usual runny nose" or something different that may require cancellation of elective surgery. The physical examination is not always conclusive; normal findings may be present during the early part of an infectious process. Chronic allergic rhinitis, on the other hand, may be associated with local infections within the nasopharynx resulting in purulent nasal discharge. A white blood cell count ≥12,000-15,000 with a shift to the left suggests an infectious process.

If surgery is postponed because of simple nasopharyngitis, it can be usually scheduled in 1-2 weeks. If a flulike syndrome that involves both upper and lower respiratory tract is present, surgery should be postponed until at least a month after the child has recovered.

THE CHILD WITH A HEART MURMUR

A previously undiagnosed cardiac murmur may often first be heard during the preanesthetic examination. Even if such a child shows no signs of cardiac disease, it is imperative that the cause of the murmur (organic vs. innocent) be diagnosed prior to anesthesia and surgery.

A child with a confirmed cardiac lesion may not require specific preoperative cardiac therapy or even a modification in the selection of anesthetic agents and technique. Antibiotic prophylaxis is, however, recommended to prevent subacute bacterial endocarditis (JAMA 264:2919-2922, 1990).

PREOPERATIVE PREPARATION

The time between the patient's arrival at the hospital and the induction of anesthesia is usually quite short. There is little time to orient the child to all the events that will take place during his/her stay. Most centers, therefore, encourage children and families to participate in presurgical preparation programs a few days before surgery; and studies have shown that children who attended those programs were much more cooperative during induction than those who did not. Such findings, however, must be interpreted carefully, since parental motivation, traveling distance, socioeconomic conditions, and the child's age—the forces that motivate parents to bring their children to these programs—are the same factors that may in themselves lead to better cooperation.

PHARMACOLOGIC PREMEDICATION

The value of, and need for, pharmacologic premedication in pediatric ambulatory surgical patients is very controversial. With modern anesthetic agents and techniques, a majority of children do not need preoperative sedation, provided that they have received proper psychological preparation and established a good rapport with the anesthesiologist. When premedication is not used routinely, the anesthesiologist must be prepared to administer a preinduction agent to the occasional difficult or extremely frightened child.

PREINDUCTION AGENTS

Preinduction of anesthesia refers to the use of such drugs as ketamine or other rapidly acting medications for last-minute premedication.

Rectal administration of methohexital is a commonly used technique in preschool children. A dose of 25 mg/kg (10% solution) has an onset time of 6-10 minutes and produces enough sedation to peacefully separate an upset child from his/her parents. Intranasal administration of midazolam (0.2 mg/kg) also has been reported to produce anxiolysis and sedation in preschool children with a rapid onset (5-10 minutes) and no evidence of delayed recovery.

Low-dose (2 mg/kg) intramuscular ketamine can be used in young children who do not cooperate with other methods of induction. The onset time is short (2-3 minutes), and recovery is not prolonged.

ANESTHETIC AGENTS AND TECHNIQUES

Smooth induction of anesthesia in the unpremedicated child is probably the most difficult aspect of pediatric ambulatory surgery. No single approach is effective for all children in all situations. The choice of agent and technique must be based on the needs of the individual child; it should not be used merely because it is the routine choice in a particular institution or because it is the only method with which the anesthesiologist is comfortable.

INHALATIONAL INDUCTION

Inhalational induction is the most commonly used technique in pediatric anesthesia. Halothane offers the advantage of a rapid onset and smooth induction. Recovery after brief halothane anesthesia is usually rapid and uneventful. Nausea and vomiting are not common. With prolonged administration of halothane, recovery time is longer than when isoflurane is used. Techniques that reduce the anxiety associated with gas induction, and therefore promote patient cooperation, include the use of transparent masks, painting the inside of the mask with a drop of food flavor of the child's choice, and allowing the child to sit up during the induction.

INTRAVENOUS INDUCTION

Intravenous induction is the method of choice in most older children. When thiopental sodium is used in healthy unpremedicated children, a relatively large dose (5-6 mg/kg) may be required in order to ensure smooth and rapid transition to general inhalational anesthesia. At CNMC, the drug is usually injected directly into a vein on the dorsum of the hand via a 25-gauge butterfly needle. Children who receive barbiturate induction tend to be sleepier and require more airway support for the first 15 minutes of the recovery period than those who have received halothane. This difference disappears by 30 minutes.

Recent studies on the use of propofol in children indicate that it results in smooth induction with a lower incidence of side effects and faster recovery than thiopental. Pain on injection can be minimized by using the large antecubital veins for injection. The incidence of nausea and vomiting is greatly decreased following propofol anesthesia.

PERIOPERATIVE FLUID MANAGEMENT

PREOPERATIVE FASTING

The need for a prolonged period of fasting (e.g., NPO after midnight) before anesthesia induction in otherwise healthy children has been recently questioned. Several studies have shown that ingestion of clear liquids up to 2-3 hours prior to scheduled induction does not increase the risk for pulmonary aspiration syndrome; consequently, some anesthesiologists have altered fasting guidelines to allow clear liquids 2-3 hours prior to surgery. It is important to note that these guidelines apply to *clear liquids only* (not solids) in otherwise healthy children. Possible benefits of shorter fasting times include minimizing thirst and discomfort while awaiting surgery, less hypovolemic-induced hypotension during induction, and less concern about hypoglycemia.

The need for routine administration of intravenous fluids during pediatric ambulatory anesthesia is controversial. If the procedure is of short duration and the anesthetic technique is one that ensures rapid recovery and return of normal appetite with minimal nausea and vomiting, many believe that the patient does not require infusion of fluids. If fluids are not administered intravenously, the period of preoperative fasting should be minimized to avoid possible dehydration and hypoglycemia.

Intravenous fluid therapy during and after surgery is specifically indicated in longer operations (over 30-60 minutes); in procedures known to be associated with a high incidence of postoperative nausea and vomiting (e.g., strabismus surgery); and in young children who have been fasting for a prolonged period of time.

POSTOPERATIVE ANALGESIA

The need for analgesics following surgery depends on the nature of the procedure and the pain threshold of the patient. It does not depend on whether the child is an ambulatory or an inpatient. Postoperative pain or discomfort can be managed by one or a combination of the following methods.

MILD ANALGESICS

For infants under 6 months of age, a combination of care and nursing (or a bottle) is all that is usually needed following a procedure that is not associated with severe pain.

For older infants and young children, acetaminophen (Tylenol®)) can be used either orally or rectally in a dose of 60 mg (1 grain) per year of age.

For more persistent, moderately severe pain a Tylenol/codeine combination is available in an elixir form containing 120 mg Tylenol plus 12 mg codeine/5 ml. The recommended dose is 5 ml of the elixir for children 3-6 years of age, and 10 ml for those between the ages of 7 and 12.

POTENT NARCOTIC ANALGESICS

When narcotics are indicated in the recovery period, a short-acting drug should be chosen. Intravenous use allows more accurate titration of the dose and avoids the use of "standard" dosages based on weight, which may lead to a relative overdose. Fentanyl, up to a dose of 2.0 µg/kg, is our drug of choice for intravenous use. Meperidine (0.5 mg/kg) and codeine (1.0-1.5 mg/kg) can be used intramuscularly if an intravenous route is not established.

REGIONAL ANALGESIA

Regional anesthesia can be combined with light general anesthesia to provide excellent postoperative pain relief and early ambulation, with minimal or no need for narcotics. By placing the block before surgery starts but after the child is asleep, one can reduce the requirement for general anesthetic agents during surgery, which in turn may result in a more rapid recovery, earlier discharge, more rapid return of normal appetite, and less nausea and vomiting.

The types of blocks that can be used safely in the pediatric ambulatory surgical patient are limited only by the skill and interest of the anesthesiologist. Generally, the techniques chosen should be simple to perform, should have minimal or no side effects, and should not interfere with motor function and early ambulation.

Ilioinguinal and iliohypogastric nerve block can be performed by infiltration of 0.25% bupivacaine solution (in doses up to 2 mg/kg) in the region medial to the anterior superior iliac spine. This block has been used successfully to provide excellent postoperative analgesia for pediatric ambulatory patients following elective inguinal herniotomy or orchiopexy.

Dorsal nerve block of the penis can be performed by simple injection of 1-4 ml of 0.25% bupivacaine without epinephrine deep to Buck's fascia 1 cm from the midline. This has been shown to provide over 6 hours of analgesia following circumcision with no complications. Alternate approaches to penile block are a midline injection or subcutaneous infiltration, which presumably blocks the nerve after it has ramified into the subcutaneous tissue. Topical application of lidocaine on the incision site at the conclusion of surgery has also been shown to be effective.

Caudal block provides excellent and reproducible postoperative analgesia following a wide variety of surgical procedures such as circumcision, hypospadias repair, orchiopexy, and herniotomy. By using bupivacaine, 0.25% solution in a dose of 0.5-0.7 ml/kg, no motor paralysis is produced. Caudal block has been extensively used in our ambulatory surgical unit, with most children discharged home free of pain 1-2 hours postoperatively. Analgesia (as measured by subsequent need of a mild oral analgesic) lasts 4-6 hours with this technique.

DISCHARGE CRITERIA

Rapid recovery and early ambulation are major objectives in ambulatory surgery. When dealing with pediatric ambulatory patients, we must guarantee safe discharge not only from the recovery room but also from the hospital. In our institution, all children recover from anesthesia in the same recovery area. Ambulatory patients are then transferred to a special short-stay recovery unit.

In order to provide uniform care and to ensure a complete legal record, many institutions have developed specific discharge criteria for ambulatory patients. At CNMC, discharge criteria include the following: appropriateness and stability of vital signs; absence of respiratory distress; ability to swallow oral fluids, cough, or demonstrate a gag reflex; ability to ambulate consistent with the developmental age level; absence of excessive nausea, vomiting, and dizziness (preferably including ability to retain oral fluids); and a state of consciousness appropriate to the developmental level.

Every child, regardless of age, must have an escort home. The escort is given written instructions concerning the child's home care and a telephone number to call to request further advice or to report complications. Staff counsel all parents about postoperative care; many units have also designed handouts that specify the care that should be provided and the signs that might herald a complication.

SUMMARY

Successful anesthetic management of children undergoing ambulatory surgery requires that the anesthesiologist be actively involved in all aspects of management. Guidelines should be established in consultation with the surgeons, nurses, and administrators to ensure proper selection and preoperative preparation of patients. The psychological evaluation and preparation of the child, and the use of pharmacologic premedication when indicated, will ensure a pleasant experience for all involved. The anesthesiologist should choose a specific anesthetic agent and a technique that is appropriate for each individual child. Use of "routine" induction techniques is rarely, if ever, appropriate. Early ambulation and discharge are very desirable in ambulatory patients. Long-acting drugs and techniques that are associated with excessive drowsiness or nausea and vomiting should not be used. Special attention must be paid to the analgesic requirements of the child. Regional blocks should be used whenever possible to supplement general anesthesia and to limit the need for narcotics during recovery. Specific criteria for discharge ensure the safety and protection of the child and staff.

FURTHER READING

1. Hannallah RS, Epstein BS: Outpatient anesthesia. In Gregory G, ed. Pediatric anesthesia. 3rd edition. New York, Churchill Livingstone, 1994, pp 781-782
2. Hannallah RS, Epstein BS: Management of the pediatric patient. In Wetchler BV, ed. Anesthesia for ambulatory surgery. 2nd edition. Philadelphia, JB Lippincott Company, 1991, pp 131-195

ANESTHETIC CONSIDERATIONS IN CONGENITAL HEART DISEASE

P. R. Hickey

The approach to anesthesia in the child with congenital heart disease (CHD) is the same whether the heart has been reconstructed or the congenital heart disease has not been surgically treated. In both cases, the current clinical status of the child's cardiac pathophysiology must be understood. When anesthesia is being given for noncardiac surgery, cardiopulmonary bypass is not available for support if surgical and anesthetic intrusions overwhelm circulatory homeostasis. During noncardiac surgical procedures, surgeons unfamiliar with the physiologic limitations imposed by congenital heart disease may place substantial burdens on the circulation in the course of their procedures. Since the anesthesiologist must maintain the often fragile circulatory balance in spite of surgical trespass, destabilizing surgical insults must be anticipated in the anesthetic plan. Familiarity with the child's pathophysiology, the details of any reparative cardiac surgery, and the planned noncardiac operative procedure should avoid major problems in anesthetic management. Evaluation, preoperative preparation, choice of monitoring, induction, maintenance, emergence, and plans for postoperative care all are predicated on this familiarity.

STATUS OF REPAIR: THE RECONSTRUCTED HEART VS. THE UNRECONSTRUCTED HEART

Children with heart disease may present before cardiac surgical treatment, after palliation, or after "repair." Palliated patients still have a distinctly abnormal circulation but, hopefully, severe consequences of pediatric heart disease (severe congestive heart failure, severe hypoxemia, polycythemia, and pulmonary vascular disease) will not be a problem during anesthesia. It is important to note that, even with a reconstructed heart in patients whose heart disease has been surgically "corrected," the circulation must still be considered abnormal in the majority of cases. Arrhythmias, ventricular dysfunction, residual shunts, residual valvular

335

T.H. Stanley and P.G. Schafer (eds.), Pediatric and Obstetrical Anesthesia, 335-343.
© 1995 *Kluwer Academic Publishers.*

stenosis or regurgitation, and residual pulmonary hypertension all may remain or develop after surgical "repair" of pediatric heart disease. The most important aspects of the pathophysiology and the common circulatory abnormalities in the unreconstructed heart, or in the reconstructed heart after repair or palliation of common lesions, are outlined below.

EFFECTS OF ANESTHESIA AND SURGICAL PROCEDURES ON PATHOPHYSIOLOGY

Knowledge of the effects of anesthetic and operative manipulations on the pathophysiology of pediatric heart disease is necessary for optimal anesthetic management. Such manipulations may have a potent influence on cardiac function, venous return, and the ratio of pulmonary-to-systemic vascular resistance (PVR/SVR), which is particularly important in the pathophysiology of pediatric heart disease. Although anesthesiologists are familiar with manipulations of SVR, manipulations of PVR are less well understood. In lesions with inadequate pulmonary blood flow and hypoxemia, such as tetralogy of Fallot or a long-standing VSD-producing pulmonary vascular disease and high PVR with R-L shunting, anesthetic and surgical manipulations should be directed towards increasing pulmonary blood flow by decreasing PVR. At the same time, systemic vascular resistance (SVR) ideally is maintained or even increased to further favorably alter PVR/SVR. Although hyperventilation is the most reliable and efficacious way of decreasing PVR in children, it is pH and not pCO_2 that controls pulmonary vasoconstriction. Additionally, use of 100% O_2 is effective in decreasing PVR, as is optimizing FRC by avoiding PEEP and adjusting ventilation patterns to avoid hyperinflation of the lungs. Unfortunately, although many drugs are still touted as selective pulmonary vasodilators, none of these drugs reduces elevated PVR without also decreasing systemic vascular resistance. Nitric oxide (an investigational inhalation agent) administered to the lungs in a range of 10-80 ppm has specific pulmonary vascular dilating properties but has not been effective in all patients with increased PVR in early studies. Equipment for its administration is not yet commercially available, so its therapeutic usefulness in patients with congenital heart disease has yet to be defined.

Distention of the abdomen and collections of blood or fluid in pleural spaces also can substantially increase PVR, so drainage of these collections may be necessary. These maneuvers can have substantial beneficial effects on cardiac output in Fontan operations, for example, in which the right atrium and pulmonary artery are directly anastomosed because of the absence of a pulmonary ventricular pump.

Less commonly, relative increases in PVR during cardiac operations may be beneficial, as in truncus arteriosus or hypoplastic left-heart syndrome, in which low resistance in the pulmonary circulation may "steal" flow from the systemic circulation through a large, nonrestrictive communication (a patent ductus) between the great vessels, resulting in systemic perfusion. Likewise, the same pathophysiology is seen in large VSDs requiring pulmonary artery bands to restrict pulmonary blood flow and augment systemic blood flow. Similar pathophysiology is seen when an excessively large shunt is created between the pulmonary and systemic circulations in Blalock-Taussig or other shunt operations, allowing pulmonary "steal." In these situations, increasing PVR by using FiO_2 of .20, adjusting ventilation to a slightly acidotic pH, and using PEEP to hyperinflate the lungs and increase airway pressure can appreciably decrease pulmonary blood flow and increase systemic blood flow until pulmonary flow can be surgically restricted, if necessary. Only by understanding the pathophysiology in each case can these kinds of anesthetic techniques effectively be used to optimize the overall circulation and oxygen delivery to the tissues.

CHOICE OF ANESTHETIC AGENT: HOW PATHOPHYSIOLOGY AFFECTS INDUCTION

In the past 10 years, much information has accumulated about the effects of anesthetic agents in congenital heart disease. This information allows rational planning of anesthetic management, based on many studies of anesthetic agents in infants and children with congenital heart disease. Many different techniques can be used successfully to anesthetize children with congenital heart disease, but if the effects of anesthesia on the pathophysiology are well understood, an anesthetic technique can be selected to compensate for the individual pathophysiology and the destabilizing effects of the planned procedure. The full range of inhalational, intravenous, and regional anesthetic techniques can be employed in patients with CHD when the anesthetic care plan is carefully tailored to the patient's CHD. However, the effects of individual anesthetic agents and techniques on myocardial contractility, overall cardiac performance, and both systemic and pulmonary vascular performance must be carefully considered in the light of specific limitations of cardiopulmonary reserve imposed by both the patient's CHD and the anticipated impact of the proposed operative procedure on that already compromised reserve.

GENERAL CARE OF PATIENTS WITH CONGENITAL HEART DISEASE

An important aspect of care in children with CHD undergoing noncardiac surgery is a cardiology consultation. Most cardiologists have little concept of the kind of physiologic stresses that major noncardiac surgical procedures can impose on the cardiopulmonary system. When major blood loss; intrusion into the airway, peritoneal cavity, thoracic cavity, or cranial cavity; or any very prolonged operative procedure is planned, a cardiology consult often can be helpful *if* the cardiologist is informed in detail of the anticipated perioperative physiological stresses.

Systemic air emboli are a constant danger in children with CHD, regardless of their usual shunting pattern, because of the dynamic nature of shunts during anesthetic and surgical manipulations. A recent case report documents hypoxemia from transient right-to-left shunting across a persistent or "probe patent" foramen ovale in a "normal" child during routine anesthetic emergence. Air traps are advisable for all intravenous lines, but these do not substitute for meticulous attention and constant vigilance.

Cyanotic, polycythemic children are at risk for strokes and other thrombotic problems in the perioperative period, particularly during periods of dehydration. Polycythemia is also associated with poorly understood coagulopathies. Both of these problems are more severe when hematocrits are greater than 60%. Unless oral intake is assured, adequate intravenous hydration before and *after* operation is important to prevent further increases in blood viscosity and potential thrombotic problems. When major blood loss is anticipated, especially in thoracic operations, blood products adequate to deal with the coagulopathy should be available. If preoperative hematocrits are over 60-70%, erythropheresis should at least be considered, in consultation with cardiologists and surgeons.

Cardiac medications such as digitalis, diuretics, beta-blockers, and antiarrhythmics should be continued preoperatively and anesthetic plans adjusted accordingly to compensate for known interactions between specific anesthetic agents and these medications. Prevention of bacterial endocarditis is an important consideration in pediatric heart disease patients undergoing noncardiac surgery. The only pediatric heart patients for whom antibiotic prophylaxis is not recommended are those with isolated secundum atrial septal defect (unrepaired), the same defect repaired without a prosthetic patch or with a transcatheter device closure, and a previously ligated patent ductus arteriosus. Details of recommendations for antibiotic prophylaxis of all pediatric patients are given in the references.

SPECIFIC LESIONS: CRITICAL ASPECTS OF PATHOPHYSIOLOGY BEFORE AND AFTER RECONSTRUCTION

TRANSITIONAL CIRCULATION IN THE "NORMAL" NEONATE

The transitional circulation present in all neonates immediately postpartum is a form of CDH. Shunting occurs dynamically in either direction through both the ductus arteriosus and the foramen ovale until these structures later close, first functionally and then anatomically. In addition, high pulmonary vascular resistance (PVR) promotes right-to-left ductal and foramen ovale shunting, with resultant hypoxemia. When undergoing any major noncardiac operation, neonates may revert to this transitional circulation, despite previous *functional* closure of the ductus arteriosus and foramen ovale. The anesthetic plan should anticipate this possibility, and each neonate should be considered to have potentially active intracardiac shunting. Once the period of perioperative stress is over, normal developmental changes modify and functionally eliminate the ductus, foramen ovale, and high PVR.

PALLIATIVE SHUNTS FOR REDUCED PULMONARY BLOOD FLOW

Systemic-to-pulmonary artery shunts supply pulmonary blood flow in cases of pulmonary atresia or other obstructive lesions in which pulmonary blood flow is limited. These shunts are inherently inefficient because blood from the pulmonary veins, which has already passed through the lungs, is freely mixed with systemic venous return and recirculated through the lungs. Problems include congestive heart failure when flow is too large and severe hypoxemia with cyanosis when flow is inadequate. Pulmonary blood flow must be several times the systemic flow for adequate oxygenation in these patients. This usually requires normal systemic arterial pressure. Any substantial degree of systemic hypotension causes marked decreases in pulmonary blood flow, thus worsening hypoxemia. Maintenance of normal levels of systemic arterial blood pressure is thus critical to preserving the patient's usual mild-to-moderate levels of hypoxemia. Decreases in systemic arterial pressures or, alternatively, any encroachment on normal FRC by positioning, diaphragmatic packing, lung retraction, pleural or peritoneal collections, or loss of airway will increase PVR, decreasing pulmonary flow and rapidly leading to severe hypoxemia. Increasing systemic perfusion pressure and thus shunt flow may compensate to some degree for these events.

FONTAN PROCEDURE (SINGLE VENTRICLE PHYSIOLOGY)

Prior to their Fontan repair, these children have a complete mixing physiology in a parallel circulation depending on balanced pulmonary and systemic blood flow. After the Fontan procedure (direct connection of right atrium and pulmonary artery), they lack a pumping ventricle for the pulmonary circulation. Pulmonary perfusion pressure is provided by the difference between central venous and left atrial pressure. Unless high right atrial pressures are maintained, cardiac output will immediately decrease. Similarly, PVR must be minimal to allow adequate cardiac output, since there is no ventricular pump to buffer surges in PVR. The anesthetic and surgical manipulations described above that increase pulmonary vascular resistance will be especially poorly tolerated after a Fontan procedure. In more recent Fontan procedures, a "fenestration" in the atrial septum is created to act as a pop-off valve and allow right-to-left shunting when PVR increases for any reason. Although this communication between the systemic and pulmonary venous circuits allows right-to-left shunting and arterial desaturation of some degree when PVR increases, cardiac output will be maintained because blood shunted into the systemic atrium and ventricle will maintain adequate cardiac output in the face of PVR increases. The status of the fenestration (open or closed) should be known prior to the anesthetic, so that alterations in pulse oximeter readings can be properly interpreted.

INCREASED PULMONARY ARTERY BLOOD FLOW AND PULMONARY ARTERY BANDS

Pulmonary artery bands protect the pulmonary vasculature from the consequences of high flow and pressure until a physiologic repair is done. The cost of this reduction of pulmonary blood flow is a hypertensive right ventricle that is prone to failure when PVR is increased. Systemic perfusion pressures adequate for coronary perfusion of the hypertensive right ventricle are essential. In the presence of a mixing type of congenital heart disease, a pulmonary artery band may result in moderate-to-mild hypoxemia. After banding, pulmonary blood flow may decrease abruptly during periods of systemic hypotension, and maintenance of adequate systemic arterial perfusion pressures is important.

TETRALOGY OF FALLOT

Agitation or stimulation that increases catecholamine levels increases PVR and spasm of the right ventricular outflow tract, increasing right ventricular pressures and right-to-left shunting (a "tat spell"). Classic treatment includes sedation and hyperventilation with 100% oxygen to decrease outflow obstruction and PVR, pressors or aortic constriction to increase systemic vascular resistance, a beta-blocker such as esmolol to decrease outflow tract obstruction, or, when the preceding rational measures fail, epinephrine. After repair, tetralogy patients frequently have pulmonary insufficiency, residual right ventricular hypertension, right bundle branch block, or accompanying right ventricular dysfunction. These problems are sometimes associated with sudden death.

TRANSPOSITION OF THE GREAT ARTERIES

Mixing (bi-directional shunting) of blood between the two circulations (pulmonic and systemic) is critical to circulatory stability in these children. This is unlike other congenital heart lesions in which shunting of blood between the two sides of the circulation causes problems. A patent ductus arteriosus or creation of a large atrial septal defect promotes mixing and generally improves the clinical status before repair. Potential problems after repair depend on the reparative operation. After atrial baffle (Mustard or Senning) repairs, atrial arrhythmias, including sick sinus syndrome and supraventricular tachycardias, inferior or superior vena caval obstructions, or systemic (right) ventricular dysfunction, may appear early or more than 10-20 years later. After great artery switch (anatomic or Jatené) repairs, problems include coronary ostial stenosis, supravalvular aortic or pulmonary stenosis, and aortic regurgitation.

COMPLETE ATRIO-VENTRICULAR CANAL

Large left-to-right shunts with very high pulmonary flow and pulmonary hypertension are the chief pathophysiological problems. Pulmonary vascular disease tends to develop early. After repair, problems of pulmonary hypertension and mitral regurgitation can occur in some children and can markedly limit cardiovascular reserve. In children with Down's syndrome, especially, reactive pulmonary vascular beds and airways can complicate anesthetic management for years after repair of the atrio-ventricular canal.

VENTRICULAR SEPTAL DEFECT

Shunt flows are determined largely by the size of the septal defect and the ratio of pulmonary and systemic vascular resistance. With large ventricular septal defects (VSD) allowing large shunts, particularly those of long-standing pulmonary hypertension and sometimes elevated pulmonary vascular resistance, may be a problem. After repair, residual pulmonary hypertension, residual ventricular septal defects, heart block, and occasional aortic regurgitation may be a problem. Some degree of left ventricular dysfunction may remain for many years after repair of large VSDs, particularly those repaired later in childhood. Thus normal cardiovascular and pulmonary reserve cannot be assumed in patients who have had repair of a VSD.

SUMMARY

The goal of anesthetic care in pediatric patients with heart disease is maintenance or even improvement in the patient's preoperative hemodynamic status in the face of destabilizing surgical manipulations. Understanding the status of the individual cardiac pathophysiology and probable intraoperative events should permit a rational selection of anesthetic techniques that minimize operative risk in pediatric patients with congenital heart disease. New developments in this area promise to make such a goal easier to achieve.

REFERENCES

1. Shulman ST, Amren D, Bisno AL et al: Prevention of bacterial endocarditis. Circulation 70:1123A-1127A, 1984

2. Campbell FW, Schwartz AJ: Anesthesia for noncardiac surgery in the pediatric patient with congenital heart disease. ASA Refresher Courses in Anesthesiology, Philadelphia, Lippincott, 14:75-98, 1986

3. Hickey PR, Wessel DW: Anesthesia for congenital heart disease. In Gregory GA, ed. Pediatric anesthesia. 3rd edition. New York, Churchill Livingston, 1994 (in press)

4. Hickey PR, Streitz S: Preoperative cardiac assessment in the patient with congenital heart disease. In Mangano DT, ed. Preoperative cardiac assessment in heart patients. Phildelphia, WB Saunders, 1990, pp 85-135

5. Hickey PR: Anesthesia for the reconstructed heart. In Stolting RK, ed. Advances in anesthesia, Vol VIII. Chicago, Year Book Publishers, 1991, pp 91-113

6. Hickey PR: Anesthesia for treatment of congenital heart disease. In Rogers MC, Tinker JH, Covino BG, Longnecker DE, eds. Principles and practice of anesthesiology, St. Louis, Mosby-Year Book, 1993, pp 1680-1718

7. Moore RA, Nicolson SC: Anesthetic care of the pediatric patient with congenital heart disease for noncardiac surgery. In Kaplan JA, ed. Cardiac anesthesia. 3rd edition. Philadelphia, WB Saunders, 1993, pp 1296-1328

8. Hickey PR, Wessel DL, Reich DL: Anesthesia for treatment of congenital heart disease. In Kaplan, ed. Cardiac anesthesia. 3rd edition. Philadelphia, WB Saunders, 1993, pp 681-757

9. Wessel DL, Adatia I, Thompson J et al: Delivery and monitoring of inhaled nitric oxide in patients with pulmonary hypertension. Crit Care Med 22:930-938, 1994

KETAMINE: FROM "STAR WARS" TO DINOSAUR IN 25 YEARS?

L. J. Rice

Ketamine was released for use in the United States in 1970 (1). It was hailed at that time as the "perfect" complete intravenous anesthetic agent. Ketamine induces a dissociation between the thalamoneocortical and limbic systems, preventing the higher centers from perceiving visual, auditory, or painful stimuli (1). Association areas of the cortex and thalamus are depressed and create a "sensory isolation" (2). In addition, ketamine can produce both motor and sensory block and has been employed for spinal anesthesia, as well as intravenous regional blockade (4,5). The mechanism by which ketamine produces this effect is uncertain.

In other words, ketamine produces a state of catalepsy, catatonia, amnesia, and analgesia. This "dissociative" state was a new frontier in the provision of anesthesia; and the increased muscle tone, occasional nonpurposeful movement, and frequent nystagmus that occurred caused some anesthesiologists to discard this new agent.

Those who continued to explore the frontiers of this unique anesthetic agent stated that it preserved airway reflexes and blood pressure, did not depress respirations, and provided analgesia that far outlasted the anesthetic effects. However, "emergence phenomena" began to be noted in up to 30% of unpremedicated adults and up to 5% of children (5). These phenomena appear to be similar to a "bad LSD trip" and are decreased by inclusion of a benzodiazepine. They are also very infrequent in children, with IM or PO use, as opposed to IV, and with smaller doses, as used in preinduction in the pediatric patient (5-9).

ABOUT KETAMINE

Ketamine has a high bioavailability following IV or IM administration (10). First-pass metabolism and lower absorption require higher doses when ketamine is administered by the oral or rectal routes. Biotransformation takes place in the liver, and multiple metabolites have been described. The most important pathway involves N-demethylation

345

T.H. Stanley and P.G. Schafer (eds.), Pediatric and Obstetrical Anesthesia, 345-356.

to norketamine, an active metabolite with anesthetic and hypnotic potency one-third that of ketamine. Following intravenous administration, less than 4% of a dose of ketamine can be recovered from urine as either unchanged drug or norketamine, and only 16% appears as hydroxylated derivatives (11). Norketamine appears to be 20-30% as potent an anesthetic as ketamine; however, little is known concerning other metabolites (12).

Although it is water soluble, ketamine's lipid solubility is 10 times that of thiopental. The molecular structure contains a chiral center at the C-2 carbon of the cyclohexone ring, so that two enantiomers of the ketamine molecule exist: s(+) ketamine and r(-) ketamine (13). Commercially available ketamine preparations are racemic, with equal concentrations of the two enantiomers; the s(+) isomer is 3 times more potent as an anesthetic and 1.5 times more potent as a hypnotic than is the r(-) isomer. In addition, the s(+) isomer has less stimulation of locomotor activity and is associated with less excitation than its racemate.

Peak blood levels of ketamine occur 1 minute after an IV dose of 1 mg/kg and 5 minutes after an IM injection of 5-10 mg/kg, with dissociation lasting for 15-30 minutes at this dose. The elimination half-life of ketamine is 2-3 hours in adults, and 1-2 hours in children (14).

Analgesia from ketamine is associated with a plasma concentration of 0.15 µg/ml following IM administration, but only 0.04 µg/ml following oral administration (10). This difference may be explained by the higher norketamine concentration associated with oral administration contributing to the analgesia. This higher norketamine level is probably associated with first-pass metabolism. Awakening from ketamine anesthesia takes place at plasma concentrations of 0.64-1.12 µg/ml.

HOW DOES KETAMINE WORK?

The anesthetic state produced by ketamine has been described as a functional and electrophysiological dissociation between the thalamoneocortical and limbic systems (1). Ketamine as a sole anesthetic produces a cataleptic state in which the eyes remain open with a slow nystagmic gaze, while both corneal and light reflexes remain intact. Hypertonus and occasional purposeful movements unrelated to painful stimuli may be noted in the presence of adequate surgical anesthesia. Adequacy of ketamine anesthesia must be judged by presence or absence of purposeful movements to noxious stimuli.

Ketamine is a potent analgesic at subanesthetic plasma concentrations, and its analgesic and anesthetic effects may be mediated by different mechanisms (15). N-methyl-D-aspartate (NMDA) receptors are blocked in the mammalian brain by PCP and ketamine (16,17). These NMDA receptors may represent a subgroup of the sigma opioid receptors that block spinal nociceptive impulses. There is also cross-tolerance between opioids and ketamine in animal models (18). This is not surprising, since animal studies have found stereo-specific opioid receptors in guinea pig ileum (19). Unfortunately, ketamine reversal by naloxone has not been shown in humans.

WHAT ARE KETAMINE'S EFFECTS?

CNS EFFECTS

Ketamine has a reputation for causing increases in intracranial pressure (ICP). However, most of the early studies of ketamine's effects on ICP were conducted on spontaneously breathing subjects and were not controlled for ICP changes due to hypercarbia. Anterior fontanelle pressure, an indirect monitor of ICP, declined by 10% in mechanically ventilated neonates following 2 mg/kg of ketamine (20). Studies in mechanically ventilated pigs with increased ICP indicated no further increase in ICP following 0.5-2.0 mg/kg of IV ketamine (21). In addition, ketamine has been directly injected into cerebral vessels with no effect on the vasculature (22). Therefore, ketamine does not appear to increase ICP in normocarbic patients.

Early EEG studies reported depression of thalamoneocortical pathways with concomitant activation of the limbic system. However, studies have also indicated that ketamine has anticonvulsant properties, rather than stimulating seizures.

EMERGENCE REACTIONS

The ability of ketamine to stimulate dreaming is poorly understood. Psychic sensations reported during emergence from ketamine anesthesia have, more than any other factor, caused this drug to be underutilized. These sensations have been characterized as alterations in mood state and body image, dissociative or extracorporeal (out-of-body) experiences, floating sensations, vivid dreams or illusions, "weird trips," and even frank delirium (23). Although the vivid dreams and visual illusions disappear immediately upon awakening, occasional recurrent illusions (flashbacks) have been reported several weeks following ketamine administration (24). These flashbacks have rarely been reported in adults, and have been reported in fewer than 10 children (25,26).

The illusions appear to be due to ketamine-induced depression of auditory and visual relay nuclei, leading to misinterpretation or misperception of auditory and visual stimuli. Furthermore, the loss of skin and musculoskeletal sensations leads to a reduced ability to feel gravity, producing a sensation of bodily detachment or floating in space.

Contrary to popular lore, there is no evidence that covering the eyes of the patient or allowing emergence in a quiet area alters the incidence of emergence reactions. Both preoperative and postoperative discussion with the patient regarding the expected effects of vivid dreaming, floating, dizziness and blurred vision greatly reduced the incidence of these unpleasant sequelae. Modvig, in the only article in the literature that compares behavior following ketamine to other anesthetic agents in children, showed no difference in behavior between children who received ketamine and those who received halothane (27). The 107 children in this study were followed for as long as 1 month after receiving anesthesia.

The psychic disturbances following ketamine vary in incidence from less than 5% to more than 30%. Factors associated with a high incidence of emergence reactions include: age older than 16 years, females, subjects who normally dream, doses of ketamine greater than 2 mg/kg IV, rapid IV administration (>40 mg/min), and a history of personality problems. Many premedicants have been employed to decrease these undesirable reactions. Benzodiazepines appear to be the most efficacious, while droperidol increases the incidence of adverse emergence reactions.

CARDIOVASCULAR EFFECTS

Ketamine is a sympathomimetic agent that prevents reuptake of catecholamines, and can thus produce mild-to-moderate increases in blood pressure, heart rate, and cardiac output. This hypertensive response is exaggerated by rapid IV injection, and is minimal with IM administration. It is also less pronounced in children than in adults. Investigators have also reported increases in pulmonary artery pressure and pulmonary vascular resistance. Systemic vascular resistance is not significantly altered. Again, most of the early hemodynamic studies of ketamine were conducted on subjects spontaneously breathing room air, and were not controlled for the effects of respiratory depression or partial airway obstruction.

Ketamine appears to produce its sympathomimetic actions primarily by direct stimulation of CNS structures. In the absence of autonomic control, ketamine has direct myocardial depressant properties. This direct negative inotropic effect is usually overshadowed by central sympathetic stimulation. However, patients with severe hypovolemia and others who are critically ill occasionally respond to ketamine administration with a precipitous decrease in blood pressure, probably due to the inability of the sympathomimetic actions of ketamine to counterbalance its direct myocardial depressant and vasodilatory effects.

Ketamine directly dilates vascular smooth muscle while causing sympathetically mediated vasoconstriction. The net effect is that systemic vascular resistance is not significantly altered by ketamine. Even though ketamine increases coronary blood flow, it may be insufficient to meet the metabolic demands of the myocardium produced by the increase in the heart rate and cardiac work.

This agent has been widely used in children with congenital heart disease. Morray and others studied the acute hemodynamic effects of ketamine in children undergoing cardiac catheterization (28). There were only minor hemodynamic changes 2 minutes after administration of 2 mg/kg of IV ketamine. These hemodynamic changes were not associated with any difference in intracardiac shunting, $PaCO_2$ or PaO_2. Hickey and colleagues found no change in pulmonary vascular resistance, systemic vascular resistance index, or cardiac index in 13 mechanically ventilated infants who received 2 mg/kg of IV ketamine (29). There were no differences in pulmonary vascular resistance between infants with preexisting elevations (PVR) and those with normal PVR.

Several authors have compared IM ketamine with halothane/nitrous oxide for induction in cyanotic children prone to hypercyanotic episodes (29,30). Both techniques were associated with increased arterial oxygen saturation, although patients who receive ketamine demonstrated increased heart rate.

Anesthetic induction with IV ketamine 2 mg/kg resulted in a significantly lower incidence of hypotension when compared to fentanyl 20 μg/kg, halothane 0.5%, or isoflurane 0.75% in preterm infants (20). Although ketamine resulted in an average 16% decrease in systolic arterial pressure, this returned to preinduction values after skin incision.

PULMONARY EFFECTS

Bronchodilator effects of ketamine have been evident since early clinical studies of the drug (31). It is likely that circulating catecholamines are the cause of ketamine's bronchodilatory effects, because propranolol will block the protective effects of ketamine in the canine model.

In patients spontaneously breathing room air, ketamine 2 mg/kg given in a rapid IV bolus produced significant reductions in PaO_2 lasting from 5-10 minutes (32). In contrast, patients premedicated with diazepam, also spontaneously breathing room air, showed no change in PaO_2 when the same dose of ketamine was administered over 60 seconds. Ketamine does not produce significant respiratory depression, except in those situations when it is given as a rapid IV bolus. Respiratory depression is extremely rare, although it has been reported with rapid IV administration of ketamine. Functional residual capacity, minute ventilation, and tidal volume are also preserved.

AIRWAY MAINTENANCE

Spontaneous respiration and muscular tone of the tongue and pharynx are preserved. When first released, ketamine was claimed to preserve protective airway reflexes. However, tracheal soiling and aspiration have been reported following the use of ketamine. In addition, ketamine seems to increase airway reactivity, and laryngospasm can result from a combination of increased airway sensitivity and increased salivation. Salivary and tracheobronchial mucus gland secretions are increased by ketamine. Prophylactic administration of antisialogogue prior to IV administration of ketamine is prudent, although small doses of IM ketamine do not seem to produce the same sialorrhea.

Concerns have been raised regarding potential aspiration when using ketamine in an unprepared patient ("full stomach"). However, there are only a few reports in the literature where clinical aspiration was evident in patients who received ketamine sedation. Several studies have shown airway reflex impairment with tracheal soiling following placement of contrast media in the oropharynxes of patients sedated with ketamine (32-34). However, the clinical significance of these studies may be questionable, as silent gastric regurgitation has been reported in 4-26% of patients receiving general anesthesia, and we have no good comparison of ketamine and other sedatives in equipotent doses.

Emesis has been reported in 10% of children receiving ketamine. When present, emesis almost always occurs late in the recovery phase when the patient is alert and the airway is clear.

WHERE IS KETAMINE USEFUL?

ANESTHESIA FOR BURN PATIENTS

Ketamine has been extensively employed in burn units for dressing changes, debridements, and skin grafts in both children and adults (35,36). Although IM doses of 1.5-2 mg/kg have been used extensively in burn units, an apparent tolerance to ketamine frequently develops. The dose must be increased frequently for those patients who face repeated administration of the agent. Higher doses (4-6 mg/kg IM) may be necessary for more extensive eschar excision. Mild emergence reactions manifested by excitement of illusion were noted in about 10% of these unpremedicated burn patients. One advantage of ketamine over narcotics for these procedures is the lack of ileus that accompanies narcotic administration. With the use of ketamine and the avoidance of this serious narcotic effect, nutrition may be improved.

HYPOVOLEMIC AND CRITICALLY ILL PATIENTS

The role of ketamine for induction and maintenance of anesthesia in patients with pericardial tamponade, unresuscitated hypovolemia, and cardiogenic shock is well documented (37). This medication has also been widely employed in the battlefield, and in other austere conditions, where resources are severely limited (38,39).

OBSTETRIC ANESTHESIA

Initial experience with ketamine in doses of 2 mg/kg IV for vaginal delivery was notable for a high incidence of maternal complications and neonatal depression (40). When compared to thiopental in elective cesarean patients, ketamine produced a rapid induction, greater analgesia, and amnesia, with a comparable incidence of unpleasant emergence reactions. Animal studies indicate that ketamine increases uterine blood flow and does not produce deleterious effects on fetal cardiovascular or acid/base status. This agent may be of particular use in patients who are

352

suspected of being hypovolemic, or those who have concomitant bronchospasm.

PEDIATRIC ANESTHESIA

Ketamine has been widely employed for sedation in children undergoing outpatient procedures, such as radiation therapy, oral surgery procedures, and other procedures that benefit from brief, intense sedation or analgesia (41).

There is increasing use of this medication in emergency departments, where sedation for pediatric procedures is a major challenge. Green and others have reported safe use of ketamine sedation for pediatric procedures in 108 children aged 14 months to 13 years (42). These authors noted acceptable conditions for procedures that included suture of lacerations, reduction of fractures and dislocations, and other examinations for which brief, intense analgesia was desirable. They noted a mean duration to time of discharge of 82 minutes with an IM dose of ketamine 4 mg/kg, in conjunction with atropine. One 18-month old child vomited shortly after injection and experienced a brief episode of laryngospasm that did not require intubation. The authors caution that equipment and expertise for advanced pediatric airway management is mandatory when this drug is used. They also require continuous supervision by a nurse throughout the period that the child is sedated, until s/he is ready to be discharged. As with any other sedation, the AAP guidelines for conscious sedation should be followed (43). Epstein reported on 1100 children who received 3 mg/kg ketamine IM for sedation in the emergency department and reaffirmed the need for close supervision of these patients (9).

In addition to the increasing emergency department experience, ketamine has also proven useful in performance of pelvic examinations in children and mentally retarded adults. Rosen and colleagues have established a "ketamine clinic" for sedation of mentally handicapped women undergoing routine gynecologic examinations (44). These authors used oral ketamine in doses of 3.5-15 mg/kg with supplemental nasal midazolam, if additional sedation was required. Forty-two patients received ketamine on 64 occasions. Fifty percent of women were able to be examined with the initial dose of ketamine; the remainder required 1-2 supplemental sedation doses. No respiratory depression was observed, and all patients were discharged within 90 minutes of examination.

Thirty percent of patients vomited. Intravenous ketamine in doses of 1.5 mg has also been used to facilitate gynecologic examination (45).

Ketamine (supplemented with midazolam) has also been used for postoperative analgesia and sedation following pediatric cardiac surgery (46). It has also been a popular choice to facilitate cardiac catheterization and transcatheter closure of atrial septal defects (47,48).

The most popular use of ketamine outside the emergency department is for premedication of pediatric patients. This drug has been administered nasally, in doses of 6 mg/kg, orally in doses of 3-6 mg/kg, rectally in doses of 3 mg/kg and IM in doses of 2 mg/kg (49-51). Hannallah and Patel demonstrated that IM injection of ketamine allowed mask induction in the presence of parents, without delaying discharge, in ambulatory surgery patients undergoing brief procedures (52). Alderson and Lerman compared oral ketamine 5 mg/kg with oral midazolam 0.5 mg/kg and found that both drugs effectively sedated children within 20 minutes of administration (7). Children who received ketamine were discharged 20 minutes later than those who received midazolam.

SUMMARY

Ketamine is not a perfect drug. However, even in 1995, we have no alternative agent with the same versatility, ease of use, and airway management profile (53). It can be given IV, IM, PO, rectally, epidurally, or in the subarachnoid space. Used properly, preinduction doses of this agent do not increase discharge time from the PACU. Ketamine, like every other anesthetic drug, is no better than the individual administering it, and no safer than his/her use of it. Until we have a better agent that provides similar amnesia, analgesia, preservation of the airway, and respiratory status, I will consider it the "American Express card" of pediatric anesthesia—I may not always use it, but I won't leave home without it!

REFERENCES

1. Corssen G, Miyasaka M, Domino EF: Changing concepts in pain control during surgery: Dissociative anesthesia with CI-358. Anesth Analg 47:746-759, 1968
2. Corssen G: Historical aspects of ketamine—first clinical experience. In Domino EF, ed. Status of ketamine in anesthesiology. Ann Arbor, NPP Books, 1990, pp 1-10

3. Bion JF: Intrathecal ketamine for war surgery. A preliminary study under field conditions. Anaesthesia 39:1023-1028, 1984

4. Amiot JF, Bouju P, Palacci JH et al: Intravenous regional anaesthesia with ketamine. Anaesthesia 40:899-901, 1985

5. Sussman DR: A comparative evaluation of ketamine anesthesia in children and adults. Anesthesiology 40:459-464, 1974

6. Sklar GS, Zukin SR, Reilly TA: Adverse reactions to ketamine anaesthesia—abolition by a psychological technique. Anaesthesia 36:183-187, 1981

7. Aldersen PJ, Lerman J: Oral premedication of paediatric ambulatory anaesthesia: A combination of midazolam and ketamine. Can J Anaesth 41:221-226, 1994

8. Green SM, Nakamura R, Johnson NE: Ketamine sedation for pediatric procedures: Part 2, review and implications. Ann Emerg Med 19:1033-1046

9. Epstein FB: Ketamine dissociative sedation in pediatric emergency medical practice. Am J Emerg Med 11:180-182, 1993

10. Grant IS, Nimmo WS, Clements JA: Pharmacokinetics and analgesic effects of IM and oral ketamine. Br J Anaesth 53:805-810, 1981

11. Geisslinger G, Hering W, Thomann P et al: Pharmacokinetics and pharmacodynamics of ketamine enantiomers in surgical patients using stereoselective analytical method. Br J Anaesth 70:666-671, 1993

12. White PF, Johnston RR, Pudwill CR et al: Effects of halothane anesthesia on the biodisposition of ketamine in rats. J Pharmacol Exp Ther 196:545-555, 1976

13. White PF, Way WL, Trevor AJ: Ketamine—its pharmacology and therapeutic uses. Anesthesiology 56:119-136, 1982

14. Grant IS, Nimmo WS, McNicol LR et al: Ketamine disposition in children and adults. Br J Anaesth 55:1107-1110, 1983

15. Collins JG: Effects of ketamine on low intensity tactile sensory input are not dependent upon a spinal site of action. Anesth Analg 65:1123-1129, 1986

16. Thomson AM, West DC, Lodge D: An N-methylaspartate receptor-mediated synapse in rat cerebral cortex: A site of action of ketamine? Nature 313:479-481, 1985

17. Anis NA, Berry SC, Burton NR et al: The dissociative anaesthetics, ketamine and phencyclidine, selectively reduce excitation of central mammalian neurones by N-methyl-aspartate. Br J Pharmacol 79:565-575, 1983

18. Pedoe Gm, Smith DJ: The involvement of opiate and monoaminergic neuronal systems in the analgesic effects of ketamine. Pain 12:57-73, 1982

19. Finck AD, Ngai SH: A possible mechanism of ketamine-induced analgesia. Anesthesiology 56:291-297, 1982

20. Friesen RH, Thieme RE, Honda AT et al: Changes in anterior fontanel pressure in preterm neonates receiving isoflurane, halothane, fentanyl, or ketamine. Anesth Analg 66:431-434, 1987

21. Pfenninger E, Dick W, Ahnefeld FE: The influence of ketamine on both normal and raised intracranial pressure of artificially ventilated animals. Eur J Anaesth 2:297-307, 1985

22. Schwedler M, Miletich DH, Albeecht RF: Cerebral blood flow and metabolism following ketamine administration. Can Anaesth Soc J 29:222-225, 1982

23. Moretti RJ, Hassan SZ, Goodman LI et al: Comparison of ketamine and thiopental in healthy volunteers: Effects on mental status, mood, and personality. Anesth Analg 63:1087-1096, 1984

24. Fine J, Finestone SC: Sensory disturbances following ketamine anesthesia—recurrent hallucinations. Anesth Analg 52:428-430, 1973

25. Meyers EF, Charles P: Prolonged adverse reactions to ketamine in children. Anesthesiology 49:39-40, 1978

26. Hollister GR, Burn JM: Side effects of ketamine in pediatric anesthesia. Anesth Analg 53:262-267, 1974

27. Modvig KM, Neilsen SF: Psychological changes in children after anesthesia: A comparison between halothane and ketamine. Acta Anaesth Scand 21:541-544, 1977

28. Morray JP, Lynn AM, Stamm SJ et al: Hemodynamic effects of ketamine in children with congenital heart disease. Anesth Analg 63:895-899, 1984

29. Hickey PR, Hansen DD, Cramolini GM et al: Pulmonary and systemic hemodynamic responses to ketamine in infants with normal and elevated pulmonary vascular resistance. Anesthesiology 62:287-293, 1985

30. Laishley RS, Burrows FS, Lerman J et al: Effect of anesthetic induction regimens on oxygen saturation in cyanotic congenital heart disease. Anesthesiology 54:238-242, 1986

31. Rock MJ, DeLaRocha SR, L'Hommedieu CS et al: Use of ketamine in asthmatic children to treat respiratory failure refractory to conventional therapy. Crit Care Med 14:514-516, 1986

32. Zgismond EK, Matsuki A, Kothary SP et al: Arterial hypoxemia caused by intravenous ketamine. Anesth Analg 55:311-314, 1976

33. Carson IW, Moore J, Balmer P et al: Laryngeal competence with ketamine and other drugs. Anesthesiology 38:128-133, 1973

34. Yeung MI, Lin RS: Laryngeal reflexes in children under ketamine anaesthesia. Br J Anaesth 44:1089-1092, 1972

35. Corssen G, Dget S: Dissociative anesthesia for the severely burned child. Anesth Analg 50:95-102, 1971

36. Demling RH, Ellerbee S, Jarrett F: Ketamine anesthesia for tangential excision of burn eschar: A burn unit procedure. J Trauma 18:269-270, 1978

37. Corssen G, Reves JG, Stanley TH: Intravenous anesthesia and analgesia. Philadelphia, Lea & Febiger, 1988, pp 99-174

38. Restall J, Tully AM, Ward PJ et al: Total intravenous anaesthesia for military surgery. A technique using ketamine, midazolam, and vecuronium. Anaesthesia 43:46-49, 1988

39. Whitten CE: Anesthesia in distant places: Prevention of anesthesia mishaps. Sem in Anesth 12:154-164, 1993

40. Schultetus RR, Hill CR, Dharamaj CM et al: Wakefulness during Cesarian section after anesthetic induction with ketamine, thiopental, or ketamine and thiopental combined. Anesth Analg 65:723-728, 1986

41. Freisen RH, Morrison JE: The role of ketamine in the current practiceof paediatric anaesthesia. Paediatr Anaesth 4:79-82, 1994

42. Green SM, Nakamura R, Johnson NE: Ketamine sedation for pediatric procedures: Part 1 , a prospective series. Ann Emerg Med 19:1024-1033, 1990

43. Committe on Drugs: Guidelines for monitoring and management of pediatric patients during and after sedation for diagnostic and therapeutic procedures. Pediatrics 6:1110-1115, 1992

44. Elkins TE, McNeeley G, Rosen D et al: A clinical observation of a program to accomplish pelvic exams in difficult-to-manage patients with mental retardation. Adolesc Pediatr Gynecol 1:195-198, 1988

45. Haran MD: Genital examination under ketamine sedation in cases of suspected drug abuse. Arch Dis Child 70:197-199, 1994

46. Hartvig P, Larsson E, Joachimssom P-O: Postoperative analgesia and sedation following pediatric cardiac surgery using a constant infusion of ketamine. J Cardiothor Anesth 7:148-153, 1993

47. Lebovic S, Reich DL, Steinberg G et al: Comparison of propofol versus ketamine for anesthesia in pediatric patients undergoing cardiac catheterization. Anesth Analg 74:490-494, 1992

48. Hickey PR, Wessel DL, Streitz SL et al: Transcatheter closure of atrial septal defects: Hemodynamic complications and anesthetic management. Anesth Analg 74:44-50, 1992

49. Weksler N, Ovadia L, Muati G et al: Nasal ketamine for paediatric premedication. Can J Anaesth 40:119-121, 1993

50. Alderson PJ, Lerman J: Oral premedication for paediatric ambulatory anaesthesia: A comparison of midazolam and ketamine. Can J Anaesth 41:221-226, 1994

51. Beebe DS, Belani KG, Chang P-N et al: Effectiveness of preoperative sedation with rectal midazolam, ketamine, or their combinations in young children. Anesth Analg 75:880-884, 1992

52. Hannallah RS, Patel RI: Low-dose intramuscular ketamine for anesthesia preinduction in young children undergoing brief outpatient procedures. Anesthesiology 70:598-600, 1989

53. Reich Dl, Silvay G: Ketamine: An update on the first twenty-five years of clinical experience. Can J Anaesth 36:186-197, 1989

CURRENT STATUS OF INTRAVENOUS ANESTHESIA IN CHILDREN

R. S. Hannallah

Until recently, intravenous techniques have not been widely used in pediatric anesthesia. This was caused by the concern that most agents that were available resulted in longer recovery when compared to inhalational techniques, and by the unwillingness to subject awake children to the trauma of venipuncture (1).

The recent introduction of propofol, short-acting opioids, and muscle relaxants into clinical anesthesia has removed most concerns about delayed recovery. It is hoped that the availability of the eutectic mixture of the two local anesthetics lidocaine and prilocaine (EMLA), which can be used to perform painless venipuncture in children, will encourage more anesthesiologists to offer, and more children to accept, an intravenous induction (2). The use of EMLA in children requires careful planning, since at least 1 hour of contact time under an occlusive dressing is required for full effect. In most cases, EMLA should be applied to two potential intravenous (IV) sites to have a back-up site available in case the first venipuncture is not successful. In institutions where preoperative laboratory testing is required, it is appropriate to offer children the option of having their required venipuncture under EMLA, with an IV cannula left in place to be used later for anesthesia induction. Although the use of EMLA does produce skin analgesia, it does not remove the fear of needles in children who have been previously accustomed to expect pain (2). Only time and repeated successful use can remove that fear.

Other methods of reducing the pain and apprehension associated with venipuncture include the use of nitrous oxide analgesia (3) and/or the use of very small IV catheters or "Butterfly" needles.

INTRAVENOUS INDUCTION

Intravenous induction of anesthesia is the method of choice in most older children for the same reasons it is the standard in adults. It

357

T.H. Stanley and P.G. Schafer (eds.), Pediatric and Obstetrical Anesthesia, 357-361.
© 1995 *Kluwer Academic Publishers.*

ensures a rapid, pleasant onset with minimal struggling and no unpleasant memories of a suffocating mask or a smelly gas. When IV induction is used in healthy young children, the drug may be injected directly in a dorsal hand or antecubital vein, usually via a 25-gauge butterfly needle. An intravenous infusion can be started later (1).

THIOPENTAL SODIUM

Thiopental sodium (2.5% solution) is a commonly used induction agent for adult outpatient anesthesia. Healthy children require a slightly higher dose (4-6 mg/kg) to induce sleep than adults. When Steward compared the recovery times following intravenous thiopental induction of anesthesia in children with those of children who had inhalational induction, he found that by 30 minutes after surgery there was no difference in the recovery score between the two groups (4). However, the children who had barbiturate for the induction of anesthesia tended to be sleepier and required more airway support for the first 15 minutes of the recovery period. He also found that there was no difference in the eventual return to a "bright and alert" status and normal appetite at home following discharge from the hospital. Repeated doses of thiopental should be avoided, as they can prolong recovery. In addition, diazepam and opiates can also have an exaggerated depressant effect if given during the early postoperative period following anesthesia induction with intravenous thiopental.

METHOHEXITAL

Use of methohexital (1.5-2.0 mg/kg) results in a significantly shorter recovery time than that following administration of an equivalent single dose of thiopental. Induction of anesthesia with methohexital, however, is followed by a high incidence of involuntary muscle movements, hiccough, and coughing episodes that can be troublesome. Severe burning often develops along the course of the injected vein. This is particularly undesirable in children because it promotes hand movement and can dislodge the needle from the vein. Pain can be avoided by mixing a small amount of lidocaine (1 mg/ml) with the methohexital. Methohexital has also been reported to induce epileptiform convulsions in susceptible patients.

ETOMIDATE

Etomidate, a nonbarbiturate hypnotic agent, has been used extensively for intravenous induction of anesthesia in Europe. When used in an intravenous dose of 0.2 mg/kg in children, etomidate produces sleep rapidly and safely, with negligible cardiovascular system side effects and little respiratory depression (5).

Pain is common following injection of etomidate; and, unlike methohexital, it is not prevented by adding lidocaine to the solution. Myoclonia is also seen following injection of this drug. Using an analgesic (e.g., fentanyl for premedication or with induction of anesthesia) can reduce these problems.

PROPOFOL

Propofol is the most ideal drug available for the anesthetic management of outpatients. It offers many advantages, including rapid onset and very prompt and pleasant recovery with minimal nausea and vomiting.

Although there is now a tremendous experience with propofol in adults, the experience in children is still limited. The induction dose in healthy children is reported to be around 3 mg/kg (6). In a recent study comparing the recovery characteristics of propofol, thiopental, and halothane, children who received an induction bolus of propofol followed by halothane maintenance recovered significantly faster than those who received a bolus of thiopental (7). The fastest recovery, however, was seen in children who received propofol for both induction and maintenance of anesthesia (7).

Unfortunately, propofol administration is associated with a high incidence of pain and a burning sensation when the small hand veins are used for injection. This problem can be greatly minimized by using the larger antecubital veins for induction (7), or by adding lidocaine (1 mg to each 1 ml of the drug) to propofol immediately prior to injection.

Experience with the use of propofol as an induction agent in infants is even more limited. The induction dose is higher than that of older children (8). When rapid IV induction is required in infants, propofol has been shown to be more effective than thiopental in obtunding the hypertensive response to intubation and, in young infants (1-6 months), results in more prompt emergence after short surgical procedures(9).

INTRAVENOUS MAINTENANCE

Experience with intravenous maintenance techniques in children started to accumulate following the introduction of propofol to clinical practice. Propofol anesthesia (with or without nitrous oxide supplementation) has been consistently shown to be associated with fast recovery and an extremely low incidence of postoperative vomiting, even following surgical procedures that normally result in vomiting (e.g., strabismus surgery) (10-12). Recovery is fastest if propofol induction is followed by a propofol infusion for the maintenance of anesthesia (7). Because of their higher volume of distribution and increased clearance, children require a higher maintenance infusion rate (125-300 µg/kg/min) than adults (13,14). This is especially true for younger children and during the early part of maintenance (7).

The use of propofol in Total IV Anesthesia techniques in children has been extremely helpful in simplifying the administration of anesthesia/sedation to children undergoing diagnostic and/or therapeutic radiological procedures outside the operating room (e.g., MRI examination) (15).

REFERENCES

1. Hannallah RS, Epstein BS: Outpatient anesthesia. In Gregory G, ed. Pediatric anesthesia. 3rd edition. New York, Churchill Livingstone, 1994, pp 781-782
2. Soliman IE, Broadman LM, Hannallah RS et al: Comparison of the analgesic effects of EMLA (eutectic mixture of local anesthetics) to intradermal lidocaine infiltration prior to venous cannulation in unpremedicated children. Anesthesiology 68:804-806, 1988
3. Henderson J, Spence DG, Komocar LM et al: Administration of nitrous oxide to pediatric patients provides analgesia for venous cannulation. Anesthesiology 72:269-271, 1990
4. Steward DJ: Outpatient pediatric anesthesia. Anesthesiology 43: 268, 1975
5. Kay B: A clinical assessment of the use of etomidate in children. Br J Anaesth 48:207, 1976
6. Hannallah RS, Baker SB, Casey W et al: Propofol effective dose and induction characteristics in unpremedicated children. Anesthesiology 74:217-219, 1991
7. Hannallah RS, Britton JT, Schafer PG et al: Propofol anaesthesia in paediatric ambulatory patients: A comparison with thiopentone and halothane. Can J Anaesth 41:12-18, 1994
8. Westin P: The induction dose of propofol in infants 1-6 months of age and in children 10-16 years of age. Anesthesiology 74:455-458, 1991

9. Schrum SF, Hannallah RS, Verghese PM et al: Comparison of propofol and thiopental for rapid anesthesia induction in infants. Anesth Analg 78: 482-485, 1994

10. Hannallah R, Britton J, Schafer P et al: Effect of propofol anesthesia on the incidence of vomiting after strabismus surgery in children (abstract). Anesth Analg 74:S131, 1992

11. Watcha MF, Simeon RM, White PF et al: Effect of propofol on the incidence of postoperative vomiting after strabismus surgery in pediatric outpatients. Anesthesiology 75:204-209, 1991

12. Martin TM, Nicolson SC, Bargas MS: Propofol anesthesia reduces emesis and airway obstruction in pediatric outpatients. Anesth Analg 76:144-148, 1993

13. White M, Kenny GNC: Intravenous propofol anesthesia using a computerized infusion system. Anaesthesia 45:204-209, 1990

14. March B, White M, Morton N et al: Pharmacokinetic model driven infusion of propofol in children. Br J Anaesth 67:41-48, 1991

15. Frankville DD, Spear RM, Dyck JB: The dose of propofol required to prevent children from moving during magnetic resonance imaging. Anesthesiology 79:953-958, 1993

POSTOPERATIVE PAIN MANAGEMENT IN
THE PEDIATRIC PATIENT

L. J. Rice

Children do not complain of pain, or even experience pain, in the same terms that adults do. Children may cope with pain by withdrawing rather than crying or asking for medication. Many children will not complain of pain, for fear the adult answer to that pain will be the dreaded "shot," or because they believe they deserve the pain as punishment for something they did wrong.

THE PROBLEM

Infants and children usually receive less analgesic medications following surgery than do adults (1,2). Schechter and Allen's survey of pediatricians, family practitioners, and surgeons in their northeastern city showed that only 75% of these specialists believed that children experienced "adult" pain by the age of 2 years (3).

Eland evaluated the hospital experiences of 25 children between the ages of 5 and 8 years undergoing major surgery (4). Thirteen of the 25 children were never given any medication for pain relief during their entire hospitalization.

Beyer and others, in a retrospective chart review, compared analgesics administered in adults and children with identical diagnoses (1). Their analysis revealed that the 18 adults received 372 separate doses of narcotic analgesics and 299 doses of non-narcotic analgesics, for a total of 671 medications for pain. In comparison, the 25 children received 24 separate doses of analgesics. These authors suggest several misconceptions that may contribute to the differences in pain medications given: 1) because children's nervous systems are immature, they do not experience pain with the intensity adults do; 2) children recover quickly; 3) it is unsafe to administer a narcotic pain medication to a child because s/he may become addicted; 4) narcotics always depress respiration in children; 5) children cannot tell you where they hurt; 6) the child needs to experience

363

T.H. Stanley and P.G. Schafer (eds.), Pediatric and Obstetrical Anesthesia, 363-373.
© 1995 *Kluwer Academic Publishers.*

pain; and 7) the nurse who wields the needle receives the child's cry of protest.

Nurses' beliefs regarding pain management also bear consideration. In an investigation of the factors affecting nurses' decisions to medicate pediatric patients following surgery, Burokas surveyed 134 experienced pediatric nurses in critical care and surgical units (5). She discovered that demographic variables, such as age, educational background, and personal pain experience do not influence pain medication decisions. However, having offspring who previously experienced severe pain does influence pediatric nurses to medicate postsurgical patients more frequently. As might be expected, nurses in critical care units are more confident with frequent intravenous narcotic administration than are those on a ward. In a chart review of 40 postsurgical patients, these authors noted that the most significant factor influencing the amount of pain medication a pediatric patient is likely to receive is his/her nurse's perception of pain relief goals. If the goal is to completely relieve pain, the child will receive more medication than if the goal is merely to decrease pain.

HOW DO I TELL IF A CHILD IS IN PAIN?

McGrath and co-workers, as well as Thompson and Varni, have reviewed the problem of clinical measurement of pain in children (6,7). Both sets of investigators note that the problems of pain assessment are complicated by children's changing but relatively limited cognitive ability to understand measurement instructions or to articulate descriptions of their pain. Children's responses are also affected by their developing behavioral repertoire and their constantly changing psychology.

Children older than 4-6 years of age can self-report pain using either the Visual Analogue scale (VAS), a modified VAS, or another validated tool such as OUCHER or the Poker Chip Scale (8,9). All of these tools require some preoperative instruction of the children. Younger children are usually assessed using a behavioral or physiologic-behavioral scale (10,11). Pain in children is much more difficult to assess than in adults, as discrimination between pain and distress may be very challenging, particularly in the younger pediatric patient. The scope of this subject is too great to deal with in detail in this forum: the reader is directed to the several excellent recent reviews in the literature (6,7). The prevailing philosophy among pediatric anesthesiologists is as follows: if I were having the procedure/surgery that this child is undergoing, would I require pain medication? If the answer is yes, the child is assessed, pain medication is administered, and a reassessment is made. If the reassessment shows a decrease of pain behaviors, pain management is considered successful, and continued evaluations are planned. If pain behaviors persist, the child receives additional pain treatment.

In addition, it is recognized that the emotional component of pain is very strong in children. Nonpharmacologic methods of pain management are also important (12). While the most important of these is minimal separation from parents, other methods, such as reassurance, cuddling, stroking, and distraction, should also be employed.

NONOPIOID PAIN MEDICATIONS

Nonopioid analgesics, usually acetaminophen or a nonsteroidal antiinflammatory agent (NSAID), act at peripheral sites of injury by inhibiting prostaglandin synthesis and/or blocking activation of primary afferent nerve injuries (13). These analgesics are useful for the treatment of mild-to-moderate discomfort (such as in many ambulatory procedures) and for reducing the need for opioids in more severe pain.

The most common oral analgesic employed in pediatric patients continues to be acetaminophen. This medication has been shown to be safe and efficacious in neonates and older children, with similar pharmacodynamics and pharmacokinetics, in all but the youngest age groups. Doses of 10-15 mg/kg orally or 20-25 mg/kg rectally every 4 hours, with a maximum dose of 2.5 g/24 hours, produces relatively low plasma levels with good analgesia (14). Although rectal administration is less convenient and absorption more erratic than oral doses, acetaminophen suppositories can be inserted following induction of anesthesia to achieve effective blood levels soon after arrival in the postanesthesia care unit (15).

Nonsteroidal antiinflammatory drugs can cause gastritis and interfere with platelet function, as well as renal function. Ibuprofen, at a dose of 10 mg/kg, was reported to be superior to acetaminophen in reducing pain scores and the severity of other symptoms in children suffering severe tonsillitis or pharyngitis. Ketorolac has been administered by both the intravenous and intramuscular routes (16,17). Since a child will often deny pain rather than submit to an IM injection, intravenous administration of ketorolac has become very popular, in spite of the fact that it is an off-label use of the drug. Intramuscular doses of 0.75 mg/kg provide highly effective postoperative analgesia, as do IV doses of 1 mg/kg as a loading dose, with 0.5 mg/kg administered every 6 hours thereafter (18). This medication is rarely employed in children in its oral formulation.

There have been no reported problems with gastritis or renal failure in pediatric patients receiving ketorolac. Although the bleeding time is not increased following administration of this drug, there is an increasing tendency to avoid its administration in surgical procedures that place a large stress on platelets and clotting mechanisms, such as tonsillectomy and adenoidectomy.

Indomethacin is available for IV administration, and because of its use in premature infants to promote closure of the patent ductus arteriosus, there has been considerable clinical pediatric experience with this agent. Use of a continuous infusion of indomethacin has been shown to provide excellent adjunctive pain relief in postoperative patients and to provide greater patient satisfaction than prn narcotics alone (19).

Aspirin is usually avoided in pediatric patients because of the association with the use of this agent to treat febrile illness and the development of Reye's syndrome. In addition, there is a higher incidence of platelet dysfunction and gastrointestinal side effects than with other NSAIDs.

OPIOID PAIN MEDICATIONS

Conventional pain management has involved on-demand administration of oral or parenteral analgesics. Narcotics are usually given to treat, rather than to prevent, pain. The most common postoperative modality of narcotic administration is still the prn intramuscular injection. However, under-utilization of analgesics under these circumstance has been well documented, particularly in pediatric patients. Other disadvantages of this approach to analgesia include wide fluctuations in blood concentrations of analgesic medication during each dosing interval and the discomfort caused by intramuscular injections, which are painful and disliked by both children and adults.

ORAL OPIOIDS

Codeine can be administered orally or parenterally and provides effective control of mild-to-moderate postoperative pain. The bioavailabilty of codeine following oral administration is around 60%. Orally administered codeine (0.5-1 mg/kg) is often combined with acetaminophen (10-15 mg/kg). This combination reduces the overall codeine requirement, thus limiting dose-dependant side effects. Although available, this medication is rarely used in its intravenous form, as it has no advantage over morphine and may be associated with a higher incidence of nausea and vomiting. Oxycodone (0.2 mg/kg) is available only as a tablet and is also often combined with acetaminophen or an NSAID. This agent appears to cause less nausea than codeine at equipotent doses.

Methadone, in a dose of 0.1 mg/kg, has also been successfully employed as an oral analgesic postoperatively, although it is more frequently employed for the treatment of chronic pain (20). This narcotic is known for its slow elimination, prolonged duration of analgesia, and high oral bioavailability. Because a single dose of intravenous or oral methadone can provide analgesia for 12-36 hours, it is a convenient way to provide prolonged analgesic without requiring an intramuscular injection.

INTERMITTENT INTRAVENOUS OPIOIDS

Fentanyl, with its short action and quick onset, is the most frequently employed opioid analgesic for pediatric ambulatory surgery patients. It is most often titrated in doses of 0.5-1 μg/kg. The rapid onset of analgesia and short duration of actions rarely delay discharge in an ambulatory surgery setting. It is frequently employed in combination with rectal acetaminophen or regional analgesic techniques in this setting.

Morphine continues to be the most popular opioid analgesic for treatment of postoperative pain in pediatric inpatients. As with any respiratory depressant agent, preterm infants and very young infants are more susceptible to the respiratory effects of this opioid, and titration of small doses should be employed (21). Intravenous doses of 0.05-0.2 mg/kg are employed in older children, usually administered by buretrol over 20 minutes, at 4-hour to 6-hour intervals. As with any intermittently administered agent, fluctuating blood levels with concomitant fluctuating analgesia will occur.

Preliminary work by Berde and colleagues indicates that intermittent intravenous administration of long-acting narcotic analgesics, such as methadone, may provide prolonged pain relief in postoperative pediatric patients (20). Berde recommends an intravenous loading dose of 0.1-0.2 mg/kg, followed by titration of 0.05 mg/kg increments every 10-15 minutes until analgesia is achieved. Supplemental methadone can be administered by intravenous infusion over 20 minutes every 12 hours, as needed. An alternative "reverse prn" schedule has been employed as well; the nurse asks the child if he has pain and administers methadone on a "sliding scale," as needed. In theory, the choice of this opioid should provide more stable blood levels of medication, as well as more consistent analgesia, without requiring as many doses as intermittent morphine would need to achieve the same effect.

CONTINUOUS INTRAVENOUS INFUSIONS OF OPIOIDS

Millar and colleagues evaluated the use of continuous morphine infusions following major surgery in 20 children from 3 months to 12 years of age (22). After loading with intravenous fentanyl 1-2 µg/kg, an infusion of morphine 14 µg/kg/hr was begun, to be adjusted by the nursing staff for optimum pain control. Pain scores and plasma morphine levels were recorded. A mean serum level of 6.54 ng/ml provided effective pain relief in all children, but the steady-state blood concentration of morphine showed a large interpatient variation (4.67-9.58 ng/ml). A satisfactory and constant analgesic state was noted within 6 hours. No clinical signs of respiratory depression or other side effects were noted, even in the youngest child. Beasley and Tibballs evaluated the safety and efficacy of continuous morphine infusion in 121 children following major surgery with similar results (23). Neither study compared continuous infusions with other modalities of narcotic administration. Lynn and colleagues evaluated the use of continuous morphine infusion doses of 10-30 µg/kg/hr following cardiac surgery and concluded that serum morphine levels less than 30 ng/ml did not interfere with weaning from mechanical ventilation (24).

Hendrickson and colleagues compared the safety and quality of postoperative analgesia provided by intermittent IM injection with continuous intravenous infusion of morphine in children 1-16 years of age (25). As might be expected, the children in the intravenous group received greater amounts of drug but were more comfortable than those in the group who got "shots." There was no difference in complications (nausea, urinary retention, ileus, respiratory depression) between the groups. Subcutaneous administration of concentrated opioids has also proven successful.

PATIENT-CONTROLLED ANALGESIA

Patient-controlled analgesia (PCA) has received enthusiastic acceptance in both adult and pediatric populations, even though pain scores are not necessarily improved when compared to prn intravenous narcotic administration, timed intramuscular administration, or epidural local anesthetics or narcotics (26). In spite of this lack of improved pain scores, patients have uniformly preferred PCA to other pain management programs. This is particularly true in the adolescent population, where control is an important part of personality development. Patients, nurses, and parents uniformly preferred PCA to prn intravenous narcotic administration, and no adverse side effects were noted (27).

Rodgers et al reported the successful use of PCA in 15 pediatric patients and added that less nursing time was required for pain management in these patients (28). Dodd and co-workers demonstrated that PCA can safely be employed in children as young as 6 years of age (29).

With the advent of more sophisticated pumps, allowing a background continuous infusion of narcotic with the patient adding small boluses as needed, the major complaint of pain upon awakening from sleep (impossible to avoid with on-demand analgesic delivery systems) should be alleviated. In this video game era, even 5-year olds appear to understand and appreciate the chance to take care of their own pain medication. "Parent-controlled analgesia," where a parent who is rooming-in with a young child is allowed to control the PCA administration, is also under investigation.

REGIONAL ANALGESIA FOR RELIEF OF ACUTE PAIN

Although more research is required of all forms of pain treatment for pediatric patients, there exist numerous studies addressing the use of regional analgesia for acute pain in the postoperative period. This may reflect the increasing attention paid to outpatients, as regional analgesia methods are particularly applicable to this population. All regional anesthetic techniques have been successfully employed for pain relief in pediatric patients. The most common techniques were discussed in the lecture on regional anesthesia; due to space limitations, interested readers are referred to standard texts (30-33).

CONTINUOUS CAUDAL OR EPIDURAL BLOCK

Caudal and epidural blocks provide excellent continuous pain relief in the postoperative period, particularly for lower-extremity and pelvic surgery. Of course, these techniques may also be used to provide adjunct intraoperative anesthesia. Desparmet and colleagues reported on a group of 21 children who received excellent analgesia following major orthopedic or genitourinary surgery (34). They also noted that test doses of bupivacaine administered to patients anesthetized with halothane may be unreliable, particularly if atropine has not been administered, and that fractionation of the total dose of bupivacaine should be employed (35). Dalens and co-workers reported on an additional 35 infants and children who received a light general anesthetic in conjunction with epidural anesthesia (36). These children ranged in age from 2 days to 7 years. Postoperative epidural analgesia may have a distinct advantage for the child with respiratory difficulties, in whom it is desirable to avoid the respiratory depression caused by narcotics.

CENTRAL NARCOTICS

Caudal analgesia with morphine has been reported in numerous series (37-40). Krane and others compared caudal morphine with caudal bupivacaine and intravenous morphine in 46 children ages 1-16 years following orthopedic or genitourinary surgery (37). Caudal morphine produced 8-24 hours of analgesia in children. Caudal bupivacaine produced only 5 hours of pain relief, while intravenous morphine provided analgesia for 45 minutes. Although the original article indicated no incidence of respiratory depression with the dose of 0.1 mg/kg of caudal morphine, a second article reported an incident occurring 3.5 hours following caudal injection of the morphine (38). The authors conclude that this block should not be used without adequate respiratory monitoring. The same authors have evaluated three different doses of caudal morphine and recommend a dose of 0.033 mg/kg to provide the optimum balance between duration of analgesia and incidence of delayed respiratory depression (39).

Subarachnoid narcotics have been utilized in the pediatric population with the same limitations as in the adult population. Jones and colleagues reported on intrathecal morphine for analgesia following open heart surgery, with postoperative analgesia lasting more than 22 hours in 60% of the patients but with respiratory depression occurring in 9 of the 56 patients (40). Broadman and co-workers reported on the use of intrathecal narcotics for postoperative pain control in 10 children following Harrington rod instrumentation for scoliosis surgery. They noted pain relief lasting more than 18 hours with a dose of 0.01 mg/kg of morphine (41). No respiratory depression was noted.

CONCLUSION

Any method used for pain relief in the adult patient can be adapted for pain relief in the pediatric patient. Children have the same right to pain relief as adults, even if their pain is more difficult to assess. More frequent use of NSAIDs, as well as many more studies of opioid administration—especially long-acting narcotic analgesics, continuous infusions, and patient-controlled or parent-controlled analgesia—are required. An increased response to the challenge of acute pain treatment with regional analgesic techniques in the pediatric outpatient will also be useful, with more continuous catheter techniques employed in hospitalized patients. Certainly we have the responsibility to provide optimum pain relief for all patients, not just those who can complain in a way that is easy to understand.

REFERENCES

1. Beyer JE, DeGood DE, Ashley LC et al: Patterns of postoperative analgesic use with adults and children following cardiac surgery. Pain 17:71-81, 1986
2. Schechter NL, Allen DA, Hanson K: Status of pediatric pain control: A comparison of hospital analgesic usage in children and adults. Pediatrics 77:11-15, 1986
3. Schechter NL, Allen DA: Physicians' attitudes toward pain in children. Develop Behavior Pediatr 7:350-354, 1986
4. Eland JM, Anderson JE: The experience of pain in children. In Jacox AJ, ed. Pain: A source book for nurses and other health professionals. Boston, Little, Brown and Co, 1977, pp 453-473
5. Burokas L: Factors affecting nurses' decisions to medicate pediatric patients after surgery. Heart & Lung 14:373-379, 1985
6. McGrath PJ, Cunningham SJ, Goodman JT et al: The clinical measurement of pain in children: A review. Clin J Pain 1:221-227, 1986
7. Thompson KL, Varni JW: A developmental cognitive-biobehavioral approach to pediatric pain assessment. Pain 25:283-296, 1986
8. Beyer JE, Wells N: The assessment of pain in children. Pediatr Clin North Am 36:837-854, 1989
9. Hester NO, Foster R, Kristensen K: Measurement of pain in children: Generalizability and validity of the pain ladder and the poker-chip tool. In: Advances in pain research and therapy: Pediatric pain. New York, Raven Press, 1990, pp 79-84
10. McGrath PJ, Johnson G, Goodman JT et al: The CHEOPS: A behavioral scale to measure postoperative pain in children. In Fields HL, Dubner R, Cervero F, eds. Advances in pain research and therapy.. New York, Raven Press, 1985, pp 395-402

11. Broadman LM, Rice LJ, Hannallah RS: Testing the validity of and objective pain scale for infants and children. Anesthesiology 69:A779, 1988

12. Houck CS, Berde CB, Anand KJS: Pediatric pain management. In Gregory GA, ed. Pediatric anesthesia. New York, Churchill Livingstone, 1994, pp 743-772

13. Maunuksela E-L: Nonsteroidal anti-inflammatory drugs in pediatric pain management. In Schechter NL, Berde CB, Yaster M, eds. Pain in infants, children and adolescents. Baltimore, William and Wilkins, 1993, pp 135-143

14. Guadreault P, Guay J, Nicol O et al: Pharmacokinetics and clinical efficacy of intrarectal solutions of acetaminophen. Can J Anaesth 35:149-152, 1988

15. Knight JC: Post-operative pain in children after day case surgery. Paediatr Anaesth 4:45-51, 1994

16. Jung D, Mroszczak E, Bynum L: Pharmacokinetics of ketorolac tromethamine in humans after intravenous, intramuscular and oral administration. Eur J Clin Pharmacol 35:423-423, 1988

17. Maunuksela E-L, Kokki H, Bullingham RES: Comparison of intravenous ketorolac with morphine for postoperative pain in children. Clin Pharmacol Ther 52:436-443, 1992

18. Sinatra RS, Savarese A: Parenteral analgesic therapy and patient-controlled analgesia for pediatric pain management. In Sinatra RS, Hord AH, Ginsberg B et al, eds. Acute pain: Mechanisms and management. St. Louis, Mosby Year Book, 1992, pp 453-469

19. Maunuksela E-L, Olkkola KT, Korpela R: Does prophylactic intravenous infusion of indomethacin improve the management of postoperative pain in children. Can J Anaesth 35:123-127, 1988

20. Berde CB, Beyer JE, Bournaki MC et al: Comparison of morphine and methadone for prevention of postoperative pain in 3- to 7-year old children. J Pediatr 119:136-141, 1991

21. Bhat R, Chari G, Gulati A et al: Pharmacokinetics of a single dose of morphine in preterm infants during the first week of life. J Pediatr 117:477-481, 1990

22. Millar AJW, Rode H, Cywes S: Continuous morphine infusion for postoperative pain in children. S Afr Med J 72:386-398, 1987

23. Beasley SW, Tibballs J: Efficacy and safety of continuous morphine infusion for postoperative analgesia in the paediatric surgical ward. Aust N Z J Surg 57:233-237, 1987

24. Lynn AM, Opheim KO, Tyler DC: Morphine infusion after pediatric cardiac surgery. Crit Care Med 12:863-866, 1984

25. Hendrickson M, Myre L, Johnson DG: et al: Postoperative analgesia in children: A prospective study of intermittent intramuscular injection versus continuous intravenous infusion of morphine. J Pediatr Surg 25:185-191, 1990

26. Gillespie JA, Morton NS: Patient-controlled analgesia for children: A review. Paediatr Anaesth 2:51-59, 1992

27. Berde CB, Lehn BM, Yee JD et al: Patient-controlled analgesia in children and adolescents: A randomised, prospective comparison with intramuscualr morphine for postoperative analgesia. J Pediatr 118:460-466, 1991

28. Rodgers BM, Webb CJ, Stergios D et al: Patient-controlled analgesia in pediatric surgery. J Pediatr Surg 23:259-262, 1988

29. Dodd E, Wang JH, Rauck RL: Patient controlled analgesia for post-surgical pediatric patients ages 6-16 years. Anesthesiology 69:A372, 1988

30. Sethna NS, Berde CB: Pediatric regional anesthesia. In Gregory GA, ed. Pediatric anesthesia. New York, Churchill Livingstone, 1994, pp 281-318

31. Rice LJ: Pediatric regional anesthesia. In Motoyama E, Davis PD, eds. Smith's anesthesia for infants and children. St. Louis, Mosby Year Book (in press)

32. Rice LJ, Britton JT: Neural blockade for pediatric pain management. In Sinatra RS, Hord AH, Ginsberg B et al, eds. Acute pain: Mechanisms and management. St. Louis, Mosby Year Book, 1992, pp 483-507

33. Haber DW, Berde CB: Spinal opioids for pediatric pain management. In Sinatra RS, Hord AH, Ginsberg B et al, eds. Acute pain: Mechanisms and management. St. Louis, Mosby Year Book, 1992, pp 470-482

34. Desparmet J, Meistelman C, Barre J et al: Continuous epidural infusion of bupivacaine for postoperative pain relief in children. Anesthesiology 67:108-110, 1987

35. Desparment J, Mateo J, Ecoffey C et al: Efficacy of an epidural test dose in children anesthetized with halothane. Anesthesiology 72:249-255, 1990

36. Dalens B, Tanguy A, Haberer J-P: Lumbar epidural anesthesia for operative and postoperative pain relief in infants and young children. Anesth Analg 65:1069-1073, 1986

37. Krane EJ, Jacobson LE, Lynn AM et al: Caudal morphine for postoperative analgesia in children: A comparison with caudal bupivacaine and intravenous morphine. Anesth Analg 66:647-653, 1987

38. Krane EJ: Delayed respiratory depression in a child after caudal epidural morphine. Anesth Analg 67:79-82, 1988

39. Krane EJ, Jacobson LE, Tyler DC: The dose-response of caudal morphine in children. Anesthesiology 71:48-54, 1989

40. Jones SE, Beasley JM, MacFarlane DWR et al: Intrathecal morphine for postoperative pain relief in children. Br J Anaesth 56:137-140, 1984

41. Broadman LM, Higgins TT, Hannallah RS et al: Intraoperative subarachnoid morphine for postoperative pain control following Harrington rod instrumentation in children. Can J Anaesth 34:96, 1987

DEVELOPMENTS IN
CRITICAL CARE MEDICINE AND ANESTHESIOLOGY

KLUWER ACADEMIC PUBLISHERS – DORDRECHT / BOSTON / LONDON

The manufacturer's authorised representative in the EU is Springer
Nature Customer Service Centre GmbH, Europaplatz 3, 69115 Heidelberg,
Germany. If you have any concerns regarding our products, please
contact ProductSafety@springernature.com

Printed and bound by CPI Group (UK) Ltd, Croydon, CR0 4YY
29/04/2026
02099472-0007